ACCEPTANCE AND COMMITMENT THERAPY

Acceptance and Commitment Therapy

An Experiential Approach to Behavior Change

STEVEN C. HAYES
KIRK D. STROSAHL
KELLY G. WILSON

THE GUILFORD PRESS
New York   London

© 1999 The Guilford Press
A Division of Guilford Publications, Inc.
72 Spring Street, New York, NY 10012
www.guilford.com

Paperback edition 2003

Printed in the United States of America

This book is printed on acid-free paper.

Last digit is print number: 9 8 7 6

Library of Congress Cataloging-in-Publication Data

Hayes, Steven C.
    Acceptance and commitment therapy : an experiential approach to
behavior change / Steven C. Hayes, Kirk D. Strosahl, Kelly G. Wilson.
        p.   cm.
    Includes bibliographical references and index.
    ISBN-10: 1-57230-481-2   ISBN-13: 978-1-57230-481-9 (hardcover)
    ISBN-10: 1-57230-955-5   ISBN-13: 978-1-57230-955-5 (paperback)
    1. Cognitive–experiential psychotherapy. 2. Behavior therapy.
3. Self-acceptance. 4. Commitment (Psychology). 5. Values
clarification. 6. Language and emotions. I. Strosahl, Kirk, 1950–
II. Wilson, Kelly G. III. Title.
RC489.C62H39   1999
616.89'142—dc21
                                                        99-32471
                                                            CIP

To my children, Camille, Charles, and Ester:
May the illusion of a "need for control" not suffocate you.
—S. C. H.

To Patricia Robinson, PhD, for her seminal work in
advancing mindfulness and acceptance strategies and her
undying support of me personally.
—K. D. S.

To my brother Randy,
who lost his life to the word machine.
—K. G. W.

About the Authors

Steven C. Hayes, PhD, is Nevada Foundation Professor and Chair of the Department of Psychology at the University of Nevada, Reno. An author of 15 books and more than 250 scientific articles, his interests cover basic research, applied research, methodology, and philosophy of science. In 1992 he was listed by the Institute for Scientific Information as the 30th "highest impact" psychologist in the world during 1986–1990 based on the citation impact of his writings. Dr. Hayes has been President of Division 25 of the American Psychological Association, the American Association of Applied and Preventive Psychology, and the Association for Advancement of Behavior Therapy. He was the first Secretary-Treasurer of the American Psychological Society and is currently cochair of the Practice Guidelines Coalition.

Kirk D. Strosahl, PhD, is Research and Training Director for the Mountainview Consulting Group, where he provides consultation and training on integrative primary care medicine, outcomes management in applied delivery systems, clinical management of the suicidal patient, and Acceptance and Commitment Therapy (ACT). Dr. Strosahl began his career as the Director of the Suicidal Behaviors Research Clinic at the University of Washington, where, along with Marsha Linehan, PhD, and John Chiles, MD, he helped elaborate the use of acceptance and mindfulness strategies with suicidal borderline patients. From 1984 through 1998 he worked as a staff psychologist and as the Research Evaluation Manager for the Division of Behavioral Health Services at Group Health Cooperative of Puget Sound, where he became a recognized expert in integration of behavioral health services into primary care medicine, and in the dissemination of empirically supported therapies into managed care settings.

Kelly G. Wilson, PhD, is Associate Director of the Center for Contextual Psychology at the University of Nevada, Reno. He has directed a National Institute on Drug Abuse grant since 1993, examining both Acceptance and Commitment Therapy (ACT) and 12-Step facilitation treatment of substance abuse. An author of over 20 articles and chapters, his interests include the integration of basic and applied behavioral science, behavioral analysis of nontraditional behavioral topics, the interface of ACT and other acceptance-oriented traditions, and the application of acceptance strategies to substance abuse.

Preface

This book is the result of the journeys we have taken. Viewed from one perspective, it represents our personal journeys through life, learning about pain and suffering, and learning how to open up and move on. Our parents, siblings, spouses, and children are in this book. Our mistakes and blind alleys are in this book. Indeed, although we will say naught else about it, our own personal struggles with personal problems probably inform this book more than any other source. There is just no way to connect with the Acceptance and Commitment Therapy (ACT) work without connecting personally with it because the model itself will not allow a convenient division into those needing treatment and those doing the treatment.

From another perspective, this book represents our professional journeys. Each of us was trained in behavioral and cognitive-behavioral therapy and worked to find ways to link this old and honorable empirical tradition to the rich but confusing veins of thought and practice from humanistic, existential, spiritual, and human potential domains. In that we have been influenced by many fellow travelers, including Bob Kohlenberg, the late Neil Jacobson, Marsha Linehan, John Kabat-Zinn, Les Greenberg, Alan Marlatt, Michael Mahoney, and Michael Dougher. ACT is a collection, with components borrowed from many traditions, and we are encouraged by the great success others are having in related work.

If there is anything novel about ACT, it is in the specific way it combines philosophy, theory, and practice. We have little interest in our approach as a finished product or brand name, and we encourage the reader to apply and modify our work. What is most important is to move ahead, using the best of the empirical and behavioral traditions, but keeping an eye toward the prize of greater understanding of the breadth and depth of human experience. In the long run what works will become the conventional wisdom of a future day, and little will remain from any of the current therapies that is distinctive. If this book helps move that day a bit closer, we are satisfied.

This book also represents a scientific journey of psychologists, teaching, researching, and learning psychology. In the academic and research domain, we have been influenced particularly by our teachers and close colleagues, including John Cone, David Barlow, Irv Kessler, Patty Robinson, Jon Krapfl, Linda Hayes, Vic Follette, Rosemery Nelson-Gray, Aaron Brownstein, Dermot Barnes, and Sam Leigland. At the other end of this chain of knowledge stand our students, each contributing in so many ways to this work. These include (in no particular order) Rob Zettle, Jeanne Devany, Sonny Turner, Zamir Korn, Irwin Rosenfarb, David Greenway, Terry Olson, Mary Wolfe, Elga Wulfert, David Steele, Joe Haas, Norm Anderson, Terry Grubb, Rachel Azrin, Ed Munt, Robin Jarrett, Sandy Sigmon, Dave McKnight, Diane Volosin, Lee Cooper, Sue Melancon McCurry, Durriyah Khorakiwala, Regina Lipkens, Nancy Taylor, Chris Leonhard, Chris McCurry, Niloo Afari, Barbara Kohlenberg, Jacque Pistorello, Liz Gifford, Robyn Walser, Wini Ju, Adam Grundt, J. T. Blackledge, Tuna Townsend, Pat Bach, Jen Gregg, Rich Bissett, Dosheen Toarmino, Eric Fox, and David Sayrs. We thank them all.

Equally important are our clients and the many clinicians who have contributed to the work. Literally everyone we have treated from any ACT perspective and everyone we have trained clinically has contributed in some way. We acknowledge them all.

And finally, there is you, the reader. This book is an invitation to take a journey yourself. In doing so, you have a disadvantage and an advantage. The disadvantage is that it may be easier to get caught up in your own literal interpretations of what you are about to read and to miss what is transformational about an ACT model. Books are literal in a way that conversation is not, and that realization has contributed a certain amount of melancholy to the process of writing this book. We hope that what we have written is helpful, even while we fear that it may be confusing.

Yet there is also an advantage. You are dealing with the frozen verbal product of the authors. There is a path laid down here, and you can go back and forth, reread, and reconsider. You can catch inconsistencies or detect what is superfluous. You can try out something from one chapter and only much later on consider what is in another. In this process of assimilation, analysis, and use, we hope that what is truly useful will become evident. We also hope that new things will emerge. If they do, we hope you will let us know what you learn. After all, in a very important sense, we are all in this boat together.

Humanity has solved or ameliorated an impressive number of the problems faced by other living creatures, yet the tool we used to do that good work—human language—turns on us in a most insidious way every day. It may take us centuries or eons to solve the problems that language creates, but solve them we will. Behavioral scientists have something few other groups concerned with human suffering have had: the processes of scientific knowing itself. If we can get beyond mere syndromes and can focus properly on the problem of human suffering, there is much we can contribute. For the sake of our clients, it is our duty to try.

STEVEN C. HAYES
KIRK D. STROSAHL
KELLY G. WILSON

Contents

•PART I•

The Problem
and the Approach

The single most remarkable fact of human existence is how hard it is for human beings to be happy. Psychotherapists are all too familiar with the sad statistical findings, taken one at a time, that document this fact (e.g., Kessler et al., 1994; Regier et al., 1993). They already know that in any given year the overall prevalence rates for mental disorders will approach 30%. They also know that there are nearly 20 million alcoholics. They know that nearly 30,000 people will take their own lives each year and countless others will try but fail. Indeed, therapists often revel in such statistics when discussing the need for more clinicians or for more funding for mental health programs. At the same time, psychotherapists generally miss the larger message these many statistics contain when taken as a whole. Even taking into account the many areas of overlap, if we add up all those humans who are or have been depressed, addicted, anxious, angry, self-destructive, alienated, worried, compulsive, workaholic, insecure, painfully shy, divorced, avoidant of intimacy, stressed, and so on, we are compelled to reach this startling conclusion: Suffering is a basic characteristic of human life.

This book is about that fact. In Chapter 1 we try to show how our conventional assumptions have hidden this obvious truth from psychotherapists and psychopathologists. A firm grasp on the ubiquitous nature of human suffering produces a view of human change and development that is quite different than if we begin with the assumption that suffering is abnormal. In Chapter 2 we defend the importance of philosophy and theory and describe the philosophical and theoretical grounds on which our work stands. We show how functional contextual philoso-

1

phy leads to radically different ideas about the nature of the relationship between cognition, emotion, and behavior. We describe an approach to human language—Relational Frame Theory—that vitalizes our work, both technically and as an approach to human psychopathology. In Chapter 3 we describe our view of psychopathology and relate many behavioral health problems to experiential avoidance and cognitive fusion. These two phenomena then become the key targets of our therapeutic work.

•1•

The Dilemma
of Human Suffering

Dania, Fla. June 16 (AP)—A 6-year-old girl was killed today
when she stepped in front of a train, telling siblings that she
"wanted to be with her mother." The authorities said that
her mother had a terminal illness.
                        —*New York Times* (June 17, 1993, p. A12)

Happiness for a dog or a cat is straightforward. If pets are given shelter, food and drink, warmth, stimulation, play, and physical health they are contented. Without the intervention of humans, animals are often missing some of these basic things. They live, as we say, a dog's life. Many humans also are missing such basic items too, and it is not difficult to understand the misery of a person living without them.

But many humans have *all* the things a nonverbal organism would need to be happy, and yet they are not. Humans can be warm, well fed, dry, physically well, and still be miserable. Indeed, humans can have forms of excitement and entertainment unknown in the nonhuman world—color TVs, exotic cars, and airplane trips to the Caribbean—and still be miserable. Literally nothing external that you can name—great looks, loving parents, terrific children, a caring spouse—are enough to ensure that a human will not suffer terribly. Every day a human being with every imaginable advantage takes a gun, loads a bullet into it, bites the barrel, and squeezes the trigger. Every morning a successful business person gets to the office, closes the door, and reaches quietly into the bottom drawer of the desk to find the bottle of gin hidden there.

Humans as a species are suffering creatures. Yet our most popular

3

underlying models of psychological health and pathology barely touch on this fact. It is the elephant in the living room that no one seems to mention.

THE UNDERLYING ASSUMPTIONS
OF THE PSYCHOLOGICAL MAINSTREAM

The mental health community has simply not adequately explained its own data on the pervasiveness of human suffering. Drawing from medical metaphors, it seems to believe that psychological health is the natural homeostatic state that is disturbed only by psychological illness or distress. That is, there is the *assumption of healthy normality.*

This assumption is at the core of traditional medical approaches to physical health. Given the relative success of physical medicine, it is not surprising that the mental health community has adopted it as well. The traditional conception of physical health involves simply the absence of disease. It is assumed that, left to its own devices, the body is meant to be healthy, but that physical health can be disturbed by infection, injury, toxicity, decline of physical capacity, or disordered physical processes.

This assumption is quite sensible within the area of physical health. The structure of the human body should be designed to deliver a reasonable degree of physical health as the natural result of biological evolution. If particular humans do not have genes adequate for a degree of physical health sufficient to ensure successful reproduction, evolution would weed out these genes over time. Of course, even within physical medicine the assumption of healthy normality has its limits. The immune system can be strengthened by exercise, diet, and other psychological and behavioral factors, for example. Thus physical health is not *merely* the absence of disease, but also the presence of something (e.g., resistance to disease). In addition, some physical disease seems to be a side effect of successful biological evolution. Cancer is often caused by minor errors in cell replication that accidentally either turn on oncogenes or turn off growth inhibition genes. Yet this process cannot be readily weeded out by evolutionary contingencies, because if cell division were always 100% correct, evolution itself would be limited. Underlining this point, it is worth noting that seemingly pathologic physical processes are sometimes in reality adaptive, such as fever (Nesse & Williams, 1994). In regard to physical health the assumption of healthy normality works fairly well most of the time.

A corollary to the assumption of healthy normality is the assumption that *abnormality is a disease.* Diseases are functional entities: They are disturbances of health with a known etiology, course, and response to treatment. The identification of syndromes—collections of signs (things the observer can see) and symptoms (things the person complains of)—is the usual first step in the identification of diseases. After syndromes are identified, the search begins to find the abnormal processes that give rise to this particular cluster of outcomes and to find ways to alter these processes so as to alter the undesirable results.

This analytic strategy is completely sensible, given the assumptions. If health is natural and is disturbed only by illness, what we need to do is to identify those with an illness and carefully examine them for some underlying deviant etiology. Psychopathology has been completely dominated by these assumptions and the analytic strategies that result. Few modern research psychologists or psychiatrists have been able to avoid adopting them.

Considering how much attention has been afforded the medical model within psychology and psychiatry, it is a bit shocking to note how little progress has been made in establishing syndromes as disease entities. After one relates the well-worn and dated example of general paresis, there are few clear success stories to tell. The "comorbidity" rates in the current diagnostic system are so high as to challenge the basic credibility of the nosology. The treatment utility of these categories is low (Hayes, Nelson, & Jarrett, 1987) inasmuch as the same treatments work with many syndromes. In addition, they cover only a portion of clients and their problems. In fully capitated managed care settings (where "diagnosing up" to receive insurance coverage is no longer necessary) a large percentage of the clients receiving psychological treatment have no diagnosable syndromal disorder at all (Strosahl, 1994). Even if clients can be given a label such as panic disorder with agoraphobia, or obsessive–compulsive disorder, many of the issues within therapy will still have to do with other problems: jobs, children, relationships, sexual identity, careers, anger, sadness, drinking problems, or the meaning of life.

The relative lack of progress in the current model is not limited to syndromal thinking per se. Often the generalized effects of psychotherapy are small, and the largest effects tend to be observed with very specific measures. The gains that are found on narrow measures very often do not generalize to gains on other narrow measures, even when the measures seem related. Yet students of psychopathology are carefully trained to know nearly every characteristic of nearly every syndromal category. Research journals in clinical psychology and psychiatry contain little else but research on syndromes, and federal funding is almost entirely dedicated to the study of these entities.

We are raising all of these points for a pragmatic reason. The clinical establishment has been approaching the area of mental health with the assumptions of healthy normality and abnormality as a disease. If this strategy had paid off massively within psychotherapy, there would be little reason to object. "Yes," we might then say, "human suffering is ubiquitous but we must leave that to the priest, minister, or rabbi. Our job is to treat and to prevent clinical syndromes. After all, that is why people come to see us. And we do that very well indeed."

But an honest and knowledgeable clinician cannot say that today. Despite the limited success of this model, we never seem ready to back up and question whether our basic assumptions are too limited. Clinical researchers have spent perhaps too much time looking for the abnormal underpinnings of psychological difficulties, when in reality suffering seems to be so basic to human life.

The approach described in this book is called Acceptance and Commitment Therapy, or "ACT" (said as one word, not as individual letters). An ACT model traces much of psychopathology to ordinary psychological processes, particularly those involving human language. Given the traditional assumption, this strategy would not make sense, inasmuch as ordinary language can hardly be a clinical syndrome or a pathological process. The ACT model does not deny that unusual and bizarre pathological processes exist. Clearly they do. If a person suffers a brain injury and behaves inappropriately as a result, this is not due to the normal psychological process. The same may be true for schizophrenia, autism, bipolar disorder, and so on, although the actual evidence in such areas is much less robust than most clinicians and researchers seem to believe. Even with such severe mental illness, however, the ACT model holds that ordinary psychological processes may amplify the core difficulty, and thus that the assumption of healthy normality should at least be broadened.

ACT supplements the traditional view by bringing a different assumption to the study of psychological distress. It is based on the *assumption of destructive normality*: the idea that ordinary human psychological processes can themselves lead to extremely destructive and dysfunctional results and can amplify or exacerbate unusual pathological processes.

The Example of Suicide

It seems worthwhile to work through a specific clinical example to compare and contrast these working assumptions. There is no more dramatic example of the degree to which suffering is part of the human condition than suicide. Death is obviously the least functional outcome we can imagine in life, and yet a very large proportion of the human family at one time or another attempts to produce it or seriously considers producing it. We think the high rates of even the least functional outcomes should provide a clear challenge to the assumption of healthy abnormality.

Suicide is the conscious, deliberate, and purposeful taking of one's own life. Two facts are shockingly evident in regard to suicide: (1) It is ubiquitous in human societies and (2) it is absent in all other living organisms. Existing theories of suicide have a very hard time accounting for both of these facts.

Suicide is reported in every human society, both now and in the past. Approximately 12.6 per 100,000 persons in the United States actually commit suicide every year (Schneidman, 1985). It is virtually unknown in infants and very young children, but first appears during the early school years. The chilling story with which we began this chapter describes a case in which a 6-year-old child committed suicide—one of the youngest on record. Her "reasons" will resonate with numerous other examples we will describe throughout this book: Even 6-year-olds have a hard time facing loss and pain.

Suicidal thoughts and attempts are shockingly prevalent in the general population (Chiles & Strosahl, 1995). About 10% of the human population will at some time attempt suicide. Another 20% will struggle with suicidal ideation and will have a plan and a means to accomplish the act. Yet another 20% will struggle with suicidal thoughts, but without a specific plan. Thus, half of the population will face moderate to severe levels of suicidality in their lives.

Equally important for our purposes is the fact that suicide is arguably absent in nonhumans. Several exceptions to this generalization have been suggested, but they have turned out to be false. Norwegian lemmings are the classic example. When their population density reaches a point that cannot be sustained, the entire group engages in a helter-skelter pattern of running that leads to the death of many of them—usually by drowning. But suicide does not involve only death. It involves psychological activity that is oriented toward personal death as a deliberate consequence of that activity. This is part of what is meant by suicide being "purposeful." When a lemming falls into the water, it tries to climb out. But there are many cases of a person jumping from a bridge, surviving, then crawling back to the bridge and jumping again.

In humans, self-elimination can fulfill a variety of purposes, but it is clearly purposeful. For example, when suicide notes are examined, it is found that more than half of actual or attempted suicides clearly involve an attempt to flee from an aversive situation (Loo, 1985; Smith & Bloom, 1985). These aversive situations include especially aversive states of mind such as guilt and anxiety (Bancroft, Skrimshire, & Simkins, 1976; Baumeister, 1990). Persons who commit suicide evaluate themselves quite negatively, believing themselves to be worthless, inadequate, rejected, or blameworthy (Maris, 1981; Rosen, 1976; Rothberg & Jones, 1987).

These psychologically driven human purposes (e.g., to avoid a feeling of worthlessness) would be hard to imagine in nonverbal organisms. For now, however, our point is more general: The example of suicide shows the limits and flaws of the purely syndromal perspective on human suffering. Suicide is not a syndrome, and many people who kill themselves do not have a well-defined clinical syndrome (Chiles & Strosahl, 1995). If the most dramatically "unhealthy" form of activity that exists is present to some degree in the lives of most humans but not at all for nonhumans, we are drawn to an obvious conclusion: There is something basic about being human that makes it so. Put more precisely, there must be a psychological process that leads so readily to suffering— one that is characteristic of humans but not of nonhumans. The research strategy we generally follow in psychopathology will probably not detect this process, because this strategy is not designed to give us adequate understanding of the ordinary facts of human existence.

Clearly, collections of signs and symptoms do exist—that is an empirical fact. Some of these will be shown to be disease entities in that a particular collection of signs and symptoms will be associated with a distinct etiology and can be treated in a particular way. Some mental health problems are pathological in the traditional sense. But short of giving nearly every citizen one or more syndromal labels, no amount of progress in the area of psychological disease will remove our need to explain and to address the pervasiveness of human suffering. *Most* humans are hurting—just some more than others. It is, in effect, normal to be abnormal.

If we face this obvious fact squarely, we have to ask the next obvious question. Why? This volume is our attempt at an answer.

THE ASSUMPTION OF DESTRUCTIVE NORMALITY

The assumption of destructive normality is basic to many of our cultural traditions, but it is much less dominant in psychology. For example, the Judeo-Christian tradition (and indeed most religious traditions, both Western and Eastern) embraces the idea that human suffering is the normal state of affairs for human adults. It is worth examining this religious tradition both as a concrete example of how far the medical/syndromal perspective has taken us away from our cultural roots on these issues, and as a way to begin considering the role of human language in human misery.

Religious Traditions

The Bible is very clear about the original source of human suffering. In the Genesis story, "God said, 'Let us make man in our image, after our likeness.' " (Gen. 1:26), and Adam and Eve were placed in a beautiful garden. The first humans were innocent and happy: "And the man and his wife were both naked, and were not ashamed" (Gen. 2:25). They were given only one command: " 'But of the tree of knowledge of good and evil you shall not eat, for in the day that you eat of it you shall die' " (Gen. 2:17). The serpent told Eve that she will not die if she eats from that tree, but rather that " 'God knows that when you eat of it your eyes will be opened, and you will be like God, knowing good and evil' " (Gen. 3:5). The serpent turned out to be correct, to a degree, because when the fruit was eaten "the eyes of both were opened, and they knew they were naked" (Gen. 3:7).

This is a powerful story, and very instructive. Asked whether it is a good thing to recognize the difference between good and evil, most religious people would surely say that it is the very epitome of moral behavior. It may be, but the Genesis story says that this kind of evaluative knowledge is also the epitome of something else. It represents the loss of human innocence and the beginning of human suffering.

In the biblical story, the effects of evaluative knowledge are immediate and direct. The additional negative effects from God's punishment come later. Adam and Eve were already suffering the results before God discovered their disobedience. When Adam and Eve discovered that they were naked, they immediately "sewed fig leaves together and made themselves aprons" (Gen. 3:7) and then they "hid themselves from the presence of the Lord God among the trees of the garden. But the Lord God called to the man, and said to him. 'Where are you?' And he said, 'I heard the sound of thee in the garden, and I was afraid, because I was naked; and hid myself.' [And God] said, 'Who told you that you were naked? Have you eaten of the tree?' " (Gen. 3: 8–11).

There is something very sad about this story of the first instance of human shame. It touches something inside us about our own loss of innocence. Humans have eaten from the Tree of Knowledge. We can categorize, evaluate, and judge. As the story says, our eyes have been opened. But at what a terrible cost. We can judge ourselves and find ourselves to be wanting; we can imagine ideals and find the present to be unacceptable by comparison; we can reconstruct the past; we can worry about imagined futures; we can suffer with the knowledge that we will die.

Each new human life retraces this ancient story. Young children are the very essence of human innocence. They run, play, and feel—and, as in Genesis, when they are naked they are not ashamed. Yet as in William Blake's famous picture, we adults drag our children from the Garden with each word, conversation, or story. We teach children to talk, think, compare, plan, and analyze. And as we do, their innocence falls away like petals from a flower, to be replaced by the thorns and stiff branches of fear, self criticism, and pretense. We cannot prevent this transition, nor can we soften it. Our children must enter into the terrifying world of verbal knowledge.

The world's great religions constituted one of the first organized attempts to solve the problem of human suffering. It is telling that all the great religions have a mystical side and that they all share a defining feature. All mystical traditions have practices that are oriented toward reducing or transforming the domination of analytical language over experience: Silence is observed for hours, days, weeks, or years; unsolvable verbal puzzles are contemplated; nonanalytical meditation is practiced; mantras are repeated endlessly; chants are recited for hours on end; and so on. Even the nonmystical aspects of the great religious traditions—which do rely on literal, analytical language—often focus on acts that are not themselves purely analytical. Judeo-Christian theology, for example, asks us to have *faith* in God (the root of the word means something more like fidelity than logical, analytical belief). Different religions vary the details of the story, but the themes are usually the same. In their attempt to know, humans have lost their innocence, and suffering is a natural result. There is great wisdom in this perspective. By comparison, the relatively recent tradition of psychotherapy is just now catching up.

The Positive and Negative Effects of Human Language

It seems to us (as it did to the writers of Genesis) that the psychological process that most distinguishes humans from nonhumans is knowing. The core of the ACT approach is built on the idea that this ubiquitous human process gives rise to the pervasiveness of both human achievement and misery.

For reasons we will describe in detail later, knowledge can be both nonverbal and verbal, but the kind that creates such difficulties (and wonders) is based on human language. By "human language" we do not mean mere human vocalization, nor English as opposed to French. Likewise, we are not referring merely to social communication, as when our pet dog barks for food or when the prairie dog emits an alarm cry. In somewhat commonsense terms, we mean symbolic activity in whatever domain it occurs (gestures, pictures, written forms, sounds, and so on).

Somewhat more technically, humans have extensive training in learning to derive relations between events and symbols. The ability to derive and combine verbal relations enormously increases the ability of human beings to assess the impact of actions, to predict futures not yet experienced, to learn from the past, to maintain, build, and pass on knowledge, and to regulate the behavior of others and themselves. As a result, humans have a capacity for cultural development, progressivity of knowledge, and adaptation to environmental demands that so far outstrips the ability of other species that humans have virtually no effective competitors on the earth other than among themselves.

This was not always the case. The ascendancy of humankind began ever so gradually. Human verbal abilities themselves have gone through a remarkable progression. Although there seems to be wide agreement that the earliest humans could use symbols, based on their burial practices, for example, the sophisticated use of these abilities is astonishingly recent. The earliest permanent and unquestionable records of sophisticated human symbolic activity appear to be cave drawings from only 10,000 years ago. The earliest evidence for written language as we know it is 5,000 years old. The alphabet was invented only 3,500 years ago. Even within the formal, written record of human affairs, there is a clear progression of verbal abilities. Only a few thousand years ago ordinary people seemingly experienced self-verbalizations as statements from the gods or unseen others (Jaynes, 1976). Today we manipulate symbolic stimuli covertly from morning to night while simultaneously functioning in the world.

The progress of humankind can be related fairly directly to these same verbal milestones. The great expansion of human influence in the world did not really begin until the time of the cave drawings. The development of the great civilizations was fostered by written language, and the world's great religions developed not long after. The enormous expansion of the ability of the human species to alter the immediate environment through technology began with the gradual rise of science and has increased exponentially since then.

The resulting progress is astounding, outstripping our ability to appreciate the change. Two hundred years ago the average human life span in the United States was 37 years. By the year 2000 it will approach 80. One hundred years ago, a U. S. farmer could feed 4 others. Today, it is 200. Fifty years ago the *Oxford English Dictionary* weighed 300 pounds and took up 4 feet of shelf space. Today it weighs less than an ounce and can be plugged into a computer.

This kind of familiar "gee whiz" litany is easy to dismiss because the impact of human verbal abilities is so enormous as to be incomprehensible. But we cannot appreciate the human dilemma if we do not see the nature and speed of human progress clearly. Human misery can be understood only in the context of human achievement, because the most important source of each is the same: human symbolic activity. To borrow a phrase from the *Star Wars* trilogy, language is truly "The Force" in human progress. It is so enormously influential in human affairs because it has such a bright side. But The Force has a dark side too. Psychotherapists know that side well.

This dual nature of human language impacts not just at the level of the group—the human species or human civilization—but also at the level of the individual. Each individual has experienced both the bright and the dark side of The Force. To ask an individual human being to challenge the nature and role of language in his or her own behavior is tantamount to asking a carpenter to question the general utility of a hammer. But hammers are not good for everything, and language is not good for everything either. We must learn to use language without being consumed by it. We must learn to manage it rather than having it manage us. We must learn to overcome the dark side.

Preparing to Go into the Lion's Den

The Zen master Seng-Ts'an had a saying: "If you work on your mind with your mind, how can you avoid great confusion?" Many human institutions (Zen Buddhism included prominently among them) have attempted to declaw the lion of human language. It is inherently difficult to use analytic language to declaw analytic language.

Yet we are writing a book, not dancing or meditating. The readers of this book are interacting with verbal material. If human language is at the core of most human psychological suffering, this presents an extreme challenge, because attempts by both the writers and readers of this book to understand destructive verbal processes will themselves be based on verbal processes.

For that reason, we will need preparation. We must be extremely careful about our philosophical assumptions and our analytic units. The next chapter will deal directly with those. The language traps that may ensnare us will have to be identified. We will need at times to use language in paradoxical and metaphorical ways in order to avoid those traps. All of this will tend to create occasional confusion, more so than in a typical book that is about something more removed from verbal processes themselves.

These are difficulties we need to face. The responsibility for altering the process of destructive normality lies in those cultural institutions designed to alleviate human suffering. In the modern era, these include most especially the behavioral sciences and psychotherapy. It is the job of psychotherapists, in part, to understand these destructive verbal processes and to work to alter them or better contain them for our clients and ourselves.

•2•

The Philosophical and Theoretical Foundations of ACT

Many therapists are impatient with philosophy and theory, wanting to get on to the practical details of how to help others. They want to know the specific techniques to use, believing that this is the practical thing to do.

The ACT approach was built over the last 18 years as much by basic philosophical and theoretical work as by technical development (for a few examples see Hayes, 1984, 1989; Hayes & Hayes, 1992; Hayes, Hayes, Reese, & Sarbin, 1993; Hayes & Wilson, 1993; Hayes, Wilson, Gifford, Follette, & Strosahl, 1996). Even clinical researchers may find this strange. The usual approach is to develop and test a technique, then to dismantle it, and only then—many years into the treatment development process—to ask basic scientific (never mind philosophical) questions about processes or mechanisms of action. We think that is a mistake. Convincing readers of that will be our first task in this chapter.

WHY THE LEVEL OF TECHNIQUE IS NOT ADEQUATE

It is worth thinking about the roles of technology, theory, and philosophy in the abstract before considering these levels concretely. The direct products of clinical science are statements: descriptions, theories, and interpretations. Even an actual technique, say, systematic desensitization, cannot be disseminated in a scientific sense. What is communicated in our research journals are statements *about* this technique.

If scientific knowledge is in the form of statements, we should ask ourselves, "What *kinds* of statements are most likely to be most valuable to clinicians?" There is good reason to think that the answer is *not* simply "descriptions of techniques."

An example may help. Suppose a cook experiments for several years and finally develops a wonderful new bread recipe. A recipe is a kind of technological statement. It is highly precise, but it has no scope. Bread recipes do not tell us how to bake pies or make beer. Because recipes have little scope, cookbooks are merely collections, with little coherence among the recipes. There are no systematic and fundamental means to relate one recipe to another. For all these reasons bakers are not scientists, even if they back up their recipes with careful data collection.

Advances in clinical science are severely limited when they are based solely on specific formally defined techniques, for three major reasons:

1. *Without statements that have broad applicability, we have no basis for using our knowledge when confronted with a new problem or situation.* Descriptions of technique, devoid of underlying theory, have little to say about novel situations. As a result, when new situations present themselves many clinicians simply throw old techniques at new problems just to see what happens. An example is the rather pathetic way certain core techniques, such as relaxation training, are included in almost every package for almost every disorder. For practical reasons we need to develop and use statements that have broad applicability, while maintaining a high level of precision. That is exactly what theory and philosophy are all about.

2. *Without statements that have broad applicability, we have no systematic means to develop new techniques.* Technology is a poor source of entirely new technology, because true innovation is generally the result of theoretical and philosophical shifts of perspective. Most of the well-known clinical techniques were developed many years ago—very few are truly new. Over time, with more emphasis on technology and less on theoretical principles, we are seeing an almost self-stimulatory concern for technological refinements and little genuine technological innovation.

3. *A discipline based purely on statements that are high in precision, but with narrow applicability, becomes increasingly disorganized and incoherent.* Disorganization and shallowness are the natural concomitants of narrow constructions. We see the products all around us. Applied psychology is fracturing into subareas organized by common-

sense categories such as patient population or clinical procedure—even though everything we know about basic psychological processes suggests that these divisions are scientifically trivial. Without an emphasis on philosophy and theory no other result is possible, because it is difficult to assimilate the mountain of seemingly disconnected bits of information that science-as-technology presents. The field becomes an incoherent mass, impossible to master and impossible to teach. In addition, the shallow level of analysis means that other areas of science cannot be related to clinical techniques. A hole in the fabric of science opens that cannot be filled. The solution to this incoherence is the organizing force of well thought out theory and philosophy.

Technological statements alone can work quite well in limited situations. There is nothing wrong with writing food recipes. But psychotherapy is *not* a very limited situation. We need to do more than collect a recipe book of psychological procedures; we need to understand human suffering and how best to treat it. Neither the history of other disciplines nor that of our own suggests that applied psychology can advance rapidly as a discipline without a comprehensive worldview and theory.

ACT as a Technology

Like all psychotherapy approaches, ACT can be understood at the level of technique as a collection of exercises, metaphors, procedures, and so on. Although ACT is an interesting collection, it is clearly only one of a myriad of therapeutic techniques. Indeed, many or even most of the techniques in ACT have been borrowed from elsewhere—from the human potential movement, Eastern traditions, behavior therapy, mystical traditions, and the like.

Unless one is approaching therapy as an aesthetic exercise, eclecticism is the only thing that makes much sense at the level of technique. If it is defined purely as a technique, one can use ACT—or any therapy—the way one uses a hammer or a drill: as a specific means to get a specific job done.

But considering ACT *solely* at the level of technique limits its possible value and misses the larger point. For one thing, even well-developed treatment approaches evolve. Almost every week we add, subtract, or refine the technical elements of ACT. As more and more therapists develop an interest in the approach, this process seems to be accelerating. We encourage ACT therapists to add techniques, develop their own metaphors, and so on. Many of the techniques in this book originated with other ACT therapists or even ACT clients.

In addition, we have evolved several flavors of ACT to fit various disorders or settings. In our work in a health maintenance organization, with four or five sessions as an average for an entire case, some elements of the approach are emphasized and others are greatly diminished. In a 24-week research protocol, the picture looks different than it does in a private practice setting. The ACT approach has also been refined and tested in a primary care setting (Robinson & Hayes, 1997). If ACT is *just* a technique, which one is it?

When ACT is approached solely as a technique, there is also a tendency to apply it "by the book." We use manuals to train ACT therapists, but experienced ACT therapists often modify the procedures or sequences of topics to fit the needs of a particular client at a particular moment. If ACT is just a set of techniques defined topographically, we seemingly have to claim that an experienced therapist dancing through our set of procedures is not doing ACT, whereas a new therapist going by the book is doing the real thing. That is patent nonsense. The effective ACT therapist uses ACT as *functionally defined*, not merely as *topographically defined*. There is another way to say this. The effective ACT therapist needs to do ACT in a way that is consistent with its theory and philosophy, not in a way that is mechanically consistent with its procedures per se.

Finally, ACT should not be viewed merely as a technology, because it integrates diverse ideas into a coherent and innovative theoretical and philosophical framework. ACT is not easily pegged as behavioral therapy, cognitive-behavior therapy, experiential therapy, humanistic therapy, existential therapy, or other such therapies. We think it not only offers something to all these traditions, it also provides an underlying theory and philosophy of the human condition.

THE NEED FOR PHILOSOPHY

If theory is necessary, is philosophy also? It is. Indeed, it is not possible to have theory without philosophy, for at least two reasons. First, as Gödel proved in the field of mathematics, it is not possible to have a symbolic system that is not based on analytic assumptions and postulates that go beyond the reach of that symbolic system. You must start with postulates or assumptions, and, thus, theory is never enough. Second, in order to assess theoretical systems, there must be some rules of evidence or criteria for truth that allow us to say that one statement or set of statements is better or truer than another. But these rules of evidence are necessarily preanalytic—they enable analysis, they are not the result of analysis. We can ignore philosophy only by mindlessly and implicitly assuming a philosophy, but it seems much better to own up to our assumptions consciously.

As a metaphor, imagine that a person stands in a place and looks out at the world. That person sees the world from a particular angle—a particular point of view. If the person stands somewhere else, the angle and field of view would change. Here is the first question: Can you avoid first standing somewhere in order to look? It seems that you cannot. If you stand here or there, you are standing here or there. If you straddled both positions, as a person might if one foot was here and one there, the resulting view would be a third view (in between here and there), not a summary of here and there. In the same way, we have to stand on our assumptions to look at the world, and we cannot avoid having only a limited set of assumptions. In principle and necessarily, each set is limited.

The philosophy of science involves explicating the assumptions that undergird scientific activity. The goal of examining the philosophical level is not to *justify* one's own philosophy, but to specify and integrate analytic assumptions. Put another way, the goal of philosophizing is nothing more than clarity and responsibility. It is to say, "This is what I assume. Precisely this. I cannot justify it, but I can own it."

It is important to keep this goal in mind, because there is an enormous temptation to use philosophy to bludgeon those outside one's own philosophical camp. This is an especially delicious form of useless activity if you criticize the *assumptions* and *values* of your intellectual adversary, because you are then in the untouchable position of laying waste to others' assumptions and values by virtue of empirical/logical analysis secretly based on your own assumptions and values. It is the adult equivalent of the children's taunt "Nah nah nah *nah* nah." This taunting can be great fun, but it is dishonest. The basic analytic units and truth criteria of scientists are not the *results* of analysis—they are the *means* of analysis. One cannot honestly say, in effect, "My assumptions and values meet my standards better than your assumptions and values meet my standards; therefore, my assumptions and values are best." All one can honestly say is, "These are my assumptions and standards. Descriptively (not evaluatively) here is what happens when you have these, instead of those." When alternative assumptions and standards are encountered, the differences can be pointed out nonevaluatively or one can temporarily take on the assumptions of the other to see whether they are being applied consistently or to see what consequences they have relative to their own purposes. Anything else is dogmatic and dishonest. In that context, then, we wish in this chapter merely to describe the philosophical assumptions of the ACT work. They are not right, true, or correct. Instead, they are "where we stand."

This book is based on a particular philosophy and a set of theoretical concepts that differ notably from those within the psychological mainstream. If the core philosophies of ACT are understood, many techniques can be added to it and it will still be ACT. ACT is an approach, based on a theory and set firmly within a philosophical tradition. It is to that tradition that we now turn.

FUNCTIONAL CONTEXTUALISM

ACT is based on functional contextualism (Hayes, 1993; Hayes, Hayes, & Reese, 1988; Biglan & Hayes, 1996). The core analytic unit of contextualism, or pragmatism, is the ongoing act in context: the commonsense situated action (Pepper, 1942). Another term might be the *historical act*, but not as a dead description of a thing done. It is doing as it is being done, in both a historical and situational context, such as in hunting, shopping, or making love.

The core components of contextualism are a (1) focus on the whole event, (2) sensitivity to the role of context in understanding the nature and function of an event, and (3) a firm grasp on a pragmatic truth criterion. There are various forms of contextualism (Hayes, Hayes, Reese, & Sarbin, 1993; Rosnow & Georgoudi, 1986). The distinctive features of a *functional* contextualist approach are its unique goals. In both its general and specific features, functional contextualism is a radical departure from the dominant view in applied psychology today.

The Whole Event

As psychologists, we wish to understand whole organisms interacting in and with a historical and situational context. That is the psychological level of analysis. To a contextualist psychologist, a psychological act-in-context cannot be explained by an appeal to actions of various parts of the organism involved in the interaction (e.g., its brain, glands, etc.). Legs do not walk, brains do not think, and penises do not make love. People do these things, and people are integrated organisms.

This is not to say that biology or anthropology or other fields are not relevant to the psychological level. These other levels of analysis are legitimate in their own right and provide a context for psychological analyses. But we do not explain one level by an appeal to another—reductionism and expansionism are rejected.

Similarly, we cannot break an act-in-context into pieces and retain the quality of the event. The unit of analysis is an interactive whole. Specifically, an act alone and cut off from a context is not viewed as a psychological event at all. The environment is not an object, and actions in and with it are not separate things from it. We are dealing with an interaction in which each participant to the interaction defines the qualities of the other participants, much as the front of a coin implies a back and vice versa.

What integrates a behavioral event as a whole event is, at one level, the purpose of the persons doing the analysis, and at another, the purpose of the behaving organism. It is common for ACT therapists to respond to a client's statement by saying, "And that is in the service of . . . ?" If the actual process in therapy seems important at that moment, the ACT therapist might instead say, "And saying that to me right now is in the service of . . . ?" By focusing the client on the implicit consequences of an ongoing action in context, the therapist is trying to organize that action into functional units. Put another way, the purpose of the analysis is to find how best to construct a stream of behavior into whole units, and these units are organized in terms of the way the behavior seems to change the situation from one state of affairs to another. Thus, the philosophical concern for the whole event, organized in terms of its consequences, is reflected directly in the course of ACT.

The Role of Context

All concepts within our approach are contextually defined and delimited. If a statement about an event is made, the next question will be "And in what context does that occur?" This does not mean that a comprehensive list must be made in answer to that question—such a list would always eventually devolve into the universe of possible events. The totality is the ultimate context, but the totality is not something that can be described. Rather, because of the pragmatic purpose of analysis in this approach, the contextual features to be abstracted are those that contribute to the achievement of the goals of the therapist or scientist.

The ACT therapist is exquisitely sensitive to the role of context. Indeed, as will be shown later, ACT is essentially a contextual therapy in that it attempts to alter the social/verbal context rather than the form or content of clinically relevant behavior.

The Pragmatic Truth Criterion

The truth criterion of contextualism is *successful working*. Analyses are true only in terms of the accomplishment of particular goals. Thus, truth is always local and pragmatic. Your truth may not be mine, because we may have very different goals. No provision is made for the evaluation of the goals themselves.

The pragmatic truth criterion stands in stark contrast to the more usual correspondence-based criteria that dominate in both academic training and in the lay culture. The most commonly held worldview in academic psychology is surely mechanism. A mechanist tries to interpret the world as if it is a giant machine of unknown design. In understanding a simple machine, the task is to analyze its parts, the relations between the parts, and the forces that operate through them. We know that the machine is understood if our model of it corresponds to what we see. Implicit in a mechanistic view, the parts, relations, and forces are already preorganized in the world and are waiting to be discovered (in the quite literal sense of taking the cover off and seeing them). Thus, mechanism in epistemology is based in realism in ontology: We can know what is because what is is real.

Functional contextualism is, by contrast, peculiarly a-ontological—we can never go from workability to issues of being. We do not assume that the world is preorganized into discoverable parts, because to do so violates our pragmatic truth criterion. Consider, for example, two different renderings of a building—one is a drawing in perspective of the building, and the other is a blueprint of the building. Which is the true drawing of the building? The functional contextualist would say that there is no "true drawing" in an objective sense. The truer drawing could be determined only in the context of purposes. If one needed a drawing in order to identify the building while walking down a street, the perspective drawing would be the more useful and thus "truer," in the sense that it is true for this purpose. In contrast, if we wanted to know about some structural aspect of the building, the blueprint would be preferred.

Consistent with this philosophy, in ACT what is true is what works. An analysis of a problem behavior is true to the extent that it helps to solve the client's problem. Clients often take a quite different approach and attempt to justify dysfunctional experiences by making ontological claims. "I'm not just thinking this," they say. "It is true." And by "true" they very often do *not* mean that it works to be guided by a particular thought. Exactly the opposite. They mean, "It exists out there, and thus I have to respond to it even though it does not work to do so."

The philosophical assumptions of the mainstream culture can thereby trap our clients into taking their own thoughts literally even when they do not work. The security provided by moving away from a pragmatic truth criterion is a false security, and it has a tremendous cost. On the one hand, it seems that we are standing on the solid ground of insight and understanding. On the other hand, we become the victims of our own unworkable strategies. In an ACT approach, clients are encouraged to stay with the experience of what works or does not work. This is how the pragmatic truth criterion is operationalized.

Some contemporary therapies are based on a mechanistic realism and attempt to deal with the problem of unworkable thoughts in another way. Some types of cognitive-behavioral therapy, for example, are based on a computer metaphor (as is much of cognitive psychology itself). Like a computer, humans are thought to store, access, and process information. In this view, the task when dealing with an unworkable thought is to change the form of the thought, just as a computer may be changed by replacing memory chips or by changing software. This "out with the bad, in with the good" mechanistic approach is quite different from a contextual perspective wherein the emphasis may be on "seeing the bad thought as a thought, no more, no less." ACT is a derivative of behavior therapy in the sense that it addresses cognitions and other forms of behavior from a contextual behavioral viewpoint. At the same time, it rejects the mechanistic content-oriented forms of many behavioral and cognitive-behavioral treatments.

Analytic Goals in Contextualism

There is a final feature of functional contextualism that is related to the pragmatic truth criterion: its goals. Clarity about the goals of analysis is critical to contextualists because goals specify how a pragmatic truth criterion can be applied. Without a verbally stated goal, successful working implies that any behavior shaped by consequences would be "true" (see Hayes, 1993, for a detailed analysis of this point). This is nonsensical philosophically. Once we have a verbally stated goal, however, we can assess the degree to which analytic practices help us achieve it. Thus, successful working can function as a useful guide for a philosophy of science.

Because successful working is the means by which contextualists evaluate events, and goals allow this criterion to be applied, analytic goals themselves cannot ultimately be evaluated or justified. They can only be stated. To evaluate a goal via successful working would require yet another goal, but then that second goal could not be evaluated, and so on ad infinitum. Of course, we do have hierarchies of goals. For example, we may have process goals that are linked to outcome goals—we seek goal x because we believe that goal y is then more likely to be reached. In such a case, goal x can be evaluated in terms of its contribution to the achievement of goal y. In this case, however, goal y cannot be justified or evaluated. Ultimate analytic goals are thus the foundation of contextualism. Such goals must simply be stated and owned—naked and in the wind, so to speak.

Many contextualists have erred on this point. They have argued that *their* goals are *the* goals, but this is an inherently dogmatic position (see Hayes, 1993, for a discussion and several examples). Skinner, for instance, argued that the goals of science are prediction and control, but it is truer to a contextualistic approach to say that these were *his* goals for *his* science (Skinner, 1953, p. 35).

Understanding the importance of goals to contextualism helps us understand why there are different types of contextualistic theories. For example, some contextualists seek a personal appreciation of the whole by an examination of its participants. They are like historians, wanting to appreciate a unique historical event by examining closely all the strands that make up the whole story. Dramaturgy, hermeneutics, narrative psychology, interbehaviorism, and social constructionism are all examples of this type of contextualism (e.g., see Rosnow & Georgoudi, 1986; Sarbin, 1986), which we have termed "descriptive contextualism" (Hayes, 1993).

The Goals of Functional Contextualism

In contrast, functional contextualists have an intensely practical goal for analysis: the prediction and influence of events as an integrated goal. What we mean by "integrated" is that the position seeks concepts that can help in the achievement of all aspects of this goal at once, and with both precision and scope. Parenthetically, *influence* is a better word than *control* (even though "prediction and control" is a more common phrase) because *control* also refers to the elimination of behavioral variability in an absolute sense. To accomplish a particular end, some forms of behavioral variability may be undesirable, but that does not mean that action without variability in an absolute sense is better understood. The issue is not elimination of all variability, but rather the production of specified response functions, and thus *influence* is a better term (Biglan & Hayes, 1996).

The Practical Impact of These Goals

The choice of a goal in contextualism is *arbitrary*—not in the sense that it makes no difference (it makes an enormous difference), but in the sense that the choice is preanalytic. It is a means of analysis, not the result of analysis. Thus, neither descriptive nor functional contextualists can claim that their goal is the "right" goal or the only goal one might choose. But we can examine what happens when these different goals are adopted.

Of all the goals of functional contextualism, the most important is "influence." The contextual features to be abstracted in any contextualistic analysis are those that contribute to the achievement of the goals of the analysis. If we want analyses that achieve prediction and influence as *integrated* goals, then we cannot accept analyses that point to features that can only help us achieve prediction but cannot (in principle) directly achieve influence.

The environmentalism inherent in functional contextualism is a direct result. Verbal analyses generate rules for people, not rules for the world. If we seek prediction *and* influence, we must have rules that start with the environment, in the sense of the "world outside of the behavior." That is where we—the rule followers—are: in the potentially manipulable world outside the behavioral system being examined. To influence another's action, one must thus manipulate context—it is never possible to manipulate action directly (Hayes & Brownstein, 1986a). B. F. Skinner said it this way: "In practice, all these ways of changing a man's mind reduce to manipulating his environment, verbal or otherwise" (Skinner, 1969, p. 239).

This is one of the profound implications of functional contextualism and it dominates many aspects of ACT. Only contextual features that (1) are external to the behavior of the individual being studied and (2) are manipulable, at least in principle, could possibly lead *directly* to behavioral influence as an outcome. In other words, given the goals of functional contextualism, all analysis must trace phenomena back to the environmental context, both historically and situationally.

Contrast this with dominant mechanistic accounts that have little need for influence as a goal. In applying the machine metaphor, mechanism can seem to give the analyst a way of standing outside the system to be explained. The elements of the machine can seemingly be observed dispassionately, much as a spark plug sitting on a table can be examined. A mechanist explains a behavioral system by specifying its structure and the nature of its orderly operation, much as a person examining a car would readily explain its action by an appeal to way the pistons and spark plugs are put together. The contexts that gave rise to this structure or the ways we can manipulate it are irrelevant to the operation of the machine or the ontological reality of the pieces that are identified.

For example, it is completely sensible for a mechanist to say, "My client did this because he thought that." When a functional contextualist examines this statement, the objectionable word is *because*. One act can allow us to predict another, but we cannot directly take advantage of this observation *to accomplish the united goal of prediction and influence* until we are also told (1) the context in which both forms of activity occurred and (2) the context in which one form of activity was related to another. This is true for a simple reason: Thinking is also an act-in-context, and so the statement "My client did this because he thought that" is really the same as saying "My client did this because he did that." Acts can be changed only by changing context. Thus, a relationship between one form of action and another (e.g., between cognitions and motor behavior) can be useful for predicting behavior, but is not alone enough to influence it.

This is one of the philosophical cornerstones of ACT. It is what distinguishes it from cognitive therapy, much of traditional behavior therapy, and many other perspectives. Rather than trying to change the *form* of private experience, ACT therapists attempt to change the *functions* of private experiences by manipulating the context in which some forms of activity (e.g., thoughts and feelings) are usually related to other forms (e.g., overt actions).

This focus on goals of analysis is reflected in ACT as well. ACT places a very strong emphasis on specifying values at the individual level. All actions are evaluated relative to the client's chosen values and goals, and the issue is always workability, not objective truth. Thus, the four major philosophical characteristics of functional contextualism described here (the whole event, context, truth, and goals) are not empty abstractions when it comes to actual therapy; they are the implicit assumptions at the heart of ACT.

The Fit between Functional Contextualism and the Clinical Agenda

Because of their applied role and purpose, most clinicians want an analysis that does the following:

1. It explains why people are suffering.
2. It allows us to predict what people with particular psychological problems will do.
3. It tells us how to change the course of events so that this particular person with this particular psychological problem can achieve a better outcome.

These three goals (interpretation, prediction, and influence) are the clinician's *natural analytic agenda*. Clients, too, want these things from professionals. The individual client coming into psychotherapy usually wants to know, "Why am I like this and what can I do about it?" Thus, clinicians have a natural need to interpret, predict, and influence psychological problems. Practical reality forces them to embrace certain analytic values.

Functional contextualism fits hand in glove with these clinical purposes because their goals are identical. This is not true of other philosophical approaches, which seek understanding, coherence, prediction, or correspondence and see influence as a purely indirect or technical matter. For example, there is nothing in the truth criterion of mechanism that *demands* that the goal of influence be met, and often it is not. Mechanists believe that when a system is fully understood, it will be obvious how to change it if indeed it is changeable. This assumption is plausible if you assume that all the world is a machine and that only one model ultimately will be shown to be true. In this approach, the better our models are, the better we are mapping reality. Mechanists hope we will be able to do something practical with this knowledge, but whether we can or not does not change the soundness of what we know. For this reason, mechanists commonly emphasize a prediction goal. Prediction is scientifically fundamental in their system because it is how correspondence between a model of the world and the actual world is assessed. Mechanists deemphasize an influence goal, which is viewed merely as an applied extension of fundamental knowledge.

You can see this process clearly in the way cognitive scientists generally turn up their noses at cognitive therapy. Although they are somewhat flattered by the attention, basic cognitive psychologists see cognitive therapy as "merely an applied activity"—its success or failure says nothing about the truth of basic cognitive models of human functioning even if it is based on these models.

For the functional contextualist, influence is not an afterthought or merely an applied extension of basic knowledge. It is a metric for both applied and basic psychology. Thus, the practical concerns of the clinician are no longer separate from the analytic concerns of the researcher. This is one reason that we have moved so easily in the development of ACT from extremely basic research about such arcane matters as "what is a word" to extremely practical matters such as how to sequence specific techniques in ACT. The manipulable events that are involved in these levels of analysis often apply, one to the other.

The a-ontological stance and heavy contextual emphasis of functional contextualism casts a very new light on old issues. The most mundane clinical statement now leads to a very different sequence of questions. For example, suppose a client says, "I can't leave my home or I will have a panic attack." A mechanistic therapist would wonder why the person is panicky, or how the panic can be alleviated. Functional contextualism encourages many other options. Among many other steps, the clinician may (1) think of this statement as a doing—as itself an action—and examine the context in which the client would say such a thing, (2) note the construction of the world into units (leave home = panic) without ascribing reality status to the events described or to their supposed causal link, (3) look for environmental contexts in which "panic" is functionally related to "not leave home," with a view toward altering these contexts rather than necessarily trying to alter the panic itself, or (4) see this statement as a part of multiple strands of action and thus look for strands in which this same statement can be integrated into a positive process. In other words, instead of entering immediately into the literal content of the statement, a functional contextualist approach moves the attention of the clinician to the act and its context and harnesses all analyses to the analytic and pragmatic goals of the clinician and client.

As alluded to in the first chapter, we believe that language is at the heart of much human misery. Having sketched the philosophical underpinnings of ACT, we can now begin to examine the theoretical basis of the therapy. In what follows, we outline the progression of the theoretical development of our understanding of language processes and their role in human suffering.

RELATIONAL FRAME THEORY AND RULE GOVERNANCE: THE VIEW OF LANGUAGE UNDERLYING ACT

Emphasizing the importance of human language is not unique to ACT. It has been recognized throughout the history of humankind and in all cultures. For example, in the Book of Genesis, God creates the world by his utterance. The Yanomamo of South America are not only obliged by taboo not to speak the name of a prominent living person, but also mandated to permanently discontinue use of the names of dead persons (Chagnon, 1983). In a number of cultures "the link between a name and the person or thing denominated by it is not a mere arbitrary and ideal association, but a real and substantial bond which unites the two in such a way that magic may be wrought on a man just as easily through his name as through his hair, his nails, or any other material part of his person" (Frazer, 1911, p. 318).

The importance ascribed to language extends to scholarly and scientific domains. The last century has witnessed the emergence of a number of schools of philosophy and psychology that have been focused on language as a key to understanding human activity and the world that surrounds us (e.g., ordinary language philosophy, logical positivism, narrative psychology, psycholinguistics).

Although many of these approaches are quite interesting, few have been driven by a clinical agenda, and thus the analyses are often not of obvious relevance to the clinical environment. Unlike many groups doing basic scientific research on language, our interest in the basic analysis of verbal behavior stemmed directly from our interests in psychological well-being and clinical work. Beginning with questions about how it may be that a conversation between a client and a therapist could possibly lead to pervasive changes in the client's life, we became increasingly interested in experimental analyses of fundamental questions about human language. We started our basic research program with an attempt to understand how verbal rules guide human behavior. We ended up with an analysis of the nature of human language itself.

In what follows we present a summary of our theoretical approach to verbal behavior. We tell the story in the same sequence in which it was constructed, beginning with the more applied issues and moving toward the more basic. In the next chapter we apply our analysis more specifically to experiential avoidance and its treatment. This is highly technical, basic experimental work. Because of the complexity of this area of theory and research, we attempt only a brief, general, and relatively user-friendly summary here. Periodically we will summarize major points that guide the ACT work in the form of basic principles.

Rule-Governed Behavior

Although most of the technical sources of ACT derive from the interface between behavior therapy and the human potential movement, its intellectual foundation comes almost entirely out of a contextual behavior analytic perspective. Within behavior analysis there has long been a distinction between contingency-shaped behavior and rule-governed behavior, and understanding that distinction is of fundamental importance clinically. "Contingency-shaped behavior" is behavior that has been established by a gradual shaping of successive approximations, such as learning to catch a ball by trial and error. Many forms of human behavior are acquired this way, but many others are based on verbal formulations of events and the relations between them. This kind of behavior is said to be "rule governed." According to Skinner (1969), rule-governed behavior is behavior governed by the specification of contingencies rather than by direct contact with them. Rule-governed behavior allows human beings to respond in very precise and effective ways where contingency-based learning may be ineffective or even lethal, such as when the consequences of behavior are subtle, small, temporally remote, cumulative, or probabilistic. For example, one would not want to engage in a shaping process to learn to avoid high-voltage electrical wires. Similarly, we know from basic experimental work that consequences that are greatly delayed are usually ineffective. Humans may, however, respond effectively to a description of enormously delayed consequences such as "Be nice to your uncle, and in 20 years he will remember you in his will."

Skinner's discussion of rules points to many of the adaptive features of this kind of verbal behavior. But rules are not without cost. We quickly discovered this in our own experimental work and that of our colleagues. It turns out that when behavior is controlled by verbal rules, it tends to be relatively insensitive to changes in the environment that are not contacted by or described in a rule itself (Hayes, Brownstein, Haas, & Greenway, 1986; Hayes, Brownstein, Zettle, Rosenfarb, & Korn, 1986; Matthews, Shimoff, Catania, & Sagvolden, 1977; Shimoff, Catania, & Matthews, 1981; see Catania, Shimoff, & Matthews, 1989, and Hayes, Zettle, & Rosenfarb, 1989, for reviews of this literature). When their behavior is guided by verbal rules, humans often track changes in the environment with less precision than do nonhumans. For example, a person told to "push this button rapidly to make points" may now be less likely, because of this instruction, to stop pushing when the points no longer occur (Hayes, Brownstein, Haas, & Greenway, 1986; Matthews et al., 1977; Shimoff et al., 1981), to push more slowly when there is no longer a need to push rapidly (Galizio, 1979), or to change patterns of button pushing to make more points (Shimoff et al., 1981).

The data shown in Figure 2.1 illustrate the problem. In this study (Hayes, Brownstein, Haas, & Greenway, 1986) subjects learned a task either by directly following a rule or by experience. Later, the task requirements were changed, without any notice being given to the subjects. All of the subjects who learned the task by experience were sensitive to the change, as compared with only half of the subjects who originally learned the task by following verbal rules.

This "insensitivity" effect excited us in part because many forms of clinically significant behavior seem to exemplify the same overall pattern: Practices persist despite their directly experienced or potential neg-

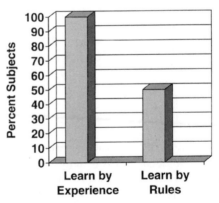

FIGURE 2.1. The sensitivity to changing task requirements when the original task was learned by direct experience or by following a rule.

ative consequences. It led us to this basic principle that guides much of the ACT work: *Establishing behavior by direct rules can induce rigidity and should not be done lightly.* Sometimes it is helpful to induce rigidity, but very often it is not, and therapists should not just rush into direct instruction without careful forethought. We conducted a series of studies trying to understand why rules worked this way (see Chapters 5, 6, and 10 in Hayes, 1989) and eventually organized what we had learned into a functional taxonomy of rule-governed behavior that allowed more precise principles to be derived.

Varieties of Rule-Governed Behavior

In our attempts to examine the effects of rules theoretically and empirically, three functionally distinct varieties of rules emerged: pliance, tracking, and augmenting (Hayes, Zettle, & Rosenfarb, 1989). These three forms of rule governance are all useful and important, but they can also produce behavioral problems.

Pliance

Pliance (taken from the word *compliance*) involves following a verbal rule based on a history of socially mediated consequences for the correspondence between the rule and the rule-follower's behavior. Suppose a child were told by a parent to "wear a coat—it is cold outside." If the child responds based on a history of pleasing or displeasing the parent, that is pliance. Developmentally, pliance is probably the first variety of rule following that individuals learn (Hayes & Hayes, 1989). There is a lot of evidence that pliance is a very pervasive form of rule-governed behavior, even in clinical situations (see Hayes, Zettle, & Rosenfarb, 1989, for a review of several studies of that kind).

Tracking

Tracking is rule-governed behavior under the control of a history of a correspondence between the rule and "natural" social or nonsocial contingencies. Natural contingencies are those produced entirely by the exact form of the behavior in a particular situation (Hayes & Wilson, 1993; Hayes, Zettle, & Rosenfarb, 1989).

Before we give examples of tracks, it is important to be clear about the nature of natural contingencies. For example, suppose a person kicks in a window. Whether the kick results in a cut is 100% dependent on the exact form of the behavior in that particular situation. The cut is a natural consequence. Other consequences are not natural in this sense, because the consequence depends on the discrimination of others about the historical factors, motivation, or other features of the behavioral episode beyond the simple form of the response. For example, whether kicking in a window results in a legal fine is dependent on whether it was "accidental" or "deliberate"—that is, whether the social community determines that the behavior was rule governed. That consequence is inherently arbitrary and conventional because it is determined by more than the exact form of the behavior in that particular situation (e.g., the opinion of the community about its history).

For an example of tracking we return to the child who is told, "Wear a coat—it is cold outside." If the child puts on a coat to get warm, under the control of a history of such rules accurately describing the likely temperature, then the behavior is tracking.

The Pliance–Tracking Distinction

Developmentally, tracking is more subtle than pliance, inasmuch as no new consequences are added to the ongoing situation by the rule. In the case of pliance, new speaker-mediated consequences are suddenly present once the rule is given. In the case of tracking, they were there all along. This is probably why young children tend to follow commands like "No!" before they learn to react to tracks that dispassionately orient them to the environment, such as "Your ball is in the bedroom." If the child fails to comply with the command "No," immediate additional consequences will be applied. If the child fails to understand or follow a track, no new consequences will be added, and, furthermore, the described consequences may appear anyway (e.g., when the child wanders into the bedroom, the ball may be found).

Pliance involves the verbal community making a discrimination about the source of the behavior seen. In that sense, the contingency involved in pliance is always arbitrary. Conversely, tracking puts rule followers in contact with the natural contingencies, and once it is established, the natural contingencies will determine whether the behavior is maintained. Parenthetically, the natural/arbitrary distinction is not the same as a nonsocial/social distinction. A rule that tells a person how to be liked by others may still be a track.

The distinction between plys and tracks is thus functional, not formal. A rule can be in obvious track form and still evoke pliance. For example, a teenager accurately told, "Your friends will get you in trouble," may respond by telling the parent to "stop trying to control what I do." The parent's rule is in track form, but it is probably functioning as a ply—as if consequences for following or not following the rule are arbitrary rather than as a description of natural consequences.

Behavior that is rebellious or resistant (what we call "counterpliance") may still be pliance, so long as the function of the rule is dependent on a history of socially mediated consequences for a correspondence between the rule and relevant behavior. Rebellion of this kind has probably been consequated in the past by the social withdrawal of the parent or other rule giver. Said another way, complying or rebelling are functionally similar. This is a pattern that child and adolescent therapists know only too well.

Augmenting

Augmenting is rule-governed behavior that alters the extent to which some event will function as a consequence. There are two subvarieties of augmentals (see Hayes & Ju, 1997). The first consists of *motivative augmentals*. These are rules that increase the value of an event that is already a functional consequence. Advertisers utilize this form of rule governance in powerful and profitable ways. An example is, "Wouldn't a big juicy Whopper taste good right now?" If an individual already valued this kind of hamburger, this description may serve to increase the probability of the person's going out for a Whopper, even though the rule does not signal any change in the *availability* of such hamburgers. The person is simply temporarily motivated to secure the consequence of interest, probably because some of the stimulus functions of the consequence are brought into the present by the verbal rule (how that happens is discussed later).

A second variety of augmental is the *formative augmental*. Formative augmentals establish some new event as an important consequence. Suppose, for example, you are told for the first time that *bon* in French is the same as *bueno* in Spanish, and that *bueno* in Spanish is the same as *bra* in Swedish, and that *bra* in Swedish is the same as *good* in English. If *good* already functions as a reinforcer, this rule alone may make it possible to teach new skills by consequating appropriate performances with *bon, bueno,* or *bra*. This process has been shown empirically in several studies (e.g., Hayes, Devany, Kohlenberg, Brownstein, & Shelby, 1987; Hayes, Kohlenberg, & Hayes, 1991).

Augmenting is the most difficult form of rule-governed behavior, because it is used dominantly to establish the control of abstract, imagined, or previously inexperienced consequences. For example, children have a hard time learning to work for such described consequences as future good grades, future good jobs, avoidance of hell, or access to heaven. Loosely speaking, we say, "They have a hard time imagining it," and what we mean is that the child's history has not yet established the influence of such verbal rules.

Some Clinical Implications of the Functional
Analysis of Rule Governance

A number of behavior problems have been analyzed in terms of problematic rule governance (see Hayes, Kohlenberg, & Melancon, 1989; Poppen, 1989; Zettle & Hayes, 1982). Moral behavior, for example, seems to depend on the gradual acquisition of more and more complex forms of rule-governed behavior (Hayes, Gifford, & Hayes, 1998), from pliance, to tracking, to augmenting, to concern over such behaviors in others. Similarly, it is known that impulsive and hyperactive behavior is more likely when rules are not functional (Barkley, 1997). ACT seeks to establish verbal control in some areas (e.g., commitment to chosen values), but it also seeks to undermine it in others. This is because of certain problems with rules that often occur. Thus, understanding the structure and purpose of ACT is easier if you understand the strengths and weaknesses of different kinds of verbal rules.

Problems with Pliance

Research has shown that the insensitivity produced by rules is largely, though not exclusively, the result of pliance (Barrett, Deitz, Gaydos, & Quinn, 1987; Hayes, Brownstein, Zettle, et al., 1986). We know that rule-induced insensitivity correlates fairly highly with psychological rigidity as a psychological trait (Wulfert, Greenway, Farkas, Hayes, & Dougher, 1994). In other words, obsessive and rigid styles of interacting with the world can be thought of as a kind of excessive pliance in which wanting to "be good" or to please others (or to offend or maintain independence from others) dominates over one's direct, personal experience of what works. It is hard to do what works if one is too focused on simply being "good" or on rebellion. Establishing behavior by pliance in therapy is particularly risky as it can lead to reduced sensitivity to other environmental contingencies or can produce counterpliance (i.e., resistance). A good example is the therapist who teaches and strongly reinforces "appropriate assertion" in a dependent female client, only to find that the client is not really becoming more independent but instead is now looking for approval from the therapist for this new behavior.

In an ACT model, many forms of psychopathology are based on destructive types of pliance. Not all forms of pliance are destructive (it seems to be especially important in childhood, for example), but in adulthood the good that comes from pliance can almost always come more efficiently from tracking and augmenting. For example, adults do not need to show compassion in order to be praised by others; they can show compassion as an expression of chosen personal values (augmenting) and doing what works in regard to those values (tracking). For these reasons, ACT is often focused on the reduction of pliance.

This value is carried over into the therapy process. The ACT therapist is very much interested in using the social context of therapy to induce change, but is quite cautious about using the therapeutic relationship to induce specific forms of rule following. As will be seen later, ACT undermines pliance in therapy in part by its paradoxical and confusing style—it is very hard to know how to please or offend an ACT therapist, and any attempts to do so are more likely to produce unexpected than predictable reactions from the therapist.

Problems with Tracking

Detecting and undermining ineffective tracking is one of the key concepts in ACT. ACT therapists spend a fair amount of time detecting "strange loops"—instances in which following an apparent track produces the opposite effect to that specified by the rule.

Tracks are problematic when they are inaccurate, untestable, self-fulfilling, or are applied to situations that can only be contingency shaped. If tracks are inaccurate, they can produce dysfunctional behavior. If they are untestable or self-fulfilling, the natural feedback loop between following a rule and the consequences of doing so will be absent or misleading. This can easily produce a strange loop. For example, tracking the rule "I am worthless" will almost inevitably lead to behavior that confirms the rule, because the actions taken will retain some of the functional properties of the rule itself. If a person says, "I pretend to be smart because I'm really worthless," the praise from others will connect the person with his or her assumed worthlessness, the praise will appear to be manipulated, the person will feel as though others are fools, and so on. The end result is likely to be *continued* feelings of worthlessness, despite the signs of objective success.

Overexpansive tracks are those that are applied to situations that can only be contingency shaped. When following overexpansive tracks, a person is likely to behave ineffectively but will not know why. An example of the latter is hitting a baseball. Yogi Berra used to say, "Don't think; just hit." The speed and coordination required in seeing a ball and swinging at it can be disrupted by trying to do so under the control of a rule (e.g., "Swing level and let your wrist break just as you hit the ball"). Overexpansive tracks are perhaps the most common form of strange loops. An example is a person with panic disorder trying to avoid panic by verbal threats ("You have to stop this or else!"). Threats elicit anxiety, and thus the attempt to regulate it verbally through threats can elicit it.

Cognitive therapy has paid considerable attention to altering the form of inaccurate tracks such as "I cannot be happy if anyone is unhappy with me" (see Zettle & Hayes, 1982). Other theorists, such as Albert Bandura, have focused attention on the effects of inaccurate "efficacy expectations." Such expectations as "No matter how hard I try, I can't stop drinking" may be thought of as inaccurate tracks. These therapeutic approaches, however, do not attempt to reduce tracking per se in given situations. Rather, they attempt to replace "bad" tracks with "good" ones.

ACT likewise focuses on a major class of inaccurate tracks: those related to private events (things that only the person having them can experience directly, such as thoughts, feelings, memories, bodily sensations, and the like) and the need for their modification, such as, "If only I could get rid of the memories of my incest history, I could become more intimate with my partner." These tracks are most problematic, however, because they tend to be self-fulfilling and thus are difficult to test.

What is unique about ACT is the attempt to weaken tracking per se in some contexts in order to bring it under better contextual control based on workability as the unit of analysis. Weakening tracking is difficult because tracking is so massively useful in most areas of living. Thus, it does little good to argue rationally for the limits of tracking: This amounts to the construction of a track about the need not to track. Even if the rule is understood or followed ("Oh, I see, Doctor. I should not be so rational. Hmmm. That is very rational."), it is unsuccessful because it strengthens the verbal process that one is trying to weaken.

In ACT, excessive tracking is addressed by undermining the literal coherence of language itself, in combination with an increased sensitivity to the workability of various rule-governed responses. Many of the more unusual techniques in ACT (such as the use of inherent paradoxes, deliberate confusion, cognitive defusion exercises) are designed to undermine excessive tracking via an alteration of literal language. The theoretical basis for this approach will be addressed in more detail shortly, when our approach to verbal meaning is described.

Problems with Augmenting

ACT also focuses on problematic augmenting. A common problematic form of augmenting occurs when a track specifies that a process goal is linked to an outcome goal. In this case, the outcome goal will function as an augmental for the process goal. The problem is never in the ultimate outcome goal—recall that within contextualism such goals can only be specified, not evaluated. The problem is that the process goal may be an innocent psychological bystander that is not necessarily related to the outcome goal.

The most important clinical manifestation of this problem is the tendency to link the form and quality of private experiences to the goal of being a success in life. If it is true that one can live a vital and committed life only if bad thoughts or feelings disappear, then this process goal assumes great psychological importance. Consider the example of a person who is trying to get rid of painful memories in order to relate intimately. Perhaps the person was raped or molested, and these memories have made it hard to develop and maintain intimate adult relationships. It is likely that such a person will work all the harder to get rid of the bad memories whenever anything occurs that highlights the benefits of an intimate relationship or the pain associated with lack of such relationships. For instance, a person's seeing a happy couple holding hands, or seeing signs of a partner's frustration after this person's refusing to have sex, could increase motivation to eliminate the memories. In this case, it is not the ultimate outcome goal (itself a formative augmental) that is the problem. Wanting an intimate relationship, for example, is not unhealthy. The problem is that an inaccurate track ("I have to control my bad thoughts and feelings to find real intimacy") is now an augmental for a struggle with thoughts and feelings. Changing problematic memories and the emotions associated with them is now even more important than before—in our view, needlessly.

ACT seeks both to undermine augmentals that lead to useless struggle and to use augmentals linked to experiential openness and chosen values. A wide variety of experiential exercises are used in ACT as motivative augmentals to sensitize the client to the suffering caused by self-struggle. The client's psychological pain is a major ally in ACT (indeed, "Your pain is your greatest ally" is a common ACT phrase), and we return to it for augmenting purposes when the going is particularly tough.

As with any contextualistic system, outcome goals are also of key importance. ACT is thus extremely focused on the client's ultimate values. Values are brought out and clarified for their augmental functions, either formative or motivative. It helps a client to let go of struggle if it can be remembered that the larger purpose is to love, or participate, or share, or contribute to others. In ACT, augmentals linked to chosen outcomes should be strengthened; those linked to process goals should be strengthened or weakened, based on their proven impact on outcome goals (i.e., their workability).

The Nature of Verbal Events

As we continued our research into rule-governed behavior, we needed to learn more about how to undermine the control of rules of any kind. As discussed earlier, in some situations it seemed as though a direct, literal, verbal solution to the problems of excessive verbal control could not work because direct, literal, verbal solutions were the very problem we were trying to undermine. This was particularly true in the area of tracking. Even accurate tracks—that is, even rational rules—are still rules. But there are some areas in which rules do not belong. Letting go of such rules seemed to require a deeper understanding of such language processes because the obvious courses of action (e.g., telling people not to be so rational) seemed internally inconsistent. After several years of work on rule governance and after producing the first book focused entirely on that topic (Hayes, 1989), we began to turn to an analysis of the nature of human language itself.

Despite our interest in contextual behavior analysis, we did not find Skinner's specific approach to be adequate in this area. The reasons for our concern have been detailed elsewhere (e.g., Hayes & Hayes, 1992), but the core concern was that traditional behavior analytic conceptions of language missed the essence of symbolic activity. Because of this mistake, the central role of language-involved actions such as cognition and emotion was denied in behavior analysis, even though the phenomena themselves were viewed as legitimate.

Stimulus Equivalence

We began working on derived stimulus relations and stimulus equivalence as a jumping-off point for an empirical attack on the essence of human verbal behavior. The fundamental phenomenon of stimulus equivalence is usually examined in what is called a matching-to-sample paradigm. In a visual example of such a paradigm, an unfamiliar visual stimulus (such as a graphical squiggle or a series of three consonants) is presented at the top of a computer screen. A set of perhaps three novel comparison stimuli is provided. The subject is then reinforced for selecting the "correct" comparison stimuli. Comparison stimuli are arbitrarily assigned as either correct or incorrect by the experimenter. There is no formal property of the stimuli that provides a basis for correctness. In this way, the subject is taught that given stimulus A1 (we are using the label "A1" for ease of understanding, but in fact the actual stimulus would be an arbitrary one such as a graphical squiggle) and comparisons B1, B2, and B3, to pick B1, not B2 nor B3. In further training, the subject may be taught that given the stimulus A1 and another set of comparisons, C1, C2, and C3, to pick C1. The stimuli that are incorrect would be correct in the presence of other samples. Given stimulus A2 and the comparisons B1, B2, and B3, for example, the subject would be taught to pick B2, not B1 or B3.

Such conditional discriminations can be trained in any complex organism (e.g., rats, pigeons, or people). What is striking, however, is the derived performances that result in people but seemingly not in nonhumans. A nonhuman exposed to a trial in which B1 is presented for the first time as the sample stimulus, with the previous samples—A1, A2, and A3—as the comparisons, will select A1 only at the level of chance. The discriminations taught do not automatically reverse. Verbally competent humans, on the other hand, will readily select A1 without explicit feedback or training, exhibiting what is called "symmetry." This occurs in human children as young as 17 months old (Lipkens, Hayes, & Hayes, 1993). Similarly, if presented with a trial with B1 as the sample and C1, C2, and C3 as the comparisons, humans will readily select C1, whereas nonhumans will again respond at chance levels. Note that in this equivalence trial, the subject has never before even seen the B and C stimuli together at the same time. We can think of equivalence classes this way: Train two sides of a triangle in any one direction; as a result, humans will show all sides in all directions.

The basic arrangement is shown in Figure 2.2. Training two stimulus relations to a nonhuman generates two stimulus relations. Training two stimulus relations to a human generates six stimulus relations. As a result, there is an inherent economy of learning that gives humans a great advantage over nonverbal organisms.

Equivalence classes provide a ready model of word-referent relations. If a child is taught to relate a written word to an oral name, and a written word to a class of objects, then all the other relations will emerge without further training. This is part of what we mean when we say that a child "understands" what a word means. The child, without explicit

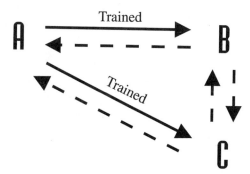

FIGURE 2.2. An example of stimulus equivalence. Training is indicated by the solid arrows, and derived stimulus relations are indicated by the dashed arrows.

training in this specific case, will be able to say the name of the object, for example.

This arrangement is shown in Figure 2.3. Suppose a child is taught that the three letters C - A - T are called "cat." Furthermore, the child is taught that these three letters go with a class of furry animals with four legs and a tail who meow. So far we have two stimulus relations (written word–oral name; written word–class of objects). But now we show such an animal to the child and say, "What is this?" The child will probably say "a cat." Similarly, if we say, "Where is the cat?" the child may point toward a furry animal with four legs and a tail. These performances are represented by the vertical dashed arrows in Figure 2.3. Although almost all humans (except the most severely retarded) show such derived relations readily and very early, after 20 years of searching there are still no convincing data for such an ability in nonhumans.

This remarkable behavioral performance opens up whole new ways of establishing and altering behavior. What makes stimulus equivalence clinically relevant is that functions given to one member of an equivalence class tend to transfer to other members. Let us consider a simple example. Suppose the child trained in the way shown in Figure 2.3 has never before seen or played with a cat. After learning the word → object, and word → oral name relations, the child can derive four additional relations: object → word, oral name → word, oral name → object, and object → oral name. Now suppose that the child is scratched while playing with a cat. The child cries and runs away. Later the child hears Mother saying, "Oh, look! A cat." Now the child again cries and runs away, even though the child was never scratched in the presence of the word.

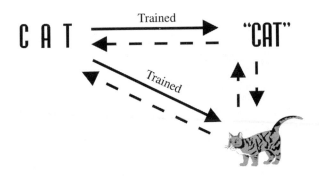

FIGURE 2.3. How derived stimulus relations establish literal meaning. Training is indicated by the solid arrows, and derived stimulus relations are indicated by the dashed arrows.

These kinds of processes are not based on the simple and familiar processes of stimulus generalization, because there are no formal properties that bring these stimuli together. These new forms of behavior are established through very indirect means. Such effects may help explain why, for example, people with agoraphobia can have an initial panic attack while "trapped" in a shopping mall and soon find that they are worrying about being "trapped" in an open field, in a marital relationship, on a bridge, or in a job. What brings these situations together is not their formal properties in a simple sense, but the verbal classes in which they share membership.

Relational Frame Theory

Equivalence is a beginning model of word-referent relations, but it is not enough to explain the functions of verbal rules nor the complexity of human language. Relational Frame Theory (RFT) (Hayes, 1991; Hayes & Hayes, 1989, 1992; Hayes & Wilson, 1993; Hayes & Barnes, 1997) expands stimulus equivalence into the larger, more general case.

RFT begins with the idea that organisms can learn to respond relationally to various stimulus events. This is not an entirely odd idea inasmuch as we know that nonarbitrary stimulus relations can be learned by almost any complex organism (Reese, 1968). For instance, a rat can be trained to turn down the least brightly lit of two alleys. With sufficient history, such a rat could negotiate a maze in which it was required to choose directions based on the relative brightness of the alternatives, even if the particular levels of illumination had never been used before. We reasoned that if such nonarbitrary stimulus relations can be learned, perhaps subjects can also learn to treat arbitrary stimulus combinations as if they are related in particular ways. Because the pairs would be arbitrary, these relational responses would have to be under the control of cues other than simply the form of the related events. For example, could humans learn to relate the two words *dim* and *bright* much as they would an actual dim and bright stimulus, given some contextual cue that would define the comparative relation between them?

Such contextual control has often been demonstrated in stimulus equivalence research (Bush, Sidman, & deRose, 1989; Gatch & Osborne, 1989; Wulfert & Hayes, 1988), and it is obvious in natural language. The spoken word *bat* has a different meaning when a person is in a dark cave, as opposed to being at a baseball game.

This simple idea has wide implications. It means that it may be possible to learn to relate events arbitrarily and in a large number of ways, and then to apply these learned relational patterns to new stimuli based simply on the proper arrangement of contextual cues. In this perspective, stimulus equivalence is a learned class of behaviors, and it is only one of many kinds of derived stimulus relations. For example, stimulus relations such as more–less, before–after, opposite, or different are all examples of learned and arbitrarily applicable stimulus relations.

This more flexible concept views the action of relating stimuli as a kind of learned overarching behavioral class. Such classes have been identified before in behavioral psychology. Generalized imitation can be viewed as an example of such a class. If a generalized imitative repertoire has been trained (the basic components of which seem to be inborn), a virtually unlimited variety of response topographies can be substituted for the topographies used in the initial training (e.g., Baer, Peterson, & Sherman, 1967; Gewirtz & Stengle, 1968). A child who has learned to smile when a mother smiles, and clap when the mother claps, may also now wave when the mother waves, even though this specific topography has never been trained. There are other examples of these kinds of learned overarching behavioral classes, such as learned creativity (Pryor, Haag, & O'Reilly, 1969) or learned randomness (Neuringer, 1986; Page & Neuringer, 1985).

There are three main properties of relating as a learned class of behavior. First, such relations show mutual entailment. That is, if a person learns in a particular context that A relates in a particular way to B, then this must entail some kind of relation between B and A in that context. For example, if Alan is said to be larger than Bob, then Bob must be smaller than Alan. We will also call this property "bidirectionality." Second, such relations show combinatorial entailment: If a person learns in a particular context that A relates in a particular way to B, and B relates in a particular way to C, then this must entail some kind of mutual relation between A and C in that context. For example, if Bob is larger than Charlie, then Alan is also larger than Charlie. Finally, such relations enable a transformation of stimulus functions among related stimuli. If you need a person to arm wrestle an enemy, and Charlie is known to be valuable, Alan is probably even more valuable. Derived stimulus functions of this kind have been demonstrated with conditioned reinforcing functions (Hayes, Devany, et al., 1987; Hayes, Kohlenberg, & Hayes, 1991), discriminative functions (Hayes, Devaney, et al., 1987), elicited conditioned emotional responses (Dougher, Augustson, Markham, & Greenway, 1994), and extinction functions (Dougher et al., 1994). Verbal relations can even actively transform functions based on the relational network involved (see Dymond & Barnes, 1995, 1996, for empirical examples). For example, suppose a person is told that a tone precedes a shock and a buzzer will follow it. The tone will now elicit arousal. The buzzer will occasion calm.

We now know that once stimulus relations are derived, they are extraordinarily difficult to break up, even with direct contradictory training (Saunders, 1989). Furthermore, even if they are changed by direct training, they will later show "resurgence" if the new pattern itself no longer works (Wilson & Hayes, 1996). In other words, once verbal relations are derived, they never seem really to go away. You can add to them, but you cannot really eliminate them altogether. Even if they disappear functionally, they may reappear if newly learned verbal behavior is disrupted.

We also now know that one of the major consequences for derived relational responding is "sense making." Even without any external feedback, subjects will create orderly stimulus relations between arbitrary stimulus sets (Saunders, 1989), and one of the most effective ways to prevent the derivation of stimulus relations is the use of occasional incoherent and confusing tests items (Leonhard & Hayes, 1991). Once we learn how to derive relations between events, we do so constantly as long as we are able to make order of our world by doing so. Whereas direct shaping gradually establishes generalized patterns of responses, the formation of sets of derived stimulus relations is more categorical—more all or nothing. Elements are either in or out, in a given context.

We are now ready to define the term *relational frame*. This term is used to specify a particular pattern of contextually controlled and arbitrarily applicable relational responding involving mutual entailment, combinatorial entailment, and the transformation of stimulus functions. This pattern of responding is established by a history of differential reinforcement for producing such relational response patterns in the presence of relevant contextual cues, not on a history of direct nonrelational training with respect to the stimuli involved (see Hayes, 1991, and Hayes & Hayes, 1989, 1992, for further elaboration). Although the term *relational frame* is a noun, it always refers to the situated act of an organism. That is, the organism does not respond to a relational frame. It responds to historically established contextual cues—and the response is to frame these events relationally. Although *framing relationally* may be preferred from a technical perspective (see Hayes & Hayes, 1992, and Malott, 1991, for further discussion), we will use the less cumbersome noun form. Relational Frame Theory is still new, but there is an array of basic behavioral evidence in support of it (see Hayes & Barnes, 1997). Even quite young children can show astoundingly complex forms of behavior based on a small number of trained relational responses (Barnes, Hegarty, & Smeets, 1997). For example, a relational network composed of just a dozen trained uni-directional relations will yield hundreds of derived relations.

So What Is a Verbal Event?

Having defined relational frames, we are finally ready to define a verbal event. A verbal event is simply one that has its psychological functions because it participates in a relational frame. This elegantly simple definition brings good order to the line of cleavage between verbal and nonverbal events. For instance, verbal rules are "verbal" because their effects depend on their elements being in relational frames. Gestures, signs, and pictures are "verbal" if their effects depend on their participation in relational frames, but they are "nonverbal" if that is not true. It is a core position of ACT that the literal nature of human language is based on relational frames. Thus, weakening the literal functions of language requires the weakening of relational frames in specific contexts.

Suppose I tell you, "After you read this book, you will understand ACT a little differently." This sentence has meaning because the various elements of the sentence are in relational frames with other events and because the elements serve as cues for new relational actions and the functions that can be transformed by them.

"After" is a relational term. It is in an equivalence class with a particular relational frame (namely, the temporal frame of before and after) and serves as a cue for the application of that relational frame. That term puts "read this book" before the consequence of that action, namely, what you understand about ACT.

By now "ACT" is in an equivalence class with "Acceptance and Commitment Therapy" for readers. The phase "you read this book" is also a sequence of stimuli in equivalence classes that specify who and what are being spoken about (e.g., "you" is in an equivalence class with the conscious organism gazing at these pages), but "read" further serves as a particular cue that brings a previously established psychological function to bear on what was just described. Thus, this part of the sentence specifies an antecedent condition (this book) and a function to apply to that condition (you read).

"You will understand ACT a little differently" also has stimuli in equivalence classes ("understanding" is in an equivalence relation with the very act of deriving stimulus relations) and stimuli that serve as relational cues ("little" and "differently"). The phrase establishes a relation of difference between the derived relations that exist now in the reader and those that will follow reading, and limits those difference relations by the comparative relation of big and small, or more and less.

Given this reformulation, the sentence is a contingency specification. It tells the reader how to respond to an antecedent and what to expect as a consequence of that action. Several different relational frames (coordination or equivalence; difference; comparison; temporal relations) are applied to a set of terms that are already in equivalence classes with various events, and contextual cues are provided for specific psychological actions that are to be brought to bear on the situation.

If you have derived the stimulus relations properly (if you understand the sentence), we could enter into the resulting relational network in any one of several ways. We could ask, for example, "What will happen after you read the book?" or "When will your understanding be different?" or "How different will it be?" If the relational network has been properly established, all of these questions will be answered readily, even though none of them has been trained directly in this instance.

These relational actions working together is what it means to "understand" a rule. Whether or not the rule is followed is a different matter. "After you read this book, you will understand ACT a little differently" could function as a track, for example, and if the reader has the proper history with such rules, it probably will. Or it could function as a ply—for example, the reader might now be expected to understand things differently by an instructor who is aware of the examples in the book, and the reader may modify his or her behavior for that reason.

All of these actions on the part of the listener or reader are "verbal" by our definition, because all of these actions depend on relational frames. In the same way, a speaker is speaking verbally and "meaningfully" when the act of speaking is dependent on a relational frame.

It is worth noting that, defined in this way, most human behavior is verbal, at least to a degree. If we look at a tree and see a T-R-E-E, a "plant" that "photosynthesizes" and has particular "cell structures" and so on—then the tree is functioning as a verbal stimulus for the observer. It is hard for humans to avoid the derived nature of stimulus functions in their world, because even "nonverbal" stimuli quickly become verbal in part when they enter into relational frames. Much of what we know we "know" only verbally.

In Chapter 1 we noted that human suffering seems to be based in part on verbal knowledge. We described the biblical story of Adam and Eve as a story with that main theme. Relational Frame Theory leads to the same conclusion. We will discuss that repeatedly throughout the book, but a brief description of the position seems worthwhile now.

Verbal and Nonverbal Knowing

The word *know* in English has an interesting etymology. It comes from two quite distinct Latin roots: *gnoscere,* which means "knowing by the senses," and *scire,* which means "knowing by the mind." In the usual human conception, knowing by the mind (knowing things consciously) is familiar and safe. It is unconscious, nonverbal processes that seem strange and hard to understand. Scientifically, it is the other way around. Knowing by direct experience, or contingency-shaped behavior, is something psychologists understand quite well. Verbal knowledge, or "knowing by the mind," is strange and hard to understand.

Relational Frame Theory views verbal knowledge as the result of networks of highly elaborated and interconnected derived stimulus relations. That is what "minds" are full of. These relational responses enable forms of activity that could not occur otherwise. It is some of these activities that are at the root of human suffering.

Let us consider an example. Almost all schools of psychology have emphasized the importance of self-knowledge. For example, B. F. Skinner suggested, "Self-knowledge has a special value to the individual himself. A person who has been 'made aware of himself' is in a better position to predict and control his own behavior" (Skinner, 1974, p. 31). We agree, but these benefits depend on relational frames.

Because of the mutual entailment quality of relational frames, when a human interacts verbally with his or her own behavior, the psychological meaning of both the verbal symbol and the behavior itself can change. This bidirectional property makes human self-awareness useful, but it also makes it potentially aversive and destructive.

A pigeon can easily be taught that kind of self-awareness or self-knowledge. For example, suppose we teach a pigeon (using food as a consequence) to peck one key after it has been shocked and another after it has not been shocked. We are, in effect, asking the pigeon whether it has been shocked, and the bird is "answering." These answers are not, however, bidirectionally related to the original condition. For that reason, the bird will as readily "report" about the shock as it will the absence of shock. These reports, after all, lead to food, not shock.

Humans are quite different, because verbal self-awareness or self-knowledge (using our definition of *verbal*) is bidirectionally related to the original condition. Thus, for example, even the very word *shock* will carry with it some of the aversive functions of shock itself. For the verbally competent human, the word *shock* and the actual shock exist in an equivalence class and therefore share some stimulus functions. This is why humans often cry when reporting past hurts and traumas even (or perhaps especially) if the report has never been made before. The crying comes because the report is mutually related to the event itself, not because the report itself has been directly associated in the past with aversive events. In addition, changes that are made in the functions of the verbal report can also change the functions of stimulus conditions similar to that being reported. For example, if the aversiveness of reporting about a past trauma with Dad diminishes (for example, by extinction and habituation), the aversiveness of Dad himself will change. Neither of these kinds of results would occur in nonverbal organisms. This bi-directional relation is the basis of a great deal of clinical work. For example, either real or imagined exposure to past trauma stimuli seem to be clinically effective with trauma survivors, as would be expected from this model.

Verbal self-knowledge thus gives us the capacity to change how we interact with the world in the future. Unfortunately, it also means that we can and will struggle with our own histories, thoughts, and emotions. That is for a simple reason: It is aversive to be verbally aware of aversive events. Thus, avoidance of aversive private experiences is the natural result of human language. We will make this case in the next chapter.

SUMMARY: IMPLICATIONS OF FUNCTIONAL CONTEXTUALISM, RULE GOVERNANCE, AND RELATIONAL FRAME THEORY

Psychology can progress rapidly only if (1) we are clear about our philosophical assumptions (metaphorically, we should look at our feet and say, "Here I stand") and (2) we base applied work on clear theoretical structures so that we can acquire the scope we need for effective and broadly applicable analyses. In that context, precise specification of techniques is needed, not just because it allows replication or ensures compliance with treatment regimens, but because it allows readers to ascertain the degree to which the techniques used fit with the underlying philosophical and theoretical position that is being tested (Follette, 1995, provides an interesting analysis of this point).

Some of the insights offered by rule governance and relational frame theory fit with the known clinical functions of language and cognition. In these areas, the work on derived stimulus relations provides a basic account and shows how primitive and early these processes are, being demonstrable even in human infants but so far not at all in nonhumans. In other areas, however, the insights are not common sense.

The following 10 generalizations can be made, based on the existing literature we have discussed so far.

Verbal Relations Dominate

1. Verbal relations in humans are primitive, dominant, and fundamental. They occur early and readily, even in infants. The basic behavioral processes involved may not occur in nonhumans and certainly do not occur as readily as in humans.

2. Much of the human world becomes verbal in our sense. Verbal stimuli include far more than words. Even the most obviously "nonverbal" event is probably at least in part functionally verbal for humans. We will call this "verbal dominance."

Context Is the Key

3. Verbal relations are contextually controlled. In some contexts they occur more than in others.

4. The stimulus functions that are transformed by verbal relations are also contextually controlled, and thus the behavioral impact of verbal relations is contextual, not mechanical. In some contexts, symbols and referents can virtually fuse together. We will call such context "the context of literality," and the effect we will call "cognitive fusion." In other contexts, the verbal relations exist but few actual stimulus functions are transferred among them.

Self-Knowledge Is a Two-Edged Sword

5. The bidirectionality of verbal relations makes self-knowledge useful, but it also makes self-criticism or self-avoidance almost inevitable. We will call this "the principle of bidirectionality."

Changing Verbal Relations through Process
or Content Differs

6. Verbal relations can occur with minimal continuing environmental support. Contexts that support sense making (in which there are payoffs for being able to draw stimuli into a coherent network of stimulus relations) are enough to maintain verbal behavior, but these direct contexts are amplified by the way the verbal community demands reasons and rationales for behavior. We will call this latter context the "context of reason giving." Contexts that do not support sense making are effective means of loosening verbal relations. This is a primary cornerstone of many ACT techniques.

7. Changing verbal relations by adding new verbal relations elaborates the existing network, it does not eliminate it. At the level of content, verbal relations work by addition, not by subtraction. Because sense making, left to its own devices, is a common context, verbal networks are ever more elaborated. The main way to weaken verbal relations effectively is to alter the context supporting the verbal process, not by focusing on the verbal content.

Rules Are Necessary and Often Useful, but They Are Tricky and Dangerous

8. Verbal rules induce relative insensitivity to the direct consequences of responding.

9. Such insensitivity is particularly likely with social pliance, tracking tied to untested or untestable rules, or augmenting linked to abstract or remote consequences. In many clinical circumstances, rule-governed behavior may continue even when it is ineffective.

10. Pliance, tracking, and augmenting are in an ascending order of complexity. All three are developmentally necessary for effective verbal regulation, but over time the less complex forms become less relevant to effective living except in specific contexts. ACT attempts to reduce excessive pliance, to enhance augmentals that are linked to desired outcomes, and to bring tracking under better contextual control. It attempts to limit rule-governed behavior to contexts that benefit from it.

An Example: Suicide

In the next chapter we will apply these insights to a clinical theory of psychopathology and its treatment. Before concluding this chapter, however, we return to the example of suicide raised in the first chapter, to show where these concepts take us.

As discussed earlier, the dominant motivation for suicide appears to be an attempt to flee from aversive states of mind such as guilt, anxiety, worthlessness, inadequacy, or blame. There is a tendency to think of such a contingency in normal escape or avoidance terms, but that is inaccurate. To train a nonverbal organism to escape or avoid aversive stimuli, the organism must be exposed to an aversive event (either directly or via cues directly associated with such an event), and then some action must withdraw or prevent the reoccurrence of that aversive event. The negative reinforcer in escape or avoidance conditioning is the reduced probability of the aversive event relative to its probability before responding.

Suicide cannot occur this way. The reduced probability of an aversive event relative to its probability before responding cannot have been directly experienced in the case of suicide. No one knows directly what it is like to be dead. Furthermore, suicide often occurs even when the action of taking one's own life produces direct and immediate exposure to aversive events well before death occurs. Suicide is purposive, but the purpose is not one that has been *directly* experienced. Rather, suicide has a *verbal* purpose. People can formulate the consequences of their own death: "If I am dead" can be placed in a class with termination of suffering, others realizing how wrong they were toward me, a better world, insurance payments to the children, going to heaven, or a thousand other such "consequences."

These various verbal events ("heaven," "suffering," and the like) have psychological functions via their participation in relational frames with other events. "Heaven" has been related to myriad positive verbal events since childhood. Similarly, "suffering" is in an equivalence class with directly experienced pain, and "no suffering" is in a frame of opposition with that very pain. Even if the person does not know directly what it is like not to suffer, this frame of opposition allows the person to imagine such a state and to feel in some ways (via a transformation of stimulus functions) what that state would be like. In this instance, rules that link suicide to a reduction in suffering can function as a formative augmental.

The sentence "If death, then no suffering" is an apparent contingency description. It is a rule, and a rule that can then be tracked. If "no suffering" has acquired positive functions, then for a person in considerable psychological pain, the formula "If death, then no suffering" will transfer these positive functions to death as a verbally constructed consequence. But the person can also construct relations between certain actions and personal death as a consequence—"If I shoot myself, I will die; and if I die, I will not suffer." Here we have an example of the final, lethal rule that leads to so much human carnage. Suicide is rule-governed behavior, based on the construction of imaginary consequences through the application of relational frames.

When people contact these rules and feel their behavior regulatory power, they often try to modify them through direct, content-based verbal means. This, unfortunately, elaborates the verbal network and can tighten the verbal noose. For example, a person may try to suppress negative thoughts or argue away negative conclusions. This will probably increase the frequency and urgency of negative thoughts and, hence, the behavioral regulatory power of the thoughts themselves. Thus, suicidality is a verbal process, but we argue that our normal methods of changing verbal content will often make the problem worse (see Chiles & Strosahl, 1995, for an interesting discussion of this paradox). ACT attempts to untangle these verbal knots by loosening the binds of language itself.

•3•

The ACT Model
of Psychopathology
and Human Suffering

Humans live in an intensely verbal world. In lay language this is well recognized, but the processes involved are not precisely described. For example, the verbal processes we are describing are often called "mental." They are said to be deposited in our "minds." Some behavioral scientists resist using such terms, and as a technical matter we agree. But there is nothing wrong with using such terms to refer to a set of verbal functions that can be technically analyzed, or with using these terms in therapy for clinical purposes. When we speak of "minds," we are referring here to an individual's repertoire of public and private verbal activities (using our technical definition of *verbal*): evaluating, categorizing, planning, reasoning, comparing, referring, and so on. Although we will use the noun form, the mind is not a thing. The brain is a thing, replete with white and grey matter, midbrain structures, and so on, but the mind is a repertoire, not a place. "Minding" would be a more accurate, if cumbersome, description.

Using these lay terms, the ACT model of psychopathology is extremely conventional: Most human suffering is due to the mind, and most psychopathology is indeed a "mental" disorder. However, the ACT model approaches mind from a technical understanding about the nature of such verbal activity. The contextual behavioral approach to language in the ACT model points to the context of verbal activity as the key element, rather than the verbal content. It is not that people are thinking the wrong thing—the problem is thought itself and how the verbal community supports its excessive use as a mode of behavioral regulation.

Verbal behavior is a wonderful tool for interacting effectively with the environment, but it tends to overwhelm all other forms of activity. As noted in the preceding chapter, it occurs with little continuous environmental support, and there is virtually nothing in the world of human experience that "the mind" cannot touch. Even the most obviously "nonverbal" event becomes, at least in part, verbal for humans. Because the contexts that support verbal behavior are ubiquitous, we tend to behave relationally from morning to night, constantly describing, categorizing, relating, and evaluating. As we do so, we tend to become fused (etymologically, "poured together with") with our cognitions (a word etymologically based on the same Latin root as "know by the mind"). The behavioral functions of our world become increasingly the product of derived stimulus relations and rules, and less based on direct experience and workability. Undermining this kind of cognitive fusion is one of the key purposes of ACT.

The contexts that weaken this process are not a major part of the dominant culture. Instead, over the last century the culture has greatly expanded the use of literal, analytical language (for example, through the media). In addition, content-oriented efforts to change verbal content are heavily promoted by the culture, including the psychotherapy culture (e.g., emotional control, cognitive restructuring). Because content-oriented efforts to change verbal relations expand and elaborate the existing relational network, humans tend to become ever more entangled in a verbal web consisting of their opinions about life, their stories about their own lives, myriad analyses regarding the need for themselves or others to change, and the value of various means to achieve these ends. We become "rational" and "reasonable" to an irrational and unreasonable degree. These self-verbalizations in turn can function as verbal rules, inasmuch as we can both speak and listen within the same skin.

As briefly mentioned in the preceding chapter, the mutual entailment aspect of relational frames readily turns self-knowledge into self-struggle. We verbally categorize our own history, physical sensations, thoughts, feelings, and behavioral predispositions. We evaluate these internal events. Those reactions produced by aversive events will, through the bidirectional transformation of stimulus functions, themselves become aversive. We will then often take direct, verbally directed action against these innocent behavioral bystanders.

In effect, a context is created in which one set of actions (emotions, thoughts, and so on) "causes" another, not because the two are mechanically linked but because the conventions of the verbal community glue them together. For example, we are told and taught that it is of central importance to feel, think, and remember "good" things, not "bad" things. Unfortunately, many of the ways we attempt to reach these ends are themselves forms of psychopathology. When the effects of rule-governed behavior of this kind are negative, the self-struggle will continue because of the insensitivity these rules induce. This is the essence of the ACT model of psychopathology, and of human suffering more generally. According to this model, most forms of psychopathology and human suffering are verbal behavior gone awry.

THE SYSTEM THAT TRAPS PEOPLE

Another way to understand the ACT approach to human suffering is to examine the actions of clients entering therapy. Entering therapy is part of a larger problem-solving strategy. Clients not only have certain problems, they also believe that their problems are caused by this or that, or that they need to solve their problems by doing one thing or another. Seeking help is as much due to these particular views of appropriate human problem solving as it is due to certain signs or symptoms. As such, the very process of seeking therapy shows how verbal systems can lead to human problems. There is a remarkable degree of consistency among people in their views of human problems and their solutions. The culture, through the vehicle of language, clearly trains people to view problems and their solutions in predictable ways. In addition, the nature of human language itself organizes and drives human problem-solving behavior. The dominant view of problem solving in psychological domains can be expressed as a logical syllogism. Clients do not normally carry this syllogism around with them in any explicit sense, but the organization of their psychological problem-solving efforts fits with the logic the syllogism expresses. The syllogism contains five components.

Human Problems Are Caused

Severe personal problems seem to make instant determinists of us all. Clients almost always come into therapy with the conviction that *human problems are caused* (the first statement of the syllogism). Despite a frequently stated belief in free will or the power of self-determination, clients in fact have usually spent hundreds if not thousands of hours analyzing the causes of their problems and trying to formulate ways of altering those causes. Problems, it seems, have to be here for a *reason*, and the context of literality and reason giving dominate as these sources of difficulties are examined. Therapy itself is cast, in most clients' minds, as a place in which the causes of suffering will be detected, challenged, and changed. When a client walks into a therapist's office, the normal agenda is, "I have a problem that has been caused by something."

Reasons Are Causes

A corollary is that because psychological pain is caused, such causes can be detected through exploration and rational analysis. Even when human problems are thought to be irrational, that very irrationality can be detected, explained, interpreted, and analyzed. Irrationality itself is, in a sense, thought to be rational. Several popular psychotherapies systematize this corollary by holding that the sources of clinical problems are irrational or distorted thinking: to be happy, one has to learn to be properly logical and analytical. It is not just scientists who formulate reasons for psychological activity. As attribution researchers have demonstrated, virtually all humans receive extensive training in formulating cause-and-effect relationships, both generally and in regard to their own behavior. As part of the socialization process, people are required and able to give verbal explanations for their behavior, even if its sources are unknown or obscure (Semin & Manstead, 1985). A person facing a psychological difficulty will, naturally, apply these analytic skills to his or her own difficulties. This will involve generating verbal explanations and justifications for disturbing actions, beliefs, feelings, bodily sensations, and other psychological events. The clear benefits of tracking in everyday life will lead the person to attempt to follow his or her own self-generated verbal rules.

Reasons provide a culturally supported view of the causes of one's behavior. For example, a person may ask someone else, "Why did you have an argument with your husband?" The answer may be, "He made me mad," or "I didn't like the way he has been treating me." An agoraphobic person, when asked, "Why did you avoid the mall?" might say, "Because I was so anxious." A depressed person, when asked, "Why are you restricting your activities so much?" might answer, "Because I don't feel like doing anything anymore." In the mainstream culture, it seems sensible to view such "good reasons" as actual causes. Thus, the second statement in the syllogism is that *reasons are causes*.

There are major problems, however, in viewing reasons to be the literal causes they present themselves to be. Verbal dominance does not mean that our verbal formulations are true in a scientific or pragmatic sense.

The Problem of Access

As a scientific matter, people do not have adequate access to much of the material that is needed to understand their own behavior. Humans have enormously lengthy and complex histories. Human freedom and mobility make easily specifiable histories highly unlikely. Much of what influences our development is out of our awareness; we are exposed to literally millions, if not billions, of "learning moments." In addition to the problem of having incredibly complex learning histories, we know very little about how most types of life experiences actually influence subsequent behavior. Given these problems with access, the idea that the verbal explanations about the causes of one's own behavior have much of a chance of being fully accurate is simply absurd.

Even if a reason is true, it is usually such a small part of the picture as to be functionally false. For example, suppose it is literally true when a person says that a fight with a spouse occurred because "he made me mad." It might well be "true" in the sense that a reaction called anger was indeed present and fighting followed. It is functionally false, however, because we don't know (1) why the anger occurred, (2) what else other than anger contributed to the fighting, and (3) how anger has come to control fighting of this sort. Presumably, a comprehensive answer might analyze the learning moments that gave rise to all these considerations. We may need to know, for example, about the person's history in regard to anger, fighting, social control, and so on. Unfortunately, most people can hardly remember what they had for breakfast last Tuesday, much less what events in the remote past constitute their learning history in regard to a given situation. The difficulty is more than just access to the events. Even if we did know *all* of the events in a person's life, we still would not know how to organize them into causal order. For all these reasons, it seems impossible that reasons could have very much to do with causes.

The Real Function of Reason Giving

This is not to say that reasons are not very interesting behavioral phenomena in their own right. Reasons undoubtedly have some important role, again no doubt owing to the powerful organizing effects of language. We spend a great deal of time teaching children to give reasons. A very young child, for example, will often answer, "Just because" in response to a request for a reason, but this would not be permitted in an older child. One must have a reason to give, in part because reasons are the way the verbal community can establish whether a person can justify his or her own behavior consistently and in terms of socially established rules of conduct. Thus, for example, if a young child is asked, "Why did you hit your sister?" and answers, "Because she made me mad," we may explain to the child what to do when he gets mad. We are not asking the child to engage in scientific speculations about what caused the behavior. This is easy to see when we examine answers that may be more scientifically correct, but that lose contact with social norms. Suppose this same child is asked the same question and responds, "Because she did things that I experienced as aversive. Aversive stimulation is an establishing operation that leads to a heightened state of reinforceability in regard to the sensory stimulation provided by forcefully striking my knuckles against her face. Furthermore, I have had extensive experience in regard to the immediate social consequences and secondary gains of aggression, which has reinforced my hitting." It seems highly likely that such an answer—even though it may be more nearly a description of causality in the situation—would secure less support from the verbal community than would the obviously inadequate former answer.

For the verbal community, the development of reason giving is desirable because it means that behavior that cannot be justified in terms of social norms is made less likely—it is not "reasonable" to do it. All of this would not be such a problem were it not for the fact that people eventually begin to take their own reasons quite seriously and treat them as if they were truly causes.

Thoughts and Feelings Are Good Reasons

Private events often precede and follow clinically significant events, and most clients explain their behavior in part based on thoughts, feelings, attitudes, memories, beliefs, bodily sensations, and so on (Addis & Jacobson, 1996). Even when clients are seemingly not trying to explain behavior per se, they evaluate their lives in terms of these same things. For example, a person's life is said to be not going well if he or she is "depressed" or "anxious." This is a kind of reason giving at a higher level. To shorten the list, let the words *thoughts and feelings* stand for all the private behaviors and private stimuli that are commonly pointed to as the reasons for human action or the bases for the evaluation of human success or failure. The third statement of the syllogism is, thus, that *thoughts and feelings are good reasons.*

Clinical experience suggests the ubiquity of this part of the system. Clients often come into therapy complaining, for example, of "anxiety" or "depression." Typically, there are real-life problems these private events are being used to explain. Such people may be withdrawing from those around them, failing in relationships, avoiding certain necessary situations, and so on. In the rarer case when a person is behaving fairly effectively at an overt level and is complaining of depression or anxiety, the person is usually not responding just to the feeling or thought, but to its meaning according to the verbal community. The presence of anxiety, for example, "means" that one's life is not going well. This general context is so pervasive in the mental health culture that we even label disorders and treatments in these terms; for example, the treatment for an "anxiety disorder" is "anxiety management." By this way of thinking, anxiety itself is the problem.

What evidence is there that people tend to use private events to explain behavior, and that these explanations are seen to be "good" reasons? Several years ago one of us (S.C.H.), along with Elga Wulfert and Suzanne Brannon, collected some data on this question. We constructed a set of several common clinical situations in which a client engaged in clinically undesirable behavior. We then asked a number of undergraduates to read the description and write down several reasons the client might be likely to give if asked why the behavior occurred. For example, if an alcoholic client got drunk, what reason might he give for his behavior? About 80% of the responses given for a wide variety of situations referred only to private events and ignored external events that might have triggered the behavior. When we asked people to write down reasons they themselves might give if they were in such a situation, the answers were similar. Even the few reasons that pointed to external events also typically included private events (e.g., "He made me mad when he did X"). We then asked the same respondents to rate the validity of each reason on a scale of 1 (low validity) to 7 (high validity). The average ratings were quite high (about 5.8) and did not differ between purely private behavioral reasons and those that involved the external environment. In short, people told us that thoughts and feelings are the most common reasons given by themselves or others for clinically undesirable behavior and that these reasons were quite valid. This type of research shows the organizing power of the social/verbal community, which alters the behavior of its participants in part through culturally supported practices in language development.

Thoughts and Feelings Are Causes

The fourth statement in the syllogism flows quite naturally from the first three: *Thoughts and feelings are causes.* This is almost universally applied by clients and therapists alike. It is why, for example, we speak of thought disorders, emotional disorders, and anxiety disorders.

As discussed in the preceding chapter, if by the word *cause* we mean something that can be used directly to *change* important psychological phenomena, then thoughts and feelings cannot cause behavior. From a functional contextualistic perspective, only events external to behavior can "cause" behavior. This is not as arbitrary as it might sound. Obviously, behavior influences the environment, which in turn influences future behavior, and in the case of behavior–behavior relationships, the first behavior can have stimulus properties that can assist in the control of the second. We can notice our own thoughts, for example, just as we

might listen to instructions given by others. However, we cannot manipulate behavior directly—we can only manipulate events external to
behavior (see Hayes & Brownstein, 1986a, 1986b, for more extended
discussion of this issue). If we say that a thought *causes* an action, we
are, in effect, saying that a dependent variable causes a dependent variable. Where is the independent variable? For this philosophical reason, if
functional contextualistic assumptions are adopted, all forms of behaviors—public and private—can participate in overall causal relationships
but should not themselves be seen as causes of other behaviors of the
same individual.

When a depressed person says he did not go to work because of his
depression, the implication is that the feeling called depression is actually causing the behavior called staying at home. Accepting this premise
puts us on very shaky ground, pragmatically speaking. The therapist or
change agent is quickly locked into a logically appealing, but relatively
ineffective, problem-solving agenda: Remove or eliminate the offending
thought or feeling, and the desired behavior will return. That, however,
is more easily said than done.

To Control the Outcome, the Cause Must Be Controlled

The fifth statement is the logical successor to the first four: *To control
the outcome we must control the causes.* For the word *cause* to mean
what is says, this is the only logical option. With this statement, the trap
is sprung, because the next statement must follow.

To Control the Outcome, We Must Control
the Thoughts and Feelings

At first it may not be obvious why this is a trap. Indeed, as noted earlier,
the field of psychotherapy (especially behavior therapy) has often
defined its procedures in terms of controlling thoughts and feelings.
Thus, for example, we speak easily of "anxiety management" or "cognitive restructuring." Psychology has almost completely bought into the
mainstream notion that one must maintain functional control over private events in order to live a successful life. There are good reasons to
believe, however, that the attempt to control thoughts and feelings is not
only often ineffective but may actually breed human misery—particularly with persons who have clinical disorders. We will spend extensive
time on this point, because it is one of the central concepts in the ACT
approach to psychopathology and human suffering.

Deliberate attempts to do anything are instances of rule-governed
behavior. When we add qualifiers to human action such as *deliberate*,

purposeful, conscious, intentional, we are doing so because we recognize that the behaviors of interest are not automatic, but are instead guided by our verbally constructed formulations. Thus, deliberate attempts to control thoughts and feelings involve a curious kind of rule generation and rule following (e.g., "Don't feel X"). In most clinical situations, the feeling, thought, memory, or other psychological event we are attempting to control is problematic, and thus the goal is to get rid of it or diminish it in some way. However, if a conscious attempt at elimination or control were workable, the client would not be seeing us in the first place. Something has gone wrong in the execution of this rule.

Some of the problems arise because the targets of these rules are not easily regulated in that fashion. In this case, overexpansive tracks are being followed, but without long-term positive result. Consider what is likely to happen if we use a rule to get rid of "Thought X." In order to do so, we must specify the thought to be eliminated. The words contained in the rule are in a bidirectional stimulus relation with the form of the thought itself. In other words, the rule contains the very content it says to get rid of. Under these conditions, the rule will probably create the very private event the person is trying to avoid. Persons with obsessive–compulsive disorder often attempt to follow rules such as "You must not think about hurting other people." A rule of this sort is itself likely to create thoughts about hurting others, because it contains events that are in an equivalence class with the thought. Thus, the more one tries to follow it, the worse things will get.

For now, it is necessary only to recognize that there is a severe problem. The system with which the client comes into therapy relies heavily on content-oriented, rule-governed change, but the client's strategy of using overexpansive tracks is often likely to amplify the unwanted experience. Moreover, trying to eliminate certain thoughts and feelings only increases the behavior-regulatory function of these thoughts and feelings, as it is a context in which the specified thoughts and feelings control avoidance behaviors. Here we have yet another context (the "context of experiential control") that needlessly links private behavior to other forms of activity, and that serves as a motivative augmental for the regulation of private experiences. The combination of these rules creates a trap that can frustrate attempts to change a person's actual life situation. Seeing thoughts and feelings as the "problem" is itself part of the problem. Furthermore, the solutions generally proposed for this problem are part of the problem.

In describing this dilemma, we do not separate people who seek therapy from those who do not. This dilemma is endemic to the culture; it is a primary culprit in our everyday struggle for life satisfaction. What we are claiming is that language itself enables humans to struggle with their own private experiences in a way that fosters the ubiquity of human misery.

THE PERVASIVENESS
OF EXPERIENTIAL AVOIDANCE

Experiential avoidance is a process recognized by a wide number of theoretical orientations. It occurs when a person is unwilling to remain in contact with particular private experiences (e.g., bodily sensations, emotions, thoughts, memories, behavioral predispositions) and takes steps to alter the form or frequency of these events and the contexts that occasion them. We will occasionally use terms such as *emotional avoidance* or *cognitive avoidance* rather than the more generic *experiential avoidance* when it is clear that these are the relevant types of private experience that the person seeks to escape, avoid, or modify.

Experiential avoidance has been implicitly or explicitly recognized in most systems of therapy. Behavior therapists recognize that "the general phenomenon of emotional avoidance is a common occurrence; unpleasant events are ignored, distorted, or forgotten" (Foa, Steketee, & Young, 1984, p. 34). Client-centered Therapy emphasizes the importance of working with a client to become "more openly aware of his own feelings and attitudes as they exist" (Rogers 1961, p. 115). Gestalt therapists suggest that "dysfunction occurs when emotions are interrupted before they can enter awareness" (Greenberg & Safran, 1989, p. 20). Existential psychologists focus on avoidance of a fear of death: "To cope with these fears, we erect defenses . . . that, if maladaptive, result in clinical syndromes" (Yalom, 1980, p. 47). Recognizing and dealing with experiential avoidance has been a central theme of modern behavioral therapies such as dialectical behavior therapy (Linehan, 1993, 1994) and revised forms of behavioral couple therapy (Koerner, Jacobson, & Christenson, 1994).

As we intimated in the preceding chapter, the principle of bidirectionality makes experiential avoidance basic to human existence. Imagine that a survivor of sexual trauma is asked to report that trauma. In so doing, there is a bidirectional transformation of stimulus functions between the report and the trauma. As we "know" verbally what has happened, some of the functions of what went before are present. The report will probably be aversive as a result—it hurts to tell about hurts. Of course, the transformation is mutual, which is why verbal self-awareness is useful. As we reformulate our experiences verbally, this process can change the stimulus functions of the events being described or of those like them. Suppose, for example, the abused person connects the fear of her husband with fear of the sexual abuse. This may then change the stimulus functions of the husband, because the source of the fear that shows up will not be related verbally to the husband in the same way ("He did not abuse me. This is just my past."). This is why insight-oriented psychotherapy may at times make sense.

What this also suggests is that human emotions that emerge from aversive events, themselves become aversive. Anxiety is a natural response to aversive things. In nonverbal organisms, because the response and the event that produces it are not bidirectionally related, anxiety is not itself bad. There is nothing in the animal experimental literature that suggests that nonverbal organisms avoid their responses to aversive events. Nonverbal organisms avoid the aversive events, and, further, they will come to avoid previously neutral events that reliably precede the aversive event. However, nonhuman organisms do not avoid events that occur after an aversive event.

This makes sense in the world of nonarbitrary relations between events. If the sound of a predator is followed by predatory attacks, it is of obvious evolutionary advantage that the sound of the predator may come to have some of the aversive stimulus functions of the predator itself. But how would it advantage an organism to avoid what followed an aversive event? Imagine that an ape becomes frightened upon hearing a lion, and runs and hides in some bushes. If it learned to avoid things that followed the aversive event, we might expect it to run and hide from the bushes—putting it back in the open savanna and subject to predation. Among humans, it is a different story. The aversive qualities of the original event transfer to our descriptions of them and to the responses we know verbally to be related to them. "Anxiety" is not just a fuzzy set of natural bodily states and behavioral predispositions (as it is in nonverbal organisms); it is an evaluative and descriptive verbal category that is highly aversive. Furthermore, these emotional events can become bidirectionally related to more and more external events.

For example, DeGrandpre, Bickel, and Higgins (1992) demonstrated that interoceptive stimuli resulting from drug ingestion could participate in equivalence relations with external visual stimuli. A drug addict walks around in a drug-relevant world, with verbal links constantly "reminding" the person of what it feels like to use. What this means is that the principle of bidirectionality leads naturally both to emotional avoidance and to the emotional relevance of the external environment. As our alcoholic and drug-addicted patients tell us, more and more of the environment seems to stimulate a struggle over using or not using.

These natural tendencies are then amplified by the verbal community. Children are told, regularly and often, that they can and ought to control negative affective states. Even babies are often evaluated according to how little they express negative affective states (e.g., "She's such a good baby, she never cries"). Punishment and reinforcement are frequently doled out according to the ability to control and suppress at least the outward signs of aversive emotional states ("Stop crying or I'll give you something to cry about"). Siblings and schoolmates support the ongoing purposeful control of thoughts, memories, or emotions. Statements such as "Don't be a baby" or "Just forget about X" will be backed up by a variety of socially mediated consequences (e.g., getting beat up, being shamed, etc.). What is going on here is that seeing negative emotion in others is aversive, so pliance is used to reduce the frequency with which children express negative emotion. In addition, the evaluative connotation of emotional labels alters the functions of private experiences that are so labeled. For example, in most contexts, anxiety is a "bad" emotion. The bidirectionality of human language can create the illusion that this "badness" is an inherent quality of the emotion itself: We say "This *is* a bad emotion," not "This is an emotion and I am evaluating it as bad."

As a result, clients often arrive in therapy focused on this agenda: "I can't control my depression" or "I'm too anxious." Even in the therapeutic milieu the therapist may overtly tell the client to emote, express, and report negative emotions, but in subtle ways may punish the client's negatively evaluated affect, thoughts, or memories. Furthermore, the therapeutic agenda itself may imply as much because a common therapeutic goal is the reduction or alteration of emotional and cognitive events. The effect of all this struggle can be detrimental. There is a profuse scientific literature that makes this clear. In the section that follows we will briefly examine some data of that kind.

THE DESTRUCTIVE EFFECTS OF EXPERIENTIAL AVOIDANCE

Thought and Emotional Suppression

When subjects are asked to suppress a thought, they later show an increase in this suppressed thought as compared with those not given suppression instructions (Clark, Ball, & Pape, 1991; Gold & Wegner, 1995; Wegner, Schneider, Carter, & White, 1987; Wegner, Schneider, Knutson, & McMahon, 1991). The rebound is greatest in contexts in which the suppression took place (Wegner et al., 1991), or while the subject is in the same mood as when the suppression occurred (Wenzlaff, Wegner, & Klein, 1991). Indeed, the suppression strategy may actually stimulate the suppressed mood in a kind of self-amplifying loop (Wenzlaff et al., 1991). Those who show thought suppression as a primary coping strategy have higher levels of depressive and obsessive symptoms (Wegner & Zanakos, 1994).

The paradoxical effects of suppression have also been shown to occur for somatic sensations (Cioffi & Holloway, 1993). In this study, subjects exposed to painful stimuli were asked to think of their home, to focus on the painful sensations, or to eliminate thoughts about pain. Those in the suppression condition later rated the pain as more unpleasant than those in the focusing condition, and recovery on discomfort ratings following withdrawal of the painful stimulus was slower.

Evidence from the Coping Styles Literature

Similar findings have been shown in the coping strategies literature. Using the Ways of Coping Questionnaire (WOC) (Folkman & Lazarus, 1988), Lazarus and Folkman (1984) identified two dominant means of coping with stressful situations: problem-focused and emotion-focused coping strategies. Problem-focused strategies involve such approaches as "I made a plan of action and followed it." Emotion-focused coping strategies involve various experiential avoidance strategies such as refusing to think about the situation, supplanting bad thoughts with good ones, or telling things to oneself to feel better. A similar instrument, the Coping Inventory for Stressful Situations (CISS), yields task-oriented, emotion-oriented, and avoidance-oriented coping subscales (Endler & Parker, 1990). Items assessing avoidance involve either distraction ("Watch TV") or social diversion ("Phone a friend").

Emotion-focused and avoidant coping strategies, as measured by the WOC, CISS, and similar instruments, predict negative outcomes for substance abuse (Ireland, McMahon, Malow, & Kouzekanani, 1994), depression (DeGenova, Patton, Jurich, & MacDermid, 1994), and sequelae of child sexual abuse (Leitenberg, Greenwald, & Cado, 1992). Those who avoid emotions as a trait tend toward increased depressive symptoms, particularly when it is combined with thought suppression as a coping strategy (Wegner & Zanakos, 1994).

Evidence from Psychotherapy Process Research

In a review of 1,100 quantitative studies of the relationships between process and outcome variables, Orlinsky and Howard (1986) found that "self-relatedness" was "the most consistently positive correlate of therapeutic outcome" (p. 366). Clients high in self-relatedness were defined as being "in touch with themselves . . . [and] open to their feelings" as contrasted with being "out of touch with themselves" (p. 359). Similarly, a high client level of experiencing has been consistently related to a good outcome in psychotherapy (Greenberg, 1983; Greenberg & Dompierre, 1981; Greenberg & Webster, 1982; Kiesler, 1971; Luborsky, Chandler, Auerbach, Cohen, & Bachrach, 1971; see Greenberg & Safran, 1989, for a review).

Experiential avoidance is an instance of rule governance, but one in which the rule contradicts the desired outcome. Avoidance rules specify the to-be-avoided event, give it key behavioral importance, and relate failure to avoid the event to possible undesirable ends. Overexpansive tracks and inappropriate augmentals will focus attention on the regulation of private experiences as an issue of critical importance. The immediate effect is often positive, because distraction or other control methods will temporarily disrupt the ongoing event. As the person begins again to self-monitor and self-evaluate, however, the avoidance rule will be recontacted and the now more powerful event-to-be-avoided will reemerge.

Of course, if avoidance rules are inherently likely to fail, those who use them as general styles of responding will be especially likely to suffer. Conversely, when therapy undermines these rules of avoidance, clients will have greater access to their own history and the "response tendency information" contained therein (Safran & Greenberg, 1988; cf. Greenberg, 1994; see Hayes et al., 1996, for a general review of these areas). Thus, these findings all seem quite predictable from the ACT perspective.

Outcomes and Processes with Clinical Disorders

A major support for the importance of acceptance and, conversely, for the toxicity of experiential avoidance are data regarding the etiology, maintenance, and amelioration of clinical disorders (see Hayes et al., 1996, for a partial review). A number of techniques other than ACT provide applied support for these concepts. For example, Marlatt has worked on the addition of techniques drawn from Eastern psychology to promote acceptance of urges (what he calls "urge surfing") as a component of relapse prevention in substance abusers (Marlatt, 1994); Linehan (1993) has improved the treatment of personality disorders by adding mindfulness strategies and work on the acceptance of aversive emotions; mindfulness training—a Buddhist tradition emphasizing emotional acceptance—has also been used successfully in the treatment of chronic pain (Kabat-Zinn, 1991); Jacobson (Jacobson, 1992; Koerner, Jacobson, & Christensen, 1994) has improved success in behavioral marital therapy by working on acceptance of the idiosyncrasies of marital partners as a route to increased marital satisfaction; emotion-focused therapy

(Greenberg & Johnson, 1988) has shown good results with couples by increasing emotional acceptance; Strosahl (1991) has improved outcomes with multiproblem clients by adding both acceptance and commitment strategies. Chiles and Strosahl (1995) have added acceptance as a major component of their model for treating suicidal behavior. In addition to these outcome data, research examining the process effect of acceptance in both analog (Cioffi & Holloway, 1993; Hayes et al., 1999) and ACT outcome studies (Bond & Bunce, in press; Strosahl, Hayes, Bergan, & Romano, 1998; Zettle & Raines, 1989) has generally supported the important role that application of acceptance strategies plays in producing positive clinical outcomes.

Controlled ACT outcome studies, although still limited, provide support for both ACT as a technology and the ACT model of psychopathology. Two small randomized trials have been carried out comparing ACT with cognitive therapy. These comparison studies were performed in part because the process mechanisms thought to underpin cognitive therapy are strikingly different from those in ACT and therefore present a unique opportunity for analyses of mode-specific change processes (cf., Zettle & Hayes, 1982 for a behavioral analysis of cognitive therapy). In the first randomized clinical trial (Zettle & Hayes, 1986), 18 depressed women were assigned to a 12-week course of either cognitive therapy (Beck, Rush, Shaw, & Emery, 1979) or ACT. In both conditions, the therapy was presented in an individual format. Results indicated that ACT produced significantly greater reductions in depression than cognitive therapy, as assessed by the Hamilton Rating Scale for Depression (HRSD); a difference existed at both posttreatment and follow-up assessment.

In a second study (Zettle & Raines, 1989), 31 depressed female subjects were randomly assigned to one of three group treatment conditions: a complete cognitive therapy package, a partial cognitive therapy package, or ACT. The complete cognitive therapy package consisted of the procedures outlined by Hollon and Shaw (1979). The partial cognitive therapy package consisted of the former, minus distancing procedures (e.g., similes, reattribution techniques, and alternative conceptualizations; see Hollon and Beck (1979) for a full description of these techniques). ACT was performed according to guidelines provided by Hayes (1987).

All three groups showed significant improvement as measured by the Beck Depression Inventory (BDI), HRSD, the Automatic Thoughts Questionnaire (ATQ), and the Dysfunctional Attitudes Scale (DAS). There were no significant differences found between the treatment conditions on any outcome measure. However, analysis of the ATQ indicated differing mechanisms of change in ACT and cognitive therapy.

Subjects in both conditions reported significant decreases in the reported frequency of automatic negative thoughts. However, unlike subjects in the cognitive therapy condition, subjects in the ACT condition reported a rapid decrease in believability ratings from pre- to posttreatment, relative to the cognitive therapy group. It is of interest that the ATQ detected differences in process moderators, even though clinical outcomes in the two treatments were similar. Furthermore, these differences are consistent with mechanisms of action that are proposed to be distinctive to the ACT approach. In ACT, the therapist teaches the depressed client to see the self-referential negative thoughts as thoughts, to be evaluated by what they do rather than by what they say. These thoughts are not what they advertise themselves to be (i.e., truth statements about the self). Thus, one can tentatively conclude that ACT performs comparably well to cognitive therapy in the treatment of major depression and that its underpinning change processes are different.

Several other controlled outcome studies have been conducted either on ACT or on modified ACT protocols in stress reduction (Bond & Bunce, in press), medical utilization (Robinson & Hayes, 1997), and chronic pain (Geiser, 1992), among other areas. ACT has always equalled or exceeded the impact of alternative empirically supported treatments, has exceeded the impact of control conditions, and has shown major differences in the predicted processes of change as compared with alternative treatments. The largest randomized controlled trial with ACT is currently under way in a federally funded study of polysubstance-abusing heroin-addicted clients, comparing ACT either to methadone and counseling or to methadone and 12-step facilitation. The early results from this study are positive, but the project is not yet completed.

Perhaps more important, ACT is one of the very few treatment approaches in the psychotherapy literature that have been examined in experimental effectiveness research (Strosahl et al., 1998), not merely efficacy research. The clinical utility of ACT provides particularly strong support for the importance of acceptance in the amelioration of psychopathology.

The design we (S.C.H., K.D.S., and others) used was innovative in that it truly met the defining criteria of effectiveness research (Seligman, 1995), but did so in an experimental, not merely correlational, fashion. In our study, we trained therapists in ACT in an HMO setting. Trained clinicians attended a didactic workshop, an intensive clinical training, and received monthly ACT supervision for a year. A control group of clinicians did not receive the additional training. Clinicians continued to receive a broad range of client assignments, covering all of the major and minor problems that come into a mental health service setting. Clinicians were free to use ACT strategies as they saw fit; they could pick or choose among ACT strategies, as the clinical situation demanded, or not use ACT at all if that seemed clinically appropriate. All of these clinicians' new clients for 1 month were evaluated prior to training and again the following year after the completion of training.

In essence, this design simultaneously evaluated acquisition of ACT skills through training and their relevance and impact. If ACT worked only with a few clients, it might have high impact but low relevance and no difference in outcomes would be found. If it seemed to apply but was not helpful, again no differences would be found. Finally, if training did not reliably lead to the acquisition of ACT skills, differences would not occur even if ACT might otherwise be useful. Only if all three worked together could differences in outcome occur. This is a fairly bold way to assess therapeutic impact in the real world, especially given the very extensive literature showing that therapist training generally does *not* improve client outcomes (Dawes, 1994) and, thus, easily obtained placebo effects are not likely.

As shown in Figure 3.1, after training, the clients of ACT-trained therapists reported significantly better coping than the clients of untrained therapists, were more likely to have completed treatment within 5 months following initiation of treatment, and were more likely to agree with their therapists about whether therapy was continuing. ACT-trained therapists also referred clients significantly less often for medication evaluations, and evidence showed that the ACT-trained therapists increased client acceptance.

So far as we know, this study is the first demonstration that general training in *any* psychosocial approach (as opposed to adherence to a specific technique) can improve general clinical outcomes across the full range of clients whom clinicians normally see (as opposed to a specific syndromal group). It considerably strengthens our view that ACT is useful with a broad range of clinical problems.

We view the initial experimental evaluations of ACT as positive but preliminary. At this point, both enthusiasm and humility seem appropriate.

WHEN EXPERIENTIAL AVOIDANCE CAN'T WORK

The conscious and deliberate avoidance of private events is highly likely to fail in several situations that are often encountered in clinical work:

1. *The process of deliberate control contradicts the desired outcome.* There are several examples of this situation. The thought suppres-

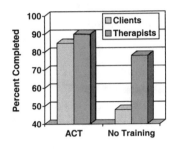

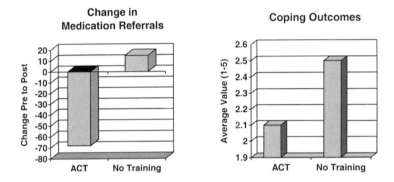

FIGURE 3.1. The broad impact of training in ACT.

sion literature just reviewed shows the phenomenon: An attempt not to think thoughts often creates these same thoughts (Wegner & Zanakos, 1994). If a subject suppresses thoughts associated with a particular mood, that very mood will later occasion the thought (Wenzlaff, Wegner, & Klein, 1991).

Emotional control may provide another example. For instance, clients with agoraphobia who made extensive use of avoidance strategies tended to develop additional anxiety over time as compared with less avoidant clients (Craske, Miller, Rotunda, & Barlow, 1990). Thus, when clients in distress attempt to suppress or control their private experiences, they may see a long-term increase in the severity of these experiences, which presumably then leads to still more avoidance and suppression.

2. *The process is not rule governed.* Many private events are conditioned directly and are not readily changed by verbal regulation. For example, if painful emotional experiences have been associated with situation *x*, it is likely that being in situation *x* will arouse negative emo-

tions by association alone. In these circumstances, attempts at purposeful control may be futile, because the underlying process is not verbally regulated. This too can lead to a vicious circle that will maintain the event the person wishes to diminish. For instance, suppose a person is extremely distressed about anxiety and tries to do everything to eliminate it. In this case, a small bit of classically conditioned anxiety will cue both purposeful attempts to reduce the anxiety and additional anxiety, because the person is distressed by anxiety. A vicious cycle is set up. Panic disorder may be an example of such a phenomenon.

3. *Change is possible, but the change effort leads to unhealthy forms of avoidance.* Suppose someone tried not to remember a given event. Memories are not simple voluntary behavior—once an event has occurred, memories will be associated with it. A memory may be avoided, however, by avoiding all situations that may give rise to it, or by dissociating. The problem with this strategy is that it can create other problems, such as limiting conscious access to life events or constricting the freedom to be in otherwise valuable situations.

4. *The event is not changeable.* Sometimes emotional control is put in the service of unchangeable events. For example, a person may take the view that "I can't accept that my dad was killed" and will consume drugs to ease his grief. Grief is a natural reaction to such losses, and no amount of drug consumption will alter either the situation or the loss. No effort to reduce or alter private events is called for here. When an unchangeable loss occurs, the healthy thing to do is to feel fully what one feels when losses occur.

5. *The change effort itself is a form of behavior contradictory to the goal of the change effort.* Confidence is a good example. Many clients want confidence, but no matter what they do, it seems to slip away. The etymology of the word helps to show why. *Con* means "with" and *fidence* comes from the Latin *fides*, which is the root of the words *fidelity* and *faith*. *Confidence* literally means "with fidelity"—being true to yourself. If that is what confidence is, we have to ask whether clients have been trying to *do* this or just to *feel* this while simultaneously doing the opposite. The act of running from scary feelings is not a confident action because it has no *fides*, no self-faith or self-fidelity. When scary feelings are present, a functionally confident action is not to get rid of them but to keep fidelity with yourself by feeling them fully, as they are and not as what they say they are. That is what feelings are for. The usual hope of the client's futile change effort is that doing non-fidelity (the change effort) will produce a feeling of fidelity. It will never happen. Feelings are side effects of historical contingencies. They are the material products of past actions and situations. All that the action of non-fidelity can possibly produce is the natural feeling associated with it. It is

possible, however, that self-fidelity will eventually lead to that feeling of self-fidelity we call confidence. We do not know if the feeling will follow the action—it depends on how strong the previous history was and how well the action of self-fidelity is being performed. Paradoxically, if the action is performed in order to get a feeling, then it is no longer truly the action of self-fidelity, by definition. Even when no emotional change occurs, however, the action of self-fidelity will produce most or all of the life benefits that the client supposed would come only through the feeling.

If all five contraindications for deliberate control as a coping strategy are added together, most clinical situations are not likely to be those in which experiential avoidance will succeed. Human emotional responses are just our own history being brought into the present by the current context. If our reactions are our history, and our reactions are our enemies, then our own history has become our enemy. There are no good technologies for removing a person's history, at least not selectively. Time and the human nervous system move in one direction—not two—and new experiences are always *added*, never *subtracted*. In order to avoid automatic emotional reactions, we have to distort our lives in such a way as to be psychologically out of contact with our own histories.

There are two notable costs of this sort of distortion. Being in contact with our history can alter future behavior in important ways, and thus diminishing that contact diminishes our experiential intelligence. Contacting our history makes our own actions more sensible. It allows us to learn. For example, it is not *bad* when a person with a sexual and physical abuse history feels nervous when similar circumstances occur; properly handled, such a process is one major way to avoid additional abuse. Naturally, such feelings are a challenge. The person may feel anxious regarding even healthy intimacy, for example. But if the person tries to remove (rather than make room for) these feelings, she risks entering into additional abusive relationships without being able to read the warning signs. Paradoxically, it is precisely the circumstances in which these feelings become overemphasized as content that feelings can no longer be used sensibly to guide behavior.

The second problem is that if avoidance is thorough, we may not even be aware that we are avoiding at all. To be aware of avoidance means that avoidance is not complete. Self-deception is necessary, but it is difficult for it to be complete if it was at all deliberate (i.e., verbally governed and therefore conscious). A subtle conflict necessarily results. Thus, successful avoidance means that a person becomes incapable of benefiting from past experience (the first problem we mentioned), and in addition, hasn't the slightest idea of what her own behavior is really about. The ACT alternative is to notice and embrace the richness of our repertoire of conditioned reactions. That is, we accept our historically established feelings and then behave in a valued direction.

HOW HUMANS GET DRAWN INTO A STRUGGLE

For reasons that we will elaborate later, people become identified with the content and process of their "mental life" to such an extent that they would usually choose to loose their arms and legs rather than "lose their minds." Disentangling people from their minds is one of the main goals of ACT. It is often therapeutically useful to refer to *minding* as if it were an entity. It helps people detach themselves from the hegemony of language to treat this behavioral domain almost as one would treat another person. It helps humans dis-identify themselves with their "minds" and thus reduces the harmful forms of social/verbal control that minds are a repository for.

Our Minds Do Not Know What Is Good for Us

Minding, as an aspect of human functioning, is like a facet of a gem. Although it is an altogether brilliant facet, we seek the gem in toto. The domination of minds over people—of this facet over all others—comes in part from the great power and utility of the stimulus relations that the social/7verbal community establishes through language. Consider the following sentence carefully (read it slowly and think about what it is talking about): "Imagine how it tastes when you bite into a juicy wedge of fresh lemon." Even though there is probably no lemon nearby, most readers salivate when reading these words, just as we did while typing and editing them. Humans are tremendously advantaged by this ability. We can create physical stability and comfort by interacting cognitively with the world. We can verbally construct dangers, needs, and futures and take action based on these formulations. But we can also struggle for no reason and hold on when we should let go.

Clients are frequently spending so much time evaluating how well they are doing, whether they are happy, and what to do about it, that they lose contact with the content about which they might be happy. In the effort to control their psychological state, they begin to lose control over their own lives. The result is that change—particularly that involving the visitation and working through of unpleasant private events—is traumatic. The individual goes through the experience unwillingly, and the negative impact of the experience is magnified by the continual self-evaluation process it occasions.

Consider, for example, chronically dysthymic clients, who on a daily basis have internal dialogues that interfere with the direct experience of living. Most of the time, these thought processes involve clients "checking in" on whether they are "feeling good." If a client goes to a social gathering, not much time will transpire before self-reflective questions will come up. For example, the client may wonder, "Well, how am I fitting in?" This question is based on certain key assumptions: That "fitting in" determines an important psychological result and thus should be tracked. A search for environmental cues begins. The individual scans the people nearby to see whether eye contact is being made, whether people are looking away, or if he is being ignored. Auditory stimuli are checked, to see whether people might be saying demeaning or ridiculing things. The client engages in additional acts of self-reflection: "How well am I relating to these people?" "Am I really being myself?" "Am I just faking being happy and normal?" "Can they really see that I'm not as happy as I pretend to be?" "Why am I pretending around people anyway?" "I thought I was coming to this party to have some fun and to be happy, but I feel worse than ever now!"

The implicit assumption, aided by a culture with the same assumption, is that there is a "right way to be," and that "right way" is happy. The internal drone caused by the self-monitoring of emotional causes and effects becomes so chronic that it is almost impossible to engage in any activity without destroying the sense of "being present" or spontaneous. For the chronically dysthymic client, the issue is feeling the right way to feel. For the client with obsessive–compulsive disorder, it is the avoidance of certain thoughts or feelings of doom. For the panic-disordered client, it is the avoidance of anxiety, death, losing control, or losing one's mind. To accomplish these goals, the client must be vigilant to the early signs that undesirable reactions are occurring. The client must examine bodily sensations, thought processes, behavioral predispositions, and emotional reactions for signs of impending failure or success. The solution to the person's problem seemingly lies in more vigilance, more scanning of the internal and external environment, and more control. But the cycle of self-monitoring, evaluation, emotional response, control efforts, and further self-monitoring is not a solution to these disorders: It *is* these disorders.

The common thread in these examples is the ever present potential for a person to live in a derived, evaluated, regulated verbal reality, rather than to experience the world as it unfolds in the here and now. The goal is happiness, but the actions are not happy ones. The goal is vitality, but the actions are deadening. Our "minds" just do not know what is good for us.

In the ACT model, the verbally established failure to accept our natural reactions to life experiences, combined with a verbally guided, resistant orientation toward inevitable and uncontrollable change, leads to many forms of psychological distress and exacerbates others. Persons with mental disorders reveal an amplified version of this normal but destructive process. Minds do not know what is good for humans for several reasons. In a general way, it is because language did not evolve for our psychological satisfaction or fun, yet is overemphasized by the culture as *the* means for achieving well-being. In a more specific sense, the problem most clients face is FEAR: *Fusion*, *Evaluation*, *Avoidance*, and *Reasons*.

Language Did Not Evolve for Fun

Although not all researchers agree, it seems highly unlikely that language evolved to promote self-actualization or happiness. No evolutionary advantage would be supplied by reminding organisms how safe and satisfied they are. Language most likely evolved as a form of social control and danger signaling. The most primitive functions of language thus are about painful things, not joy and peace of mind. Indeed, emotional talk of any kind occurred relatively late in language, as is revealed by the etymology of common emotional terms. If the avoidance of danger and deprivation through verbal means is what provided verbal behavior with its evolutionary advantage, it is not surprising that language can trigger the most primitive physiological control functions. For example, some clients with panic disorder can produce physiological arousal sufficient to induce fainting simply by imagining a panic attack in a public setting.

Here we encounter the paradox associated with having such a finely developed "mind." A mind is a wonderful tool for detecting and evaluating external dangers and developing plans for adapting to these demands, but we cannot avoid applying these same processes to the content of our private world. When we do so, we both see and produce negativity.

Language Is Sanctified by the Culture

Language is an extremely important element of human existence, but it is not everything. Perhaps more than any other behavioral domain, language products have been culturally sanctified to the point that seeing language itself as a problem is quite unlikely. For example, from childhood we are told how important an education is to our development. We cram our heads full of verbal relations in the form of facts, figures, and dates. In so doing much is gained, but it does not mean that we care more about others, that we can be a good friend, that we can remain emotionally present, or that we develop spiritually. In fact, these conditions may be all the more difficult.

All of the world's major religions have understood this dilemma and have developed mystical or meditative practices to attempt to solve it. The same cannot be said of the contemporary mental health establishment. Most of the dominant schools of psychotherapy continue to operate on the implicit assumption that cognition and emotion can be managed at the level of content. In cognitive therapy, the emphasis is on teaching the client "rational thinking." The assumption is that if we teach clients to follow the rules of logic, then they will produce more acceptable feelings and behavior will be improved. The job of therapy is to challenge and confront these beliefs and make them go away so that more rational beliefs can come in their stead. In traditional behavior therapy, negative emotions are targeted and more positive emotions are trained in the hopes that more acceptable feelings will improve behavior.

Much like the rest of the language community, the psychotherapy community has adopted the assumption that appropriate thought or emotional content may be substituted for personal experience. Therefore, if we modify the thought or emotional content, personal experience must surely follow. But this is precisely what our clients in distress have been trying to do. Mainstream therapy is simply a more systematic, planned (i.e., more verbally regulated) version. Such an approach may be helpful in some circumstances, but the benefits may be limited, precisely for those most in need of help. Clients, after all, are those for whom mainstream cultural life change methods have failed. If this content-oriented scheme were actually going to work readily and completely, most clients would not need treatment in the first place. In an important sense, clients are the culture's treatment failures.

FEAR: Fusion, Evaluation, Avoidance, and Reasons

The language and behavior of the client entering therapy reflects the culmination of FEAR as aspects of human language. It will be useful to examine how this is manifest in the transactions within the therapeutic environment.

Cognitive Fusion

Symbols are poured together with the events they describe and with the people who describe them. For example, a client will say, "I *am* depressed." The statement looks like a description, but it is not. It suggests that the client has fused with the verbal label and treated it as a matter of essence or identity, not emotion. "I am depressed" casts a feeling as an issue of being—"am" is, after all, just a form of the word "be." At a descriptive level what is happening is something more like "I am a person who is having a feeling called 'depression' at this moment."

The pouring together of verbal events and the targets of these events is even more common. We discussed the basic process when we described how relational frames operate. When we think a thought, what shows up are some of the stimulus functions of what the thought is literally about. Suppose a panic-disordered client imagines a terrible end produced by showing anxiety in a novel, high-visibility situation (e.g., losing control while being on stage giving a talk to hundreds of people). This thought will often make that bad end seem immediately present and highly likely, and anxiety is a natural response to immediately present and highly likely aversive events. As a result of cognitive fusion, the thought itself may occasion panic symptoms. The event imagined has not actually happened; however, the fusion of the symbol and the event allows the functional properties of the event to actually be present, in a psychological sense. Thus, without ever visiting the high-risk situation (e.g., the person may never have actually given such a talk) the panic-disordered client has already had a panic attack "while giving a talk," and yet another situation will be avoided in the service of controlling panic. It is not the thought itself that is the problem. It is the fusion with it and the resultant avoidance that does the damage.

As human beings become more and more indistinguishable from their thoughts and feelings, suffering tends to increase for at least two reasons. First, the act of boring in on negative thoughts or feelings is usually done with the purpose of vanquishing them and restoring health. This can never work, because our negative feelings are an instrumental part of our "health." Some people are born without a physical sensation of pain—ironically, they can be readily identified by the missing or injured digits and limbs that result. It is life threatening not to feel pain. Similarly, it is life deadening not to feel sadness, anxiety, or anger. The model of health that is implicit with our evaluative abilities is "all positive." It is "out with the bad, in with the good." But such a model is not health—it is sugarcoated madness. Second, as we have emphasized previously, when we rivet attentional processes on negative thoughts or feelings with the intent of eliminating them, we usually increase their frequency, intensity, duration, and behavioral regulatory powers.

When we simply accept the fact that a thought is a thought, and a feeling is a feeling, a wide array of response options immediately become available. We begin to notice the process of thinking and feeling, not just the content of that activity. We begin to notice the act of structuring the world, and not just the apparently "real" world silently structured by language. We begin to notice that we are wearing colored glasses, rather than simply looking at the colored environment.

This is an important cornerstone of the ACT model, and a variety of ACT interventions are designed to break up this fusion and to deliteralize language representations. To deliteralize means to disrupt ordinary meaning functions of language such that the ongoing process of framing events relationally is evident in the moment and competes with the stimulus products of relational activity. Deliteralization breaks down the tight equivalence classes and dominant verbal relations that establish stimulus functions through verbal means. Paradox, confusion, and meditative exercises are examples of deliteralization techniques.

Consider as an example the statement "This statement is false." If a person interacts with this event verbally, the relations that are established are self-contradictory. Stated another way, the relational frame cued by the word "is" transfers the functions of the word "false." But as soon as that occurs, this very transfer cancels the frame cued by the word "is," which in turn alters the functions of the word "false." If it is true that the statement is false, then the statement is true, not false. But if it is true, then it must be true that it is false. This kind of situation cannot be solved purely inside literal language. For the paradox to be solved, one must weaken rule control and the repetitive application of relational frames. And as this happens, direct contingencies—what works—can better participate in the regulation of behavior.

The press of the language community weighs heavily against readily making the distinction between language content and language processes. Literal meaning is like a magician who makes coins appear and disappear—the power of the illusion means that the secret process behind it is not readily given up.

Figure 3.2 shows the relationship we are describing. The dimension of literal meaning is referential. It always lags at least a bit behind direct experience. Any description, even of "now," is slightly removed from the exact experience described. Consider the words "I am speaking of now." The "now" spoken of when the sentence began to be uttered is not the same "now" present when the sentence is understood or even completed. Contrast this with direct perceptual experiences, which are always now (when else could they be?). Thus, as we enter into the world of literal meaning, we necessarily become just a bit removed from the ongoing flow of experience. Whereas the referential *content* of language removes the human from full connection with ongoing experience, the *process* of deriving stimulus relations is always in the "now"—a point that will provide a way out of the conundrum of literal language in the therapeutic work of ACT.

Evaluation and Self-Discrimination

Language allows events to be abstracted and treated as objects. We are taught the nature and meaning of specific "emotions," for example. A loose collection of bodily states, thoughts, behavioral predispositions, and contextual factors are gathered together under a verbal label, and we learn to call them "depression" or "anxiety." Our emotions become thing-like and verbally accessible. These are then evaluated, which gives them both conventional and valence functions. This process can lead to finer and finer discriminations about the content of private experiences. Without language it would be impossible to establish the event called, say, "existential angst," and there would be no way to recognize such an event were it to occur. This process of verbal self-discrimination is important because it allows humans to evaluate and then struggle with the internal targets that are created as a result. Now that we know what "existential angst" is, we can run from it. Virtually all of our measures of "psychopathology" are built on the assumption that to be psychologically healthy is to be free of disordered emotional and cognitive responses. According to this standard, a coma victim might be considered the ideal of psychological health.

Popular culture is relentless in its promotion of this view of health. In a recent beer commercial, a bar is filled with young, vibrant women and men having what is apparently an ideal Friday evening. The characters in the bar look quite normal, except that instead of heads they have big yellow "happy face" buttons. "Don't worry, be happy," the song

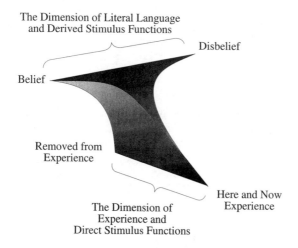

FIGURE 3.2. The relationship between literality and experiential openness.

says. The problem is that this "ideal" is a purely verbal concept. It is both unobtainable and out of contact with how humans actually can move forward with pain. Not only does no one live such a life, the effort to produce it is destructive. Yet this motivative augmental is one of the central themes of modern culture.

Evaluation is a constant. If clients are asked to look around a therapy room, literally nothing in that room can escape a negative evaluation with just a few moments' effort. Thus, this constant habit of evaluation will be applied as readily to ourselves as to our environment. But seeing an ugly door or an ugly rug—even though the seeing is "inside" the person—does not affect us the same way as does seeing an ugly thought or an ugly emotion. We are set up to struggle.

ACT undermines evaluation in an interesting way: by reducing the dominance of language itself. ACT does not evaluate evaluations. It does not say, "You shouldn't say should" or "It is bad to say bad." Instead, ACT tries to open the window and let a little (nonverbal) air in.

Avoidance

One of the most immediate ways to "feel better" when one sees an ugly thought or an ugly emotion is to escape or avoid it. This immediate "beneficial" effect is so powerful that we are all emotional avoiders to some degree. Human behavior is controlled by the immediate contingencies, even if the long-term effects are dismal, and emotional avoidance is a clear example of precisely this kind of behavioral trap. ACT undermines avoidance by encouraging acceptance, by undermining literal language, and by pointing directly to the consequences of overexpansive tracks in this area.

Reason Giving

Another reason that normal language processes lead to internal struggles is that we learn to explain and justify our own behavior in emotional and cognitive terms. As we explained earlier, our clients learn to put forward negative thoughts, feelings, memories, or physical sensations as valid and sensible causes of overt behavior—an explanation that is generally supported by the culture. A person saying, "I was too depressed to leave the house," will certainly be thought to have said something reasonable and understandable. He or she may even garner sympathy or reassurance for this formulation. "I have no idea why I didn't go" will probably receive a much less positive response, even if it happens to be a more accurate statement.

Unfortunately, people begin to believe their own reasons—their own stories. People create tracks that seem "right" but that are useless or destructive if followed. As members of a community "internalize" these cultural beliefs and practices, they become functionally true by that very process. There is growing clinical evidence for the impact of reason giving. For example, depressed clients who can give "good reasons" for their depressed behavior tend to be both more depressed and harder to treat that other depressives. Furthermore, they respond to treatment differentially as compared with depressed people who do not have as many reasons for their depression (Addis & Jacobson, 1996).

ACT tries to undermine excessive reason giving by deliteralization and by a healthy dose of honest ignorance.

ACT: ACCEPT, CHOOSE, TAKE ACTION

In the ACT approach, a goal of healthy living is not so much to feel *good*, but rather to *feel* good. It is psychologically healthy to feel bad feelings as well as good feelings. Ironically, when feelings become all important and dictate what we do—when they mean what they say they mean—then we cannot afford to feel them freely and without defense. Conversely, when feelings are just feelings, they can mean what they *do* mean: namely, that a bit of our history is being brought into the present by the current context. Feelings are interesting and important, but they do not dictate what happens next. Through language processes, clients have often come to experience their emotions as literally bigger than themselves. Each time an emotional avoidance strategy is used, this belief is given added credibility, inasmuch as the avoidance itself suggests that something must be avoided.

Acceptance: The Alternative to Avoidance

The alternative to avoidance is acceptance. Etymologically, *acceptance* comes from Latin root "accipere" meaning to receive or take what is offered. Psychologically, it connotes an active taking in of an event or situation. Psychological acceptance at its lowest level is implicit in any psychotherapy, because, at the minimum, the client and therapist must "take in" the fact that there is even a problem to be worked on. At a higher level, acceptance involves an abandonment of dysfunctional change agendas and an active process of feeling feelings as feelings, thinking thoughts as thoughts, remembering memories as memories, and so on.

Choice and Committed Action

For most people, emotional avoidance was never designed to be an end in itself. It is not an outcome goal: it is a process goal. The social/verbal community has established the idea that successful living will come when bad experiences get out of the way. If you ask a client *why* he or she should, say, avoid anxiety, the reply will usually be in terms of the effect it is having elsewhere. The person may believe, for example, that anxiety is preventing a promotion, hurting a relationship, or so on. Thus, emotional avoidance strategies promise that it is by the process of getting rid of bad feelings that commitments can be kept. This does not work for the following reason: We do not control the internal events that seemingly stand in the way of fulfilling commitments.

For example, suppose a man marries a woman and promises to love and honor her. Now suppose one day he wakes up and does not feel loving toward his partner. Without the ability to accept this feeling and maintain loving actions, the marriage commitment can become null and void. Given our usual tendency to base actions on thoughts and feelings—things over which we have only limited control—a lack of acceptance means that commitment is difficult. This is why marriage vows often mean only "until I no longer feel like it."

Acceptance applies to different areas in different ways—it is not always the appropriate action. "Taking what is offered" (acceptance) is always the best course in the area of personal history, because history is never changeable. Private experiences are a more complex case. Here both acceptance and first-order change may be relevant. Most of our clients are those for whom deliberate change has already shown itself to be problematic, but at more moderate levels the regulation of private experiences may be somewhat successful. At the other extreme, "taking what is offered" is rarely the best course in the area of overt behavior, because overt behavior is changeable and there is no reason to accept that which is negative and changeable. The ultimate test between the two is workability. As indicated by its very name, the ACT model incorporates both acceptance and change.

Reflecting the Serenity Prayer of Alcoholics Anonymous, ACT aims to teach clients how to accept the things that cannot or need not change, and how to change the things that can be changed. Unlike this prayer, ACT provides specific guidance on how to know the difference. The purpose of acceptance is not navel watching or emotional wallowing. Rather, ACT therapists recognize that in the context of making choices and taking actions, automatic reactions will appear. The client who must avoid these reactions must also avoid change. What dignifies acceptance is that it is done in the service of valued change in the client's external world, not in the world of private experiences. The client, having had verbal control weakened through willingness and cognitive diffusion, regains contact with the world. This, in turn, allows choice and committed action in realms that can be verbally regulated (e.g., overt behavior).

ACT AS A CONTEXTUAL COGNITIVE-BEHAVIORAL THERAPY

Is ACT a behavior therapy, a cognitive-behavioral therapy, a type of clinical behavior analysis, a contextual therapy, or a humanistic/existential/Gestalt therapy? It is all of these. It is based on functional contextualism, which we have argued is the underlying philosophy of behavior analysis (Hayes et al., 1988; Biglan & Hayes, 1996). Its theoretical basis is drawn from behavior analysis. In both these senses it is a form of clinical behavior analysis or a behaviorally rationalized therapy. But the content of this theory is all about cognition and emotion, even though the model is not cognitive in an information processing sense. Thus, it is reasonable to call it a cognitive-behavioral therapy. The approach, however, shares much with Gestalt therapy and emotion-focused psychotherapy (Greenberg & Safran, 1989), as well as with more Eastern meditative and spiritual approaches. We do not view the distinctions between these streams of thought to be important to the ACT work, and relish the fact that it spans several seemingly distinct traditions.

CONCLUDING REMARKS

The ACT approach follows a health, not an illness, model. In the ACT model, suffering is universal and the primary cause of suffering is the intrusion of language into areas where it is not functional. In a sense, the ACT therapist and the client are "in the same stew." They are subject to the same influences, both explicit and implicit, that emerge from both acculturation and the behavior-regulatory properties of language.

For example, ACT makes no assumption that depressed people get that way because they are "broken." Indeed, it seems quite odd to ascribe illness status to a syndrome that is experienced by approximately 30% of the population over the life span. Clients have an opportunity, through their own suffering, to learn something timeless and important about the process of being human. In that sense, people who have suffered are specially advantaged.

This does not, of course, mean that some behavioral disorders are not due to illness and disease in a physical sense. Some behavioral problems are surely due to disturbed biological conditions, for example. But even here a psychological struggle, established by human language, can make it harder for people to face their own difficulties.

The ACT approach to psychological stress and mental disorders is deceptively simple, yet complicated in the myriad ways that acceptance, fusion, emotional avoidance and commitment play themselves out in the individual case. Because the vehicle for understanding this is the language system that is the culprit in the first place, there are multiple opportunities for both effective psychological intervention and stifling impasse. The model creates a definite perspective within which the therapist can operate, often with great effect and in a very intense relational way with the client. At the same time, this approach humanizes and dignifies the client's suffering while offering a healthy alternative to a useless struggle with his or her own history. It is to the clinical practice of ACT that we now turn.

A PERSONAL EXERCISE FOR THERAPISTS

Our ACT workshops are often intensely personal. It is important that therapists have a sense of the psychological area in which ACT work is done in order to avoid using ACT as a dogmatic belief system or as a way to be clever with clients (see Chapter 10). We have found that therapists who are willing to look at themselves can move through the material more efficiently.

At the end of each of the clinical chapters (Chapters 4 to 9), there will be a short set of questions or exercises designed for therapists. We suggest you take notes on these as you try them out. The answers to each series of questions will be used in subsequent chapters.

The Problem

Take a sheet of paper and write down your answers to the following three questions. Save your answers. We will return to them later.

1. What is the main problem that stands between you and the valued direction in which you most want your life to go at this point?
2. What would tell you that this problem had been solved?
3. What do you think will have to happen, or what will you have to do, for this problem to be solved?

•PART II•

Clinical Methods

The following six chapters provide detailed information about how to perform ACT in clinical settings. ACT concepts and strategies are presented in a particular sequence that often mirrors how these content areas emerge in the course of treatment. However, the particular order in which concepts are presented is not rigid. Some clients are not struggling significantly with emotional avoidance, for example, but instead have little sense of purpose and direction. Others have strong life values but struggle to implement these goals because action precipitates distressing thoughts, unpleasant memories, or painful feelings. Some have both of these concerns. When practiced appropriately, ACT is a multifaceted and flexible set of concepts and interventions, and it is always important to match both the type and intensity of intervention to the client's clinical needs.

The essential goals of ACT are summarized simply in the acronym described in the preceding chapter: *Accept, Choose, and Take action.** ACT therapists try to help clients make room for the automatic effects of life's difficulties and to move in the direction of their chosen values. The barriers to doing this are experiential avoidance and cognitive fusion, which prevent a behavioral commitment to living a valued life. The sources of those barriers are dominantly verbal, and, thus, in a larger sense the goal of ACT is to establish a new verbal community in therapy that will foster effective action.

---

*The use of the acronym "ACT" for "Accept, Choose, and Take action" is not original to us, although our use of it for "Acceptance and Commitment Therapy" was well established before we first saw it elsewhere in the popular clinical literature. We are in the process of trying to locate the original source, however, and apologize to the author.

The stages of ACT are designed to help the client shift from overfocusing on the content of psychological experiences, to developing an understanding of the context of these experiences, both negative and positive. This is done to enable the client to pursue valued goals in life. To accomplish this shift, the ACT therapist (1) undermines the client's unworkable change agenda (Chapter 4); (2) shows how the unworkable agenda is based on emotional control and avoidance strategies (Chapter 5); (3) helps the client detect and diminish cognitive fusion (Chapter 6); (4) helps the client contact a sense of self that is distinct from programmed reactions and literal beliefs about the self (Chapter 7); (5) helps the client identify valued life directions and the goals and actions necessary to achieve them (Chapter 8); and (6) supports the client in engaging in committed action, allowing thoughts, feelings, and memories to function, not as obstacles, but as an expected part of goal-directed living (Chapter 9).

We will not present a comprehensive set of ACT techniques in these clinical chapters, because the book would become far too unwieldy if we did. Instead, we will give major examples of ACT interventions appropriate to a given purpose and will present their theoretical rationale. Where appropriate, sample clinical dialogues (usually drawn from transcripts of actual ACT sessions) will be included to show how these interventions are put into practice.

The voice of the next six chapters is quite different from that of the preceding ones. Scientific discourse is based on precise, technical description. It is dependent on literal meaning and the coherence of discourse at that level. In therapy, discourse is purely pragmatic, and any way of speaking that gets the job done—even if it is scientifically "wrong" or incompatible from one time period to another—is pragmatically "true." Indeed, ACT therapists typically warn clients of the difference between literal talk (e.g., that used by a scientist or historian) and talk to make a difference (e.g., that used by the director of a play). In the former case, the facts must be described accurately. In the latter case, the director may help the players get a feel for their characters using virtually any verbal means that accomplishes that goal. ACT uses both forms of talk, and the client has to give the therapist room to speak like a historian one moment and like a director the next, without insisting that all these forms of talk fit together into some grand literal truth.

In ACT, this is even more important than might normally be the case. For one thing, the dispersive quality of contextualism makes it easy and comfortable for contextualists to use language systems oriented toward different goals that may be incompatible at a literal level. After all, if what works is "true," and the local goals we are working toward change with context, then we can have multiple or even contradictory truths. For example, the authors' free use of "minds" as virtual entities, on one hand, and the tight behavioral analysis of the nature of "minding," on the other, are literally incompatible but pragmatically coherent. The former is designed to teach clients to approach their own verbal behavior differently; the latter is designed to orient professionals toward the mechanisms involved.

We often tell ACT clients that we are talking primarily to make a difference and to hold what we say very lightly at the level of literal truth. Like an ACT client, the reader will also have to allow us freedom in these clinical chapters to focus primarily on the deliberately loose metaphorical talk of ACT sessions, with only periodic excursions back into the technical discourse of science to show the principles involved.

This diversity of styles of discourse is also amplified in ACT because the whole approach is designed to avoid the traps of literal language. To do this, the ACT therapist tends to use verbal modalities that are inherently less literal, especially metaphor, paradox, and experiential exercises. It seems worth reviewing the theoretical rationales for this noticeable emphasis on less literal verbal modalities. For theoretical reasons, even if ACT therapists wanted to avoid verbal inconsistencies between scientific and clinical discourse, it would be hard to do.

USE OF METAPHORS

Many ACT strategies are deliberately metaphorical. Metaphorical talk has several nice features for our purposes (see McCurry & Hayes, 1992, for a review and analysis of both the scientific and clinical literature on metaphor).

First, because metaphors are not specific and proscriptive, it is more difficult for clients to show pliance to them. Pliance requires that the social community (especially the rule giver) be able to monitor the correspondence between the rule and relevant behavior. Metaphors are just stories, and thus it is never clear what would constitute compliance or resistance. The client senses this as well and knows that there is no obvious way to "be good" or "be bad" when responding to metaphors. This ambiguity keeps the coercive power of the therapeutic relationship in check and limits self-defeating client responses that are tied to histories of coercive social relationships. The social rules that ACT seeks to undermine are dominantly plys, and it makes no sense to emphasize normal pliance-based methods to undermine pliance.

Second, metaphors are not simply logical, linear forms of verbal behavior: they are more like pictures. The point of the ACT metaphors is often hard to capture in a simple moral or verbal conclusion. Instead, metaphors present a picture of how things work in a given domain. Carefully presented metaphors can be a kind of experiential exercise—as if one had actually experienced the described event or story. The event is verbal, and thus the experiences are derived and not direct, but the impact of the talk is still more experiential because the talk used is not linear, analytic, or proscriptive. This is advantageous inasmuch as ACT is attempting to ground client action in the direct experience of contingencies and in rules that track those contingencies. Metaphors help set a social/verbal context in which overreliance on rationality is questioned and where the wisdom of directly experienced contingencies is more highly valued.

Third, metaphors are easily remembered and can be used in many settings other than the specific setting in which they are learned. This makes metaphors useful if one is looking for broad-based behavior change. Metaphors can ground complex or paradoxical points to the world of common sense—they allow the client to test the possibility that a complex or paradoxical clinical situation is just like other simpler, more concrete situations. Thus, well-selected metaphors can help make the surprising aspects of the ACT approach more plausible. ACT is not a "normal" intervention model, and at times it can seem very confusing or counterintuitive. Metaphors can help clients make contact with ACT principles without having to reach them in a literal context.

THERAPEUTIC PARADOX

Paradox is an important component of ACT interventions for a simple reason: The language traps that clinical disorders represent are inherently paradoxical. Pointing to these traps will thus raise inherent paradoxes. In order to break down the language processes that set up these traps, ACT also uses logical paradox. Unlike most "paradoxical interventions," however, ACT almost never uses constructed paradoxes.

A logical paradox is the kind that is encountered in philosophy classes. In a logical paradox, contextual cues are provided for one verbal relation, but when that relation is derived it in turn becomes a contextual cue for another, contradictory relation (e.g., "This statement is false"). ACT occasionally relies on logical paradox, especially initially, because it helps break down literal language and thus permits a general loosening of derived stimulus relations and a general weakening of rule-governed behavior in areas where it does not belong.

Constructed paradox is one in which the social demands of rule following create a social system in which the person either must follow the rule or resist the rule and in either case the effects are beneficial. This is usually what clinicians mean by "therapeutic paradox," and the use of constructed paradox is common in most paradoxical interventions (Ascher, 1989). For example, a rebellious teenager with authority problems may be told by the therapist to disobey the therapist. The idea is that the adolescent either breaks the rule and thus becomes less rebellious, or follows the rule and thus becomes less rebellious. ACT generally does not use constructed paradoxes, for two reasons. First, they ordinarily have a symptom elimination focus. Even if they do work, they often leave in place the change agenda that created the problem to begin with. Second, they rely on pliance, which ACT views as a major source of clinical difficulty. Social demands that lead to compliance *or* resistance are, by definition, plys.

Inherent paradox is the dominant paradoxical mode in ACT. Inherent paradox is produced by a functional contradiction between the literal and the functional properties of a verbal event. Most forms of inherent paradox involve verbal constructions that have to do with events that are not readily verbally governed. Thus, they literally refer to a process that cannot be entirely literal or verbal in the sense described in Chapter 2. "Try hard to be spontaneous" is an example of an inherent paradox. Spontaneity has to do with contingency-shaped behavior, not rule-governed behavior. But trying to achieve something deliberately is a kind of rule following. Trying to achieve spontaneity thus undermines spontaneity. Deliberate spontaneity is an inherent paradox.

Inherent paradox is important in ACT for two reasons. First, repeated contact with inherent paradox in therapy helps loosen the grip of literal language by highlighting the fact that literal language is useful in some contexts and not in others. This is a major clinical goal of ACT because fusion with verbal events is thought to be a major source of the client's persistent use of ineffective change strategies. Second, the ACT view of psychopathology is itself an inherent paradox. ACT therapists take the view that trying to change negative content is a major source of that very content and that abandoning the effort to change is itself the biggest and most important change that can be made. This view is inherently paradoxical.

EXPERIENTIAL EXERCISES

ACT makes extensive use of experiential exercises that are designed to help the client contact potentially troublesome (and often avoided) thoughts, feelings, memories, and physical sensations, or to experience firsthand some of the odd workings of their own verbal processes. Voluntary exposure to feared experiences in therapy has a number of important functions. First, it allows the client to experience particular thoughts, feelings, or memories in a different, and safer, context. This may alter some of the verbal relations that promote experiential avoidance or escape. Undermining the overarching rule system that promotes experiential avoidance is the single most important goal of ACT, and small exposure exercises contribute substantially to this process. Second, eliciting difficult experiences allows them to be observed and studied experientially. Observing and studying a private phenomenon requires nonjudgmental detachment from that same phenomenon. Experiential exercises provide phenomenological grist for the therapeutic mill. Third, having clients participate in exercises that highlight flaws in human language is far superior to discussing those same flaws, in part because the former is not linear and analytic, and the latter can easily become so. Like metaphor and paradox, experiential exercises strengthen a social/verbal context that persistently asks, "But what does your experience tell you?"

•4•

Creative Hopelessness: Challenging the Normal Change Agenda

THEORETICAL FOCUS

When a client comes into psychotherapy, he or she is resistant to change. We do not mean resistance as a state, a trait, an intrapsychic event, nor an explanation for the failure of treatment. Resistance is merely a description of the client's predicament. Ordinarily, the client has worked, struggled, considered, planned, evaluated, contemplated, and dealt with "the problem." The client has often talked to friends, discussed it with family, prayed, read, purchased tapes, and visited therapists. Therapy is only one of a long line of change efforts and, by definition, those efforts have not solved the problem.

If a person has exerted so much effort and yet is coming for treatment, one of two things must apply: (1) The person has not found the right way to fix the problem, or (2) the model for change is flawed and unworkable. Clients typically go through many cycles of change efforts and often reach a point where the question is asked: "Why am I failing?" The usual answer clients give themselves (and the usual answer given to them by others) is, "I am failing because I need more (confidence, willpower, emotional control) or less (anxiety, depression, worry)."

From an ACT perspective, the client's problem-solving efforts are dominantly driven by culturally sanctioned, language-based rules that specify how problems are to be analyzed and solved and the rewards that await those who follow these rules. The culture instructs the client that

- Psychological problems can be defined as the presence of unpleasant feelings, thoughts, memories, bodily sensations, and so on;
- These undesirable experiences are viewed as "signals" that something is wrong with the client and that something has to change;
- Healthy living cannot occur until these negative experiences are eliminated;
- The client needs to get rid of negative experiences by correcting the deficits that are causing them (e.g., lack of confidence, mistrust in relationships); and
- This is best achieved by understanding or modifying the adverse factors that are the cause of difficulty (e.g., low self-confidence resulting from overcritical parents; mistrust caused by a sexually abusive parent).

In most empirically validated therapies, the therapist and client employ a similar model of change because they are both verbally regulated by these mainstream cultural views. The exact target or means of intervention may be different, of course. The therapist may suggest that the problem is not that the person has the wrong spouse or the wrong job, but that the client has distorted or irrational thoughts. To some degree this may be a new idea to people (few nonpsychotic persons come into therapy complaining of irrational cognitions or inappropriate cognitive schemas), but the overarching idea is entirely familiar. At a metatheoretical level, the core conception is this: "The problem is one of bad content; change the content and the problem will go away." Viewed from afar, we do have to wonder: If manipulating personal experience and history is such a powerful change strategy, why is the client coming to see a therapist in the first place? Indeed, most clinical techniques bear a strong family resemblance to advice the person has already received from Mom, Dad, the local priest, a best friend, co-workers, neighbors, or siblings.

ACT approaches the client's situation with a different assumption. Perhaps the client's change agenda itself is not very workable. Perhaps the reason intelligent and hardworking people suffer so much is that they are trapped by the normal functions of human language itself, as amplified and exacerbated by years of acculturation. The client's usual change agenda is based on rules that are so common and ubiquitous in human affairs that to challenge them can seem nonsensical at first. ACT requires that therapists go after this sense of "normality." The ACT therapist undermines resistance by exploring its nature and scope and by showing that the most natural, normal, sensible, and usual efforts to solve problems can be the source of those very problems. In other words, it is not that the problem itself is resistant to change, but rather that a direct, linear change effort can make the problem worse.

ACT attempts to clear the field of these cultural rules and instead appeal to the client's actual experience, which is quite different. In essence, ACT keeps asking the client: "Which will you believe, your 'mind' or your experience?" This general question functions as a motivative augmental that is designed to create a heighten sensitivity to the consequences of direct relevance, the client's own pain and sense of unworkability.

Typically, the ACT therapist begins this process by drawing out the system. Drawing out the system involves a dialogue focused on three primary questions: (1) What does the client want? (2) What has the client tried? and (3) How has that worked? The theoretical rationale for this approach is important. The client is operating under the influence of an overexpansive track that has a form described previously: Identify the problem ("bad" thoughts, feelings, etc.), eliminate the problem (eliminate "bad" thoughts, feelings, etc.), then life will improve (e.g., "I will have fulfilling work, marriage . . . "). From a Relational Frame Theory (RFT) perspective, this particular track involves an *if . . . then* relational frame (i.e., if *"bad" feelings* then *bad life*, and the opposite frame that is entailed, if *no "bad" feelings* then *good life*).

The goal of drawing out multiple examples from the client's own history is to help the client discern this underlying rule and contact its consequences (which are often quite painful). In the next phase, the therapist will begin to undermine this ineffective tracking, so it is important that the client is experientially connected to what is often a long series of unsuccessful attempts to forge a successful life using this strategy. In addition, the therapist wants to create a link between the general track underlying these different attempts so that functionally similar strategies will be grouped into a class of events. Drawing many instances into a larger class is useful because it makes it more likely that targeting extinction of some of them will lead to weakening the entire class (Dougher et al., 1994). When the system is challenged, ideally what is being undermined is the general track, not just a particular ineffective instance.

When the ACT therapist has organized most of the client's solutions into a "control of private experience = successful living" class, the workability of that entire class is challenged. We call this "creative hopelessness" because, as these seemingly reasonable strategies fall away under the glare of experienced unworkability, the client often does not know what to do next. This is a creative position, because entirely new strategies can develop without being overwhelmed by previous rule systems. In summary, creative hopelessness involves the weakening of both pliance and overexpansive tracks tied to ineffective and needless experiential control. This, in turn, serves as a powerful motivative augmental for fundamental change.

CLINICAL FOCUS

In this phase of ACT, the therapist focuses on the following issues:

- The client has tried everything, but the problem remains.
- The problem is not one of motivation.
- The problem is not one of specific tactics.
- This problem is not like most other areas of life. There is something inherently paradoxical about it. Whereas working hard to solve a problem normally pays dividends, in this situation working hard makes the problem seem worse.
- Perhaps the solution is part of the problem.
- The client needs to respond to direct experience and feedback from life, not to the logic of the problem-solving system.
- The client is not to blame for being stuck and is able to respond in ways that will change the situation.

Table 4.1 presents a summary of the major therapeutic goals of this phase, along with specific strategies and interventions.

INFORMED CONSENT

Before ACT begins, the client must be prepared for it. This can be an intensive intervention, and the client should not be subjected to such interventions lightly. Informed consent in ACT consists of giving general descriptions of operating principles and a frank discussion of the areas of ambiguity. In addition, alternative forms of therapy should be described.

Because ACT can raise fairly fundamental issues, it is wise to get the client to commit to a course of treatment and agree not to measure progress impulsively. This usually involves agreeing to meet a certain number of times with the client and then perform a progress review. The client is told to expect ups and downs. As treatment is unfolding, it is not unusual for clients to question their commitment to facing previously avoided experiences. Using a session-contracting approach keeps the cli-

TABLE 4.1. ACT Goals, Strategies, and Interventions Regarding
Creative Hopelessness

Goals	Strategies	Interventions
1. Gain informed consent and commitment to therapy.	Develop knowledge necessary for informed consent. Develop therapy contract.	Address alternative treatments. Address risks and benefits. Propose specific time frame to review. Orient person to therapist and client roles.
2. Describe the client's change agenda and how it hasn't worked.	Detailed discussions of client's experience with problem. Help client evaluate experience.	What do you want from life? How have you tried to get it done? How has it worked?
3. Undermine client attachment to change agenda.	Develop workability as a yardstick.	Focus on workability. Talking to describe versus talking to make a difference. Use of metaphor. Use inherent paradox.
4. Engender willingness to abandon the unworkable change agenda.	Evoke creative hopelessness. Distinguish blame from response-ability.	You are stuck. Man in the Hole Metaphor Chinese Handcuffs Metaphor Feedback Screech Metaphor Tug-of-War with a Monster Metaphor Learned skill metaphors (e.g., playing baseball, music, dancing)
5. Undermine useless "understanding."	Use paradox, confusion, and deliteralization to destabilize "understanding."	How does that work for you? Interventions tailored to client feedback.
6. Undermine client attachment to change agenda.	Distinguish current hopelessness from eventual workability. Avoid the old agenda claiming the new.	Defocus on hopelessness as belief or feeling; focus on experienced effects of change efforts. Proscribe change efforts.

ent involved in therapy while creating a mechanism for the client to withdraw if necessary.

DRAWING OUT THE SYSTEM

We begin ACT with a set of assumptions. One of the most important is the idea that what the person has been trying to do to solve the problem is itself part of the problem. This cannot be seen easily (even though the client has usually experienced the workability of stepping outside of the trap of logic), because language itself produces and supports this unworkable agenda. Directly describing the trap—as if letting go of it is a simple intellectual matter—can be counterproductive, because that effort would support the linear, literal, analytical, evaluative approach that is the core of the trap in the first place. The approach has to be less direct.

One of the first goals of ACT is simply getting clearer about what has not worked. During the initial assessment phase, this is easy to do because it looks very much like normal assessment. In the initial session(s), the therapist draws out the system that has been strangling the client by exploring several key questions.

What Does the Client Want?

The client has been struggling purposely, not randomly. Both the client's "psychopathological" behavior and the client's attempts to change this behavior are functional—both forms of behavior are attached verbally to certain consequences. The client might be asked, "What do you want from therapy?" or "If a miracle were to happen here, how would your life be different?" or any number of versions of this question ("What do you want from life?" "What will have to happen before you can get better?" "What do you think the real problem is?" etc.). Usually, the answer to such questions will be a mix of two things, and it is crucial that the ACT therapist be ready to detect and distinguish both.

The client will usually reveal certain desired goals. The person may want to travel, go to school, make a contribution to other people, have children, develop spiritually, love others, live with integrity, be more honest, and so on. We will call all of these *outcome goals*, although later in this book we will show how they actually involve two distinct aspects (goals and values). In addition, the client will reveal a second set of goals that are linked to these outcome goals, because he or she believes that they are necessary to the accomplishment of these outcomes. We will call these *process goals*. Process goals have their value in part because they will help in achieving an outcome. The system that is strangling the client is usually composed of the linkage between outcome and process goals.

For example, one of us (S.C.H.) recently had a client who was depressed, anxious, and in the middle of an unpleasant, drawn-out divorce that she initiated only after many years of a miserable relationship. When she was asked, "What do you want from therapy?" she answered, "I need to feel better about myself. Sometimes I think I almost hate myself. I am insecure most of the time. It goes back as far as I can remember—even as a little girl I remember thinking that I was bad and I would never get it right." Later she added, "I think I've never really grown up and taken charge of what is happening to me. My marriage turns out to be a sham, my kids don't want to be with me—I've made a mess of it. For years, I just dealt with it by drinking, but of course that just made it worse. But now that I've stopped drinking, I realize how bad I feel most of the time—I think if I knew how hard it would be I'd never have been able to quit."

This answer presents the usual mix of outcome and process goals. The outcome goals include taking charge of her life, having a relationship that is valid and intimate, and having a good relationship with her children. These outcomes are supposedly being interfered with because of various psychological obstacles: hating oneself, feeling insecure, feeling bad, and thinking, "I'm bad." Here we have the core of the client's unworkable system: When the insecurity and bad feeling go away, the client will be able to live a more powerful and valuable life. Changing bad feelings is a process goal. Living well is an outcome goal. The answer also reveals some of the efforts that have been used to try to make this system work—the client "felt better" when drinking. Paradoxically, although the change agenda suggested that feeling better would lead to positive outcomes, the client has experienced the exact opposite. Efforts to feel better at first (e.g., by drinking) did indeed change the process goals. The client did feel better. Drinking worked. But changing these process goals did not produce the outcome goals. Indeed, drinking made her life much less livable. The process did not work.

At this point in assessment and therapy, no intervention is called for. The system should not be challenged or even pointed out. But the therapist should be clear about what the client has been trying to do and should organize it into a coherent whole that can be linked to a powerful clinical strategy. Later on, the details of the client's struggle will be important and useful as the therapist tries to challenge the system that has been strangling the client.

What Has the Client Tried?

Most clients are working within a system in which undesirable psychological content is construed as a barrier to effective living. Based on this system, the client has been trying to change the situation so as to change the psychological content, or has tried to deal with the psychological content by avoiding it, disputing it, arguing with it, challenging it, justifying it, rationalizing it, denying it, ignoring it, tolerating it, and so on. The therapist should spend some effort (even a great deal of effort if that is what is required) trying to enumerate all of the various methods that have been used and the success they have produced. This should be done without any sense of therapeutic criticism or arrogance.

The methods the client has used may include a variety of therapy methods and other culturally supported change methods such as drugs, relaxation training, cognitive restructuring, religion, meditation, avoidance, social reassurance, distraction, and so on. In each case the ACT therapist should draw out the change method very clearly and link it back to the client's system. The following dialogue demonstrates how an ACT therapist evaluates the change agenda of a chronic worrier:

THERAPIST: What else have you tried to do?

CLIENT: Well, sometimes I try to talk myself out of it. I say, "This is silly, you are making a mountain out of a molehill."

THERAPIST: In other words, criticize and chastise yourself. And the purpose of this criticism . . . ?

CLIENT: To get me to stop it.

THERAPIST: To get yourself to change—to stop worrying.

CLIENT: Yeah. . . . The things I worry about are silly. I mean some of the things that come into my mind are just nuts.

THERAPIST: And the idea is that if you could get rid of those worries—those thoughts—then the anxiety would be less and you'd be able to face your daily situation better.

CLIENT: Right, but it is pretty hard to convince myself to stop it, so sometimes it works but sometimes it doesn't.

THERAPIST: So if you could just convince yourself that you don't need to worry, then it would work and things would start moving ahead. OK. So far we've got criticism, chastising, and attempts to convince yourself to stop. What else have you tried?

The ACT therapist is drawing out the structure of the system by this kind of questioning. The system itself isn't being challenged—indeed, the therapist takes the position that whatever the client has been doing is understandable and normal. It is not normal in the sense that it should be done or that it is workable. Rather, this is an example of exactly how the system works. The client has been following the culturally supported system. It is a good idea to include the therapy setting itself in this kind of exploration. The client can be invited to reveal how coming into therapy is itself another change effort. This can be helpful because it shows that the therapist is not defensive about being included in the client's agenda.

Here is an example from a session with a depressed client in the middle of a divorce:

THERAPIST: And this. Coming in here. Is it part of that effort to change how bad you feel as well?

CLIENT: Of course. I'm not sure what I will get out of this really, but if I could feel even a little better about myself, it would be worth it.

THERAPIST: So you're hoping to remove some of the bad feelings and get more good feelings because then you would be able to move on.

CLIENT: (*pauses*) I guess so.

THERAPIST: So this is another thing to try. Good. So let's add this therapy to the list. It is another thing you've done to feel better.

CLIENT: I've tried almost everything I know to feel better.

THERAPIST: I'm sure you have. You have indeed. And this—therapy—is yet another attempt.

CLIENT: You say it as though there is an alternative.

THERAPIST: Well. I don't know. Right now I just want to be clear about what you have tried and how it has worked.

How Has It Worked?

In ACT, the therapist is engaging the client in a kind of contest between two main players. On one side is the client's mind. By "mind," we mean the set of rules and relations that the client uses to order the world. Because so many of these are culturally established, it can be clinically useful to speak of "mind" as if it is another person or something slightly external (as indeed it is in the sense of being a cultural intrusion into the individual). On the other side, there is the wisdom of the client's direct experience. The client has directly contacted certain outcomes. The mind and experience are in fundamental conflict. The therapist's job is to challenge the client's reliance on verbal rules so that experiential wisdom can play a greater role. The challenge is to undermine ineffective rules and replace them with contingency-shaped behavior, accurate tracks, and augmentals linked to chosen values.

In this early assessment phase of therapy, the therapist comes back repeatedly to a central question: If you do what your mind tells you (if you follow the change agenda), are the consequences that are produced actually those that the rules specify? Do the rules pay positive dividends? If the answer is yes, there would be few reasons for therapy in the first place. The culture gives ample training in how to use systems of verbal rules to produce change, and if that were enough, we could all just do what our minds tell us to do and all would be well. In fact, our clients have been doing what their minds tell them to do and all is not well. But most clients do not fully appreciate the nature of the game that is being played. The system can fail to produce and still not be seen as the source of the problem. The following dialogue with the chronic worrier introduced earlier demonstrates how to evaluate how well a rule system is working:

CLIENT: Right, but it is pretty hard to convince myself of it, so sometimes it works but sometimes it doesn't.

THERAPIST: So if you could just convince yourself, then it would work. OK. Let me ask you this. Your mind says that when you convince yourself that your concerns are silly, you will stop having those concerns, you will become less anxious, and then you will do better. Right?

CLIENT: Right.

THERAPIST: OK. And does that work? What does your experience tell you?

CLIENTS: Sometimes. But I can't always talk myself out of them.

THERAPIST: And even when it does work, if we expand the time frame a bit, would you say that over time, as you've followed the rules your mind has laid out for you, that your concerns overall are less or more?

CLIENT: . . . . Overall it is more.

THERAPIST: That seems like a paradox, doesn't it? I mean, you do what your mind says, sometimes it even seems to work, and then somehow it seems as though the concerns and worries are getting bigger, not smaller. They are more important, not less.

CLIENT: So what should I do?

THERAPIST: What does your mind tell you to do?

CLIENT: Try harder.

THERAPIST: Interesting. And have you tried harder?

CLIENT: And harder and harder.

THERAPIST: And how has *that* worked? Has it paid off in a long-term or fundamental way, so that by doing it you have transformed the situation and it is no longer a problem? Or are you, unbelievably enough, sinking in deeper as you try harder and harder?

CLIENT: . . . . I'm sinking in deeper.

THERAPIST: If we had an investment advisor with that track record, we would have fired him long ago, but here your mind keeps leading you into efforts that don't really, fundamentally, pay off, but it keeps following you around with its "blah, blah, blah," and it is hard not to give it one more try. I mean what else can you do but what your mind tells you to do? But maybe we are coming to a point in which the question will be, "Which will you go with? Your mind or your experience?" Up to now, the answer has been "your mind," but I want you just to notice also what your experience tells you about how well that has worked.

Focusing on how the system is working does two things. First, it focuses attention on the consequences of the client's verbal understanding. This is a powerful place to work from, because no matter how well defended the client is, the fact of therapy itself is undeniable evidence that there is a problem, unless the client has been forced or cajoled to come and doesn't view the situation as a problem. The pain of failure is a great ally, because the place from which it is possible to try new things is the place in which old things aren't working. Thus, whenever an ACT therapist gets caught up in a fascinating life story, workability provides a reliable way to shift attention back to the contextual issues that are really more important. For example, if a client logically "explains" why things are the way they are, the therapist can pause and say, "And how has this analysis you are telling me about worked for you? What does your experience tell you?" Workability is a way out of the traps laid by the content of language, both for the client and for the therapist. In behavioral terms, what is at issue are the actual consequences of actions or strategies, not the justification or logic of them.

Second, by using the language of "your mind," the therapist is beginning to encourage the client to look at mental reactions rather than looking at the world through them. In other words, the therapist is beginning to look at the process of verbal relations, not simply at the stimulus functions that are altered by these processes. Phrases such as

"So your mind then tells you X" undermine the way verbal relations normally work, because networks of derived stimulus relations present themselves as organized "reality," not as the action of creating an organized picture. Creating an almost person-like entity called "the mind" taps the client into a history of what to do when other people talk. It is easier to separate from self-talk when it is treated as an object-like event, because we have a greater history of separating the roles of the speaker and the listener and of distinguishing rule understanding from rule following when dealing with two people.

CONFRONTING THE SYSTEM: CREATIVE HOPELESSNESS

Engendering creative hopelessness is the first major ACT intervention. If the psychological trap that underlies most psychopathology is built into human language, it will be extraordinarily difficult to dismantle. If the therapist were to point it out directly, it would have to be pointed out from within language, and if language is the problem, the therapist would be participating in the trap in the name of dismantling the trap. There is a need to confront literal language, and yet therapy involves using language with the client. Complex forms of psychotherapy are unavoidably largely verbal enterprises and cannot be done simply through music, pictures, dance, or other less verbal systems of communication.

To confront an entire system, one must act outside that system. When ACT therapists begin to believe what they are saying, they are in dangerous territory. ACT uses words to accomplish ends, and if they do not do that, they are not true, no matter how logically defensible they may be. As discussed in Chapter 2, this is the essence of the pragmatic and contextualistic philosophy underlying ACT. Thus, as ACT interventions are described, we will change "voice" from the more logical, scientific approach that has been taken up to this point to another voice in which meaning is use, and nothing more. Just as ACT clients are cautioned about overreliance on belief, the reader is cautioned as well. Therapeutic talk in ACT is tied entirely to workability, not to the logic and rationality of literal language. ACT consciously adopts contextualistic criteria for talk. No matter how rational and logical the thought, the question always is, "And does that work for you?" This applies to the client, but it also applies powerfully to the therapist.

Workability and Creative Hopelessness

In working with severely affected, multiple-problem, chronic, or personality-disordered clients, considerable emphasis must be placed on clearing away the old system so that something new can happen. This section is written with relatively severely affected clients in mind. For other clients with a more normal and limited range of problems, this set of interventions can be deemphasized, especially if therapy is occurring within a time-limited context. A much softened version, however, can be useful even in very brief clinical encounters.

Clearing away the old system is, in part, a process of confrontation, but the confrontation is not between the therapist and the client. Rather, it is between the client's change agenda and the client's experience of the workability of that system. Thus, there should be no sense of "one-upmanship." The therapist is in the same boat as the client, and while the client is hooked by his or her system, the therapist is probably hooked by one too. The therapist's advantage is not that of the smart or together person talking with the dumb or broken person. Rather, it is the advantage of the person looking at the system from the outside over the person participating inside the system. It is the advantage of perspective.

As a visual metaphor, imagine a therapist and a client sitting side by side. As the therapist talks about the system, he or she is pointing to something several feet in front of them. Indeed, ACT therapists often sit next to the client and work just this way, especially if the client is raising problems as barriers that seem to be standing between the client and the therapist. This physical posture says that the therapist is not challenging the client. Together the therapist and client are challenging the system. They have a working alliance.

One way to confront an unworkable situation is to describe it as such. Recall that the therapist has already collected a long list of things the client has tried to eliminate: emotional uneasiness, disquieting thoughts, or other psychological experiences. The therapist knows the major strategies that the client has tried in the past. The various ways in which the client has attempted to manipulate thoughts and feelings (e.g., drugs, alcohol, overt avoidance, sex, attacking others, moving away, social withdrawal, and so on) have been listed and examined in great detail. The ultimate unworkability of those strategies has been gently and directly examined. What hasn't yet been faced is that the change agenda itself is flawed. The following dialogue illustrates how the issue of creative hopelessness is introduced.

THERAPIST: You have told me a lot of things you have tried to do, and it seems to me that you have tried to do just about everything that is logically there to be done. You've done all the obvious and reasonable things. You've thought hard, you've worked hard. You've looked for the angles. And now here you are in therapy . . . still trying. But you've hired me. I work for you. So it is my obligation to point something out: "This isn't working, right?"

CLIENT: I haven't figured it out yet.

THERAPIST: Here is another way to say what you just said: Even trying to figure it out isn't working so far.

CLIENT: Not yet.

THERAPIST: Not yet. What if it won't? What if this whole thing is a setup?

CLIENT: A setup?

THERAPIST: Well, in other areas if you had worked this hard, you'd have a lot of good things to show for it. Isn't it true in your experience, although it doesn't seem that it should be this way, that the more you've struggled with emotional discomfort and disturbing thoughts—the more you have tried to get rid of them—the more difficult it has become? They don't seem to respond to conscious control. These feared reactions haven't gotten smaller, they have gotten bigger.

CLIENT: I don't know how to get rid of them. I'm hoping you can help. How should I get rid of them? What am I doing wrong?

THERAPIST: Those are important questions because they show very clearly what has been going on, but let's not get off on that issue quite yet. Let's start with what you know directly. You feel stuck.

CLIENT: Big time.

THERAPIST: It is not clear what to do next, but it doesn't seem as though there is a way out.

CLIENT: Exactly.

THERAPIST: So I'm here to say something: "You are stuck. There is no way out." . . . Within the system in which you have been working there is only one thing that can happen: what has been happening. Just consider that as a possibility. . . . Look, you know it *hasn't* been working. Now let's consider the possibility that it *can't* work. It isn't that you aren't clever enough, or that you don't work hard enough. It is a setup. A trap. You're stuck.

CLIENT: So I'm hopeless. I should give up. Why am I coming here?

THERAPIST: I don't know. But right now let's just try to see what hasn't been working. Anyway, I didn't say *you* are hopeless, I said *this* is hopeless. This whole thing that has been going on. This struggle is hopeless. And, yeah, if a struggle is hopeless, it is time to give up on that struggle.

CLIENT: Then what should I do?

THERAPIST: Well . . . first let's start from here. If this whole thing is a trick, a trap, we need to open up to that reality so that something different can happen. You came here expecting some kind of solution I might have. You've been trying to find the solution and think maybe I have it. But maybe these so-called solutions are actually part of the problem. Check and see whether this isn't true—maybe this isn't true for you, but just look and see whether it is: Deep down you don't believe that there *is* a solution. If I trotted out one more clever idea, part of your mind would be saying, "Oh, yeah. Sure. Right." Your direct experience says this situation is hopeless. Your mind says, "Of course, there is a way out. There has got to be a way out." I'm here to ask a simple question: which are you going to believe—your mind or your experience?

In common, everyday language, hopelessness is not an acceptable state of mind. Therapists often work hard to counter feelings of hopelessness and to instill optimism about the future. However, seeing a hopeless *situation* as hopeless is not a bad thing. If the client can give up on what hasn't been working, maybe there is something else to do. Thus, in this phase of ACT, the therapist tries to help the client face hopelessness, but as a kind of creative act. The goal is not to elicit a *feeling* of hopelessness or a *belief* in hopelessness; instead, the objective is to engender a posture of giving up strategies when giving up is called for in the service of larger goals, even if what comes next is not known.

When a client is caught in a self-defeating struggle, it is important to acknowledge it. Hopelessness in this case doesn't mean despair; it is creative hopelessness because it allows for new things to emerge. It is in the interest of changing the agenda in a fundamental way. Approaching the issue of unworkability from a strictly intellectual point of view is very difficult for most clients. Normally, metaphors can make the point without invoking the client's normal verbal defenses. The *Man in the Hole Metaphor* is a core ACT intervention in the early phase of therapy.

The situation you are in seems a bit like this. Imagine that you're placed in a field, wearing a blindfold, and you're given a little tool bag to carry. You're told that your job is to run around this field, blindfolded. That is how you are supposed to live life. And so you do what you are told. Now, unbeknownst to you, in this field there are a number of widely spaced, fairly deep holes. You don't know that at first—you're naive. So you start running around and sooner or later you fall into a large hole. You feel around, and sure enough, you can't climb out and there are no escape routes you can find. Probably what you would do in such a predicament is take the tool bag you were given and see what is in there; maybe there is something you can use to get out of the hole. Now suppose that the only tool in the bag is a shovel. So you dutifully start digging, but pretty soon you notice that you're not out of the hole. So you try digging faster and faster. But you're still in the hole. So you try big shovelfuls, or little ones, or throwing the dirt far away or not. But still you are in the hole. All this effort and all this work, and oddly enough the hole has just gotten bigger and bigger and bigger. Isn't that your experience? So you come to see me thinking, "Maybe he has a really huge shovel—a gold-plated steam shovel." Well, I don't. And even if I did I wouldn't use it, because digging is not a way out of the hole—digging is what makes holes. So maybe the whole agenda is hopeless—you can't dig your way out, that just digs you in.

This metaphor is extremely flexible. It can be used to deal with many beginning issues. In the interaction with the client, the therapist can fill out the metaphor to address specific issues that the client raises or that the therapist thinks are pertinent. It is also useful to try to integrate the client's responses into the ongoing metaphor, as demonstrated by the following scripting:

1. *"Maybe I should just put up with it."* "You've tried other things. You've tried to tolerate living in a hole. You sit down and twiddle your thumbs and wait for something else to happen. But that doesn't work, and besides, it's just no fun living your life in a hole. So when you say, 'Put up with it' or 'Give up,' what I hear is that you are really staying with the same agenda (digging your way out) but no longer trying, because it doesn't work. I'm suggesting something else. I'm suggesting changing the agenda."

2. *"I need to understand my past."* "Another tendency you might have would be to try and figure out how you got in the hole. You might tell yourself, 'Gee, I went to the left, and over a little hill, and then I fell in.' And, of course, that is literally true; you are in this hole because you walked exactly that way. Your exact history brought you here. But notice something else. Knowing every step you took does nothing to get you out. And besides—remember you are blindfolded—even if you had not done exactly that, you'd have gone somewhere else instead. You might have fallen into another hole anyway, because there are lots of holes to be found. So you found anxiety, someone else found drug abuse, someone else found bad relationships, someone else found depression. Now, I'm not saying your past is unimportant, and I'm not saying we won't work on issues that have to do with the past. The past

is important, but not because figuring it out lets you escape emotional pain. It is only the past as it shows up here and now that we need to work on—not the dead past. And it will show up in the context of your moving on with your life. When it does, we will work on it. But dealing with the past isn't a way out of the hole."

3. *"Am I responsible for these problems?"* "Note that in this metaphor, you are responsible. Responsibility is recognizing the relationship between what we do and what we get. Did you know that originally the word *responsible* was written *response able*? To be responsible is simply to be able to respond. So, yes, you are able to respond. And, yes, your actions put you in the hole and your actions can take you out. Response-ability is acknowledging that you are able to respond and that were you to do so, the outcome would be different. If you try to avoid responsibility, there is a painful cost: If you cannot respond, then truly nothing will ever work. But I'm saying digging is hopeless, not 'you are hopeless.' So don't back up from responsibility—if you have an ability to respond, then there are things you can do. Your life can work."

4. *"Should I blame myself?"* "Blame is what we do when we are trying to motivate people to do something—to change or to do the right thing. But you look plenty motivated to me. Do you need more? Do you need to buy 'I'm at fault'? Blaming is like standing at the edge of the hole and throwing dirt on top of the person's head and saying, 'Dig out of here! Dig out of here!' The problem with blame in this situation is that it is useless. If the guy in the hole has dirt thrown down on his head, it won't make it any easier to get out of the hole. That doesn't help. When your mind starts blaming you, does buying blaming thoughts strengthen you or weaken you? What does your experience tell you? So if you buy blame from your mind, go ahead, but then be response-able about that. If you buy into that, you will be doing something that your experience tells you doesn't work."

5. *"What is the way out?"* "I don't know, but let's start with what isn't working. Look, if you still have an agenda that says, 'Dig until you die,' what would happen if you were actually given a way out? Suppose someone put a metal ladder in there. If you don't first let go of digging as the agenda, you'd just try to dig with it. And ladders are lousy shovels— if you want a shovel, you've got a perfectly good one already."

6. *The need to give up first.* "Until you let go of the shovel you have no room to do anything else. Your hands can't really grab anything else until that shovel is out of your hand. You have to let it go. Let it go."

7. *A leap of faith.* "Notice you can't know whether you have any options until you let go of the shovel, so this is a leap of faith. It is letting go of something, not knowing whether there is anything else. In this

metaphor you are blindfolded, after all—you'll know what else is there only by touch, and you can touch something else only when the shovel is out of your hands. Your biggest ally here is your own pain. That is your friend and ally here, because it is only because this isn't working that you'd ever even think of doing something as wacky as letting go of the only tool you have."

8. *The opportunity presented by suffering.* "You have a chance to learn something most people never will—how to get out of holes. You would never have had a reason to learn it if you hadn't fallen into this hole. You'd just do the rational thing and muddle through. But if you can stay with this, you can learn something that will change your life. You'll learn how to disentangle yourself from your own mind. If you could have gotten away with it, more or less, you'd never have done that."

Metaphors such as *The Man in the Hole* serve to disrupt both the particular problematic *if . . . then* frame and, at least momentarily, sense making or rule control more generally. Again and again in this segment of therapy, ACT therapists engage the confrontation between the client's altogether sensible behavior and its fundamental unworkability in his or her life experience. A systematic battering down of sense making is intended to allow the client to make more direct contact with unworkability. Sense making is a powerful repertoire, and clients will not shed it entirely, or for long. However, even momentary direct contact with the contingencies provides a wedge that can be used to break apart the problematic control-private-events-to-control-life-quality of the *if . . . then* frame.

There are several other metaphors that can help the client face the hopelessness of winning the struggle. Some are quite short, such as the *Chinese Handcuffs Metaphor.* These can be useful as supplements, when the client needs additional ways of connecting with the issue, or as quick introductions useful in the earliest parts of treatment or pretreatment (e.g., when trying to describe the therapy as part of an informed consent procedure). Usually the therapist will use one or two such metaphors about being stuck. If the client seems to connect with one, others can be reserved in case the same point has to be revisited later in therapy. Many such metaphors have been used in ACT, and others are easily generated: Being stuck can be like wrestling with a tar baby, or like being a monkey trying to get a cookie out of a jar too narrow for his closed hand, and so on.

Metaphors such as these capture, very quickly, the essence of the client's situation. In short order, they suggest that the problem is in the system, not in the client's lack of effort. They point to the possibility that there

CHINESE HANDCUFFS METAPHOR

The situation here is something like those "Chinese handcuffs" we played with as kids. Have you ever seen one? It is a tube of woven straw about as big as your index finger. You push both index fingers in, one into each end, and as you pull them back out, the straw catches and tightens. The harder you pull, the smaller the tube gets and the tighter it holds your fingers. You'd have to pull your fingers out of their sockets to get them out by pulling them once they've been caught. Maybe this situation is something like that. Maybe these tubes are like life itself. There is no healthy way to get out of life, and any attempt to do so just restricts the room you have to move. With this little tube, the only way to get some room is to push your fingers in, which makes the tube bigger. That may be hard to do at first, because everything your mind tells you to do casts the issue in terms of "in and out" not "tight and loose." But your experience is telling you that if the issue is "in and out," then things will be tight. Maybe you need to come at this situation from a whole different angle than what your mind tells you to do with your psychological experiences.

is a counterintuitive solution to the client's problem while calling attention to the unworkability of logical solutions in some contexts. All of this is done within a context that provides a kind of common sense and experiential reality check: Life can, indeed, sometimes be just like this.

The strange verbal game that goes on in ACT has to make contact with the client's knowledge about how the world works; otherwise this looks like nothing but pointless psychobabble. ACT may be a kind of psychobabble, but it is never pointless. It is talk that is designed to make a difference, not talk that must be literally "true." Metaphors help keep the client on track without having to wrap too many words around the core perspective.

Understanding: Belief versus Experiential Wisdom

Verbal "understanding" at this stage is, as at any stage of ACT, to be looked at skeptically (by both client and therapist). There is no "right answer" in ACT. The ultimate yardstick for any new strategy is its workability in the client's life. ACT presents a fundamental challenge to decades of socialization, belief, effort, and analysis, all sitting in the repository of the client's understanding. If the client "understands," this usually means that what is being said has been recast so that it fits with the unworkable change agenda and the client's well-established system of verbal rules. Even if the client says something that is fairly close to an ACT perspective (e.g., "You're saying I just need to feel my feelings"), it is the job of the ACT therapist to detect what that verbalization is *functionally* and to speak to that function.

The goal of ACT is to weaken the excesses of literal language and the implicit assumptions and agendas that literal, linear thinking contains. The ACT therapist is attempting to open up a realm that is at a right angle to belief and disbelief. This is not a matter of persuading the client to believe in a new agenda, because the new agenda is literally beyond belief. Thus, the ACT therapist may challenge any indication of verbal "understanding," especially early in therapy. Conversely, statements of confusion may be responded to quite positively. This sort of intervention strengthens what is shaping up to be a decidedly different social/verbal context from any the client has experienced.

A graphical presentation of the field of verbal and experiential relations of normal adults was shown in Figure 3.2. As people move up into the world of literal belief and disbelief, they necessarily move down the continuum from experiencing (being present, aware, and in the moment) to nonexperiencing (living in a world of substitute stimulation that is about some other time or somewhere else; living in a world dominated by the derived stimulus functions of human language). The point is that it does not always matter who is "wrong" or "right" or what is "believed" or "disbelieved." In all of these cases, language is dominating over direct experience. That applies to both parties. The therapist's formulations are also just ongoing verbal behavior, susceptible to the same prejudices as the client's. If the therapist is willing to let go of an attachment to literal language, an opportunity is created in which it is possible to confront the client's verbal system and still remain present and equally vulnerable. ACT therapists engage in therapeutic interaction on that razor's edge in which language itself is given no firm place to stand on either side of the therapeutic interchange.

Confusing No Hope with Creative Hopelessness

The ACT therapist can make two kinds of errors in the area of hopelessness: confusing creative hopelessness with hopelessness as a negative feeling state or with hopelessness as a belief. Creative hopelessness is neither. It is an action or behavioral posture that occurs when all the behavior oriented toward a desired outcome—in this case immediate, deliberate control over negative thoughts and feelings—is experienced as unworkable. Creative hopelessness is just giving up on what experience tells you is futile. If a client directly experiences the uselessness of solutions, they lose their luster because they cannot deliver the promised rewards. Creative hopelessness has the effect of undermining the defective or overexpansive track that is keeping the client stuck.

"Hopelessness the feeling" often has a desperate quality that is connected to a magical or child-like belief that someone, somewhere will rescue the person and produce the desired outcome, because the alternative appears to be unacceptable. In other words, the feeling is being used as a kind of ply that is supposed to produce a reaction from someone (God, a spouse, the therapist, oneself). There is good clinical evidence that many clients use hopelessness and despair in exactly this socially coercive manner (Biglan, Lewin, & Hops, 1990). Experientially, this type of hopelessness is perceived as defeat or resignation to suffering. It is not really a creative state, because the client hasn't faced the futility of the agenda itself.

"Hopelessness the belief" is equally problematic, because it tends to be overexpansive. In its most pernicious form, hopelessness the belief is put forth as a state of the person: "I *am* hopeless."

The following dialogue demonstrates how the ACT therapist might respond to the issue of hopelessness, stated as a belief:

CLIENT: So why am I coming in to see you? It sounds as if you are saying I will never be successful.

THERAPIST: My purpose is not to help you win this struggle. That does not mean that *you* are hopeless or *you* can't be successful. In fact, my goal is to help you have your life work, and I 100% think I can help you do that if you are willing to face these monsters you have been running from.

CLIENT: If it is easy to have your life work, why haven't I done it?

THERAPIST: I never said it was easy. It is hard. Not hard *effortful*—it is hard *tricky*. This is a very tricky trap—one that catches us all. Look, it is absolutely clear to me that if you knew what to do, you would have done it. I don't believe for a minute that you are broken, weird, perverse, or self-destructive. You have done the absolute best you can. You have everything you need to move ahead from here to live a vital, committed, meaningful life. It is just that we have to start from here—here is where you are. So *you* look and *you* see whether your experience doesn't tell you that you are caught in a struggle you seemingly can't win. Are you willing to trust that experience, allow it to influence you, and then to move from here? That is what your life is asking of you right now.

This phase of ACT does not involve talking *about* hopelessness. It involves facing the *experienced* hopelessness of the client's situation. If there is a lot of dialogue *about* the issue of hopelessness, chances are the therapist is trying to "convince" the client, which is a certain route to trouble.

BARRIERS TO GIVING UP
THE UNWORKABLE SYSTEM

Clients usually need help getting "present" and action focused, rather than analyzing their problems to the point of paralyzing adaptive behavior. It is one thing to acknowledge that a change agenda is hopeless. It is deceptively difficult to then stop engaging that agenda. For many clients, stopping unworkable strategies is hard because previously avoided experiences will quickly be released into the client's psychological field and there often is not a clear alternative response other than avoidance. Further, most clients are skeptical of the idea that they have the ability to respond without first relying on analysis, evaluation, and rational decision making. Metaphors are very useful at making the point that less analysis and less struggle can increase adaptive responses. The *Feedback Screech Metaphor* can be of aid in this area particularly for relatively overwhelming and traumatic private events.

The therapist should present this as a learned skill that will take time to acquire. A variety of metaphors can be used that exemplify the fact that many things in life are not simply the result of having some vital bit of information. Instead, they are the result of practice and experience. Some clients may be able to relate easily to sports metaphors (e.g., "Have you ever noticed that the more you think about *how* you are hitting the ball, the harder tennis becomes?") or playing a fast piano

---

FEEDBACK SCREECH METAPHOR

You know that horrible feedback screech that a public address system sometimes makes? It happens when a microphone is positioned too close to a speaker. Then when a person on stage makes the least little noise, it goes into the microphone; the sound comes out of the speakers amplified and then back into the mike, a little bit louder than it was the first time it went in, and at the speed of sound and electricity it gets louder and louder until in split seconds it's unbearably loud. Your struggles with your thoughts and emotions are like being caught in the middle of a feedback screech. So what do you do? You do what anyone would. You try to live your life (*whispering*) very quietly, always whispering, always tiptoeing around the stage, hoping that if you are very, very quiet there won't be any feedback. (*Normal voice*) You keep the noise down in a hundred ways: drugs, alcohol, avoidance, withdrawal, and so on. [Use items that fit the client's situation.] The problem is that this is a terrible way to live, tiptoeing around. You can't really live without making noise. But notice that in this metaphor, it isn't how much noise you make that is the problem. It's the amplifier that's the problem. Our job here is not to help you live your life quietly, free of all emotional discomfort and disturbing thoughts. Our job is to find the amplifier and to take it out of the loop.

---

piece, singing, dancing, writing poetry, guitar playing, or similar activities. We may ask the client, "Suppose you read every book ever written about swimming: the physical mechanics of it, biographies of great swimmers, books on all of the strokes and styles of swimming. Would that make you a swimmer? Wouldn't you still have to practice in the water? Well, our work here is like that." The therapist should use activities that fit the client's experience and interests.

LETTING GO OF THE STRUGGLE
AS AN ALTERNATIVE

Near the end of this phase, it is helpful to expose the client to the idea that letting go of futile struggle may be a viable option. The following is a metaphor that was generated by a wonderful and courageous client with agoraphobia as a description of a breakthrough she experienced in ACT. This client abandoned a 20-year struggle with panic and started living instead, doing all the things she had always wanted to do (starting a business, going to school, leaving a destructive marriage) by including anxiety as a legitimate component of these life changes. We call this the *Tug-of-War with a Monster Metaphor.*

> The situation you are in is like being in a tug-of-war with a monster. It is big, ugly, and very strong. In between you and the monster is a pit, and so far as you can tell it is bottomless. If you lose this tug-of-war, you will fall into this pit and will be destroyed. So you pull and pull, but the harder you pull, the harder the monster pulls, and you edge closer and closer to the pit. The hardest thing to see is that our job here is not to win the tug-of-war. . . . Our job is to drop the rope.

The drop-the-rope image is a perfect one for the larger agenda of ACT, in which emotional willingness and detachment from thoughts will dominate. Sometimes clients ask, "How do I do that?" after hearing this metaphor. It is best not to answer directly at this point, because that is the whole issue that the therapy addresses. The therapist can instead say something like "Well, I don't know exactly how to answer that right now. But the first step is simply to see that you are holding the rope."

Depending on how the client reacts to metaphors, the key messages they contain can be used as a kind of new language in ACT sessions. If a client comes in with a new struggle, the therapist might describe it as digging. If a client is facing a new challenge, it might be talked about as an opportunity to drop the rope. Clients themselves—especially successful ACT clients—often start using these images in session and begin generating their own metaphors. If a client creates a metaphor that fits well, the wise ACT therapist will go with it and integrate it into the therapeutic work. Indeed, many ACT metaphors presented in this book are metaphors that have been added to ACT work over the past 15 years because clients created them.

THERAPEUTIC DO'S AND DON'TS

Am I Hurting, or Helping, the Client?

Therapists exposed to the ACT perspective at first may be concerned that clients exposed to unworkability and creative hopelessness will react with horror, will leave therapy, or will otherwise engage in dramatic negative actions. In decades of experience in developing this model, with many hundreds of clients and well over a thousand therapists who have received ACT training, we are unaware of anyone who has left therapy at this point in a crisis caused by confronting the hopelessness of their struggles. So far as we know, no one has committed suicide or entered into a deep depression. Quite the contrary: Although clients frequently express some concern, anger, or destructive forms of hopelessness, these are normal initial reactions that can easily be worked through.

If the ACT therapist does this phase well, the net result is generally calming (not that creating calm is our purpose—this is merely the effect). After all, the client's unworkable struggles have been a tremendous burden. Recognizing and letting go of the struggle can be a great relief. The mistake is to think that we are adding something to the client's distress by facing the hopelessness of the struggle. Creative hopelessness can help form a powerful connection between the ACT therapist and the client's own experience in a way that emotionally validates the client. This is not a mind game in which the therapist is trying to produce something that was not there before. The therapist is simply trying to help make evident and to normalize what the client is already in contact with.

Most clients experience this with an odd sense of relief. It is odd because the literal content seems so severe ("Yes, you are stuck"), but it is a relief because it fits the client's actual experience. The message from the therapist is very positive, even though it is superficially negative. The general message is that being stuck is not your fault. You are not to blame (although you are response-able). You have been caught up in a trap that has caught most, if not all, other humans, and now you have a chance to confront that head-on and really learn something that many people never will learn. Your experience is valid. It is OK to start from exactly where you are already—nothing needs to change first. Face the futility of the struggle, and new things can happen.

The following transcript from a successful former ACT client demonstrates the impact of creative hopelessness:

COMMENT FROM WORKSHOP AUDIENCE: I'm surprised they come back for a second session.

S.C.H.: I've never had a client drop out at this point. They're usually quite interested—they've never had anyone talk to them in this way before.

AUDIENCE: I'd hate for a client to go out and commit suicide when you say there is no way out.

CLIENT SITTING IN: But along with that rap comes a feeling of hope too. You go into therapy thinking you've done everything you can possibly do. You want the therapist to give you a trick, and yet deep down you know that can't happen. If it could have, you'd already have done it. So you sort of feel relieved to hear that you have tried everything. And with this you also feel hope, because you figure he must know something you don't. So it really wouldn't create a suicidal feeling. You can't wait to find out where he is going with this thing.

Don't Expect Anything to Change

It is usually best during this phase not to create an expectation that something "positive" will happen as a result of defining the struggle the client is in. In general, it is too early to suggest any behavior change on the part of the client. In fact, positive things often do happen, but positive movement at this phase is tricky because it can lead to an immediate reengagement with the unworkable agenda the client has been pursuing. It is an irony that progress achieved by abandoning a verbally established agenda will immediately be claimed as evidence that the agenda is workable. Thus, the expectation that no immediate change is sought or anticipated is prophylactic, as demonstrated in the following monologue:

"In the next week I don't want you to do anything different. Don't change your behavior—don't try anything new. I don't expect that what we have done here will be of any help that you will detect. If you notice positive things, file them away so that we can talk about them. In all likelihood, if such things occur they don't have anything to do with what we are doing."

Homework Assignments

It is a good idea to give homework, but not for behavior change. The client's motivations for behavior change cannot be trusted yet, as they may still be in the service of the old change agenda. Instead, self-monitoring assignments designed to gather data about situations where the client engages in struggle are most appropriate. It is usually wise to have the client keep a written record, either a self-monitoring form or a daily journal. The client should bring this material to each session, to help support therapeutic discussions, given the following instructions:

> "One thing you can do between now and when we get back together is to try to become aware of how you carry out this struggle in your daily life. See whether you can just notice all the things you normally do; all the ways you dig. Getting a sense of what digging is for you is important because, even if you put down the shovel, you will probably find that old habits are so strong that the shovel is back in your hands only instants later. So we will have to drop the shovel many, many times. You might even make a list that we can look at when we get back together: all the things you have been doing to moderate, regulate, and solve this problem. Distraction, self-blame, talking yourself out of it, avoiding situations, and so on. I'm not asking you to change these actions; just try to observe how and when they show up."

PROGRESS TO THE NEXT PHASE

The creative hopelessness phase is concluded when clients show signs that they see how the system has moved them in circles, while expressing an openness to looking at alternatives. Often, clients will begin to catch themselves "doing the problem" in session. Sentences will be half finished as they realize that they are "doing it again." Very often, the rate of client talk will decline. Clients sometimes will laugh unexpectedly or say things like, "I'm confused. I don't know what to do next." Any sense of lightness, openness, or humorous self-perspective can be trusted.

PERSONAL WORK FOR THE CLINICIAN

In the preceding chapter, you were asked to describe the main problem that stands between you and moving toward what you most value in life.

You were asked to describe what would tell you this problem had been solved and what you would have to do to make this happen. In this exercise, you will take a look at how this change process is working. Save your answers. They will be needed in the next chapter.

1. How long has this problem, or problems like it, been around in your life?
2. What types of strategies have you used to solve or eliminate this problem?
3. Think about each strategy. How well has it worked in the short run? How well has it worked in the long run?
4. Do these strategies look like the way you typically respond to other problems in your life? If so, how are they similar?

CLINICAL VIGNETTE

A 38-year-old woman, single parent of three preadolescent children, enters therapy complaining of persistent sadness and loss of interest in her friendships, leisure activities. She used to go to church regularly but has stopped in the last 6 months. Two years ago, her husband died in an automobile accident. They had been happily married for 14 years. Out of necessity, she is now working full-time. Her stated goal for therapy is, "I've been sad for too long now. It's time for me to snap out of it, but the more I push myself to snap out of it, the worse I seem to feel. I don't know how I'm ever going to get my life going if I keep feeling this way."

> *Question for the clinician:* Try to conceptualize the client's situation from the viewpoint of the change agenda. Then describe a few key strategies you might use. Take a few moments to develop your response before reading ours.
>
> *Our answer:* The client has a change agenda that looks something like this: "When my sadness goes away, then I'll be able to start my life again." This is unlikely to happen, given the tragedy of her husband's death and the massive change in her life that has resulted. We would probably focus on the specific strategies she has used to try to get control of her sadness. How have these strategies worked? We would probably emphasize that trying to overcome sadness is a "reasonable" strategy and compliment her for doing it so persistently. Our goal at this stage would be to have her experientially understand that her "stuckness" may in fact be the insistence on controlling her sadness.

APPENDIX: CLIENT HOMEWORK

What Hasn't Worked?

1. Write down everything that your problem has cost you. Be as specific as possible.

2. Now write a list of everything you have done in an attempt to solve this problem. Be thorough and specific: You should be able to come up with several examples of strategies you've used in your attempts to solve it (for example, swearing you were going to stop, using your willpower, getting furious at yourself in order to spur yourself on, avoiding, criticizing, etc.) and many specific examples of where you have used these strategies.

3. Honestly evaluate how far each of these strategies has brought you toward solving the problem.

•5•

Control Is the Problem,
Not the Solution

The significant problems we face cannot be solved on the
same level of thinking we were at when we created them.
—ALBERT EINSTEIN

If "clearing the field" has been successful, the client is intrigued, ready
for new things, and confused. The client has a vague sense of what hasn't
been working but can't quite see it clearly. For most people, this sense of
ambiguity is a powerful motivator. In this phase of ACT, what hasn't
been working is going to be given a name: Control. In the ACT model,
attempts at controlling and eliminating unwanted private experiences lie
at the heart of most unworkable change agendas. Although control-
oriented change strategies appear sensible, when they are applied to the
wrong targets they tend to engender and intensify the very experiences
that are repugnant to the client. The cost associated with putting these
experiences "in the closet" (emotional avoidance, escape, and numbing)
is greater than the damage the original experiences would have done if
they were allowed in without defense.

Four factors most clients bring into therapy seem to support deliberate control as the preferred coping strategy in the domain of private
events:

- "Deliberate control works well for me in the external world."
- "I was taught it should work with personal experiences (e.g.,
  'Don't be afraid . . . ')."

- "It seems to work for other people around me (e.g., 'Daddy never seemed scared . . . ')."
- "It even appears to work with certain experiences I've struggled with (e.g., relaxation works for a while to reduce my anxiety symptoms)."

The purpose of this phase of ACT is to begin to destabilize the client's confidence in these four rationales for control-based change efforts. The client will experience the scope and nature of the problems created by these cultural messages and will begin to examine an alternative.

Undermining the control agenda is safe to do only if it is based on the client's experience—otherwise we are merely adding a lot of verbiage to an already overloaded verbal system. Thus, this phase is initiated with the assumption that the client is very much in touch with the unworkability of current change efforts, even though the client may not be entirely clear about how these change efforts fit into a control-oriented agenda. In more seriously dysfunctional clients, this phase is not initiated unless creative hopelessness has been engendered. More functional clients can enter the present phase rather quickly if they have made experiential contact with the issue of unworkability.

Therapy at this stage of ACT is like the process experienced by a person standing a few yards offshore. Each time a wave goes out to sea, a little more sand is washed away from beneath the person's feet. Eventually, it is hard to stand without falling over. The goal of the ACT therapist at this point is to wash away the destructive ground the client has been standing on. The therapist tries gradually to remove the props that are holding up a harmful system, with the hope that the system will fall over. A variety of techniques are used to wash away the sand and weaken the foundations. Most of these do so by pointing to the client's experience of unworkability.

THEORETICAL FOCUS

Scientifically speaking, the goal of this phase is to change the context in which culturally conditioned rule systems operate. These rule systems typically treat such innocent behavioral bystanders as emotions or memories as causal cogs in a behavioral machine. In ACT it is the context of cognitive and emotional control itself that is targeted.

This phase of ACT is aimed at disrupting the client's unworkable tracks while helping to lay the groundwork for more workable ones. By giving the unworkable struggle a name and a clearer shape, clients have something verbally to do with these early stages of ACT. For example, they can consider verbally whether control in this area actually works. This obviously is itself a rule-generation process, but it is based on direct experience and is less based on pliance and overexpansive cultural tracks.

In addition to naming control as one context in a world of possible responses, we use a variety of metaphors and experiential exercises that further challenge the workability of maintaining control over private experiences. As the client makes direct contact with the unworkability of control strategies, as opposed to tightly held verbal formulations about how control *ought* to work, he or she becomes more susceptible to direct contingencies. However, great care must be taken in this segment not to *dictate* or demand that the client evaluate control strategies as unworkable. Such a posture is likely to generate either pliance or counterpliance and runs counter to the therapeutic agenda of loosening rule governance and increasing sensitivity to directly experienced contingencies.

Reduction in problems with pliance is best accomplished by the use of techniques such as metaphors and experiential exercises, rather than direct instruction. These interventions place the defective *if . . . then* track in a context in which the material is sufficiently nonthreatening that the client is not motivated to avoid, *and* which highlight the unworkability of the track. Pliance and counterpliance are minimized, because the client is allowed to experience directly how the contingencies work. There is no obvious rule to follow, or to defend against.

Another method of reducing pliance problems is by asking questions rather than stating conclusions. For example, a statement such as "Your attempts at control really didn't work in that situation" may cause the client to be defensive and to think about ways the strategy *did* work in that situation, even if it did not bring about fundamental change. Or the client may say, "Well, maybe that didn't work, but what are you offering?" Neither of these are particularly useful postures for the client. In contrast, if the therapist says, "It sounds as though in some ways this worked, at least in the short run. But I'm wondering, what is your sense about how it worked at a really fundamental level? Did it really change things in a fundamental way, in the way you have been hoping for?" There is very little to react against in this sort of formulation. Whenever possible, foster pliance by questioning rather than dictating. We are, after all, trying to help the client make closer contact with his or her own experience, not with our beliefs.

CLINICAL FOCUS

In this phase of therapy, the therapist will focus on the following issues:

- The client's change efforts are really efforts at controlling private events.
- The culture, through language, engrains control strategies.
- The client's short-term experience with control suggests that it might work, but in the long term it clearly doesn't work.
- The main manifestations of the control agenda are emotional avoidance and escape.
- The more the control strategy is applied, the more negative experiences escalate and take control of the client's life.
- The alternative to control is acceptance of uninvited experiences.

Table 5.1 presents a summary of the major therapeutic goals of this phase. For each goal, specific strategies are listed, along with ACT exercises and metaphors that can be used to implement therapeutic strategies.

TABLE 5.1. ACT Goals, Strategies, and Interventions Regarding Control

Goals	Strategies	Interventions
1. Control is the problem and leads to unworkable outcomes through emotional avoidance and escape.	Show how the control agenda creates suffering. Show how control moves seem to work in the short run, but fail in the long run. Show how the culture supports using control.	Rule of private events Polygraph Metaphor Chocolate Cake Exercise Daily Willingness Diary
2. Control moves are arbitrarily learned and maintained, apart from or despite experience.	Teach conditioning model. Elevate awareness of control instructions in language. Distinguish rule following from workability.	What Are the Numbers? Exercise Rules of the Game Exercise Identifying Programming Exercise
3. Willingness is an alternative to control, and there is a cost to being unwilling.	Teach how willingness undermines the control agenda. Teach client how low willingness creates distress.	Two Scales Metaphor Box Full of Stuff Metaphor Clean versus Dirty Discomfort Diary

GIVING THE STRUGGLE A NAME:
CONTROL IS THE PROBLEM

Usually the client will have noted normal and typical "digging" moves from the homework in the previous phase. These should be explored, without interpretation or an attempt to understand them, but with a real interest in the exact nature of these maneuvers. As demonstrated in this dialogue with a client with panic disorder, the ACT therapist first probes to elucidate the nature of the client's unworkable control strategies.

THERAPIST: What else did you observe?

CLIENT: Well, when I was about to go into the department meeting, I noticed I checked several times to see whether I still had my bottle of Valium in my purse. I knew it was in there—I always carry it anyway—but I checked it maybe four times within 5 minutes right before the meeting.

THERAPIST: What do you think the checking was in the service of?

CLIENT: I guess reassuring myself that it was there.

THERAPIST: So that you could . . .

CLIENT: Well, so that I could always quick sneak a pill if things got too bad. I have learned to open the bottle with one hand and sort of tuck a pill in the knuckle joint. Like a magician does. Then I cough or something, and I get it in my mouth. It tastes pretty bad, but actually if I just let it dissolve it works faster anyway, so I don't need water or anything.

THERAPIST: So one thing you observed is that before you go into the department meeting you make sure you have a way of dealing with your anxiety. And you check for the bottle to reassure yourself that you have that way out even if you can't just leave the room.

CLIENT: Yeah.

THERAPIST: And that is in the service of keeping the anxiety away.

CLIENT: For sure.

THERAPIST: Can I say it this way?: Access to tranquilizers is probably one way you dig.

What the ACT therapist is doing is revealing the form (the client's behaviors) and purpose (the immediate goals) of the client's behavior and is linking them to client's change agenda (using the metaphor of "digging"). At this point, no big deal is made of any of this—it is touched on, clarified, formulated in fairly commonsense terms, and then just left on the shelf. Eventually, the goal is to lump this set of responses into a single class—emotional control—along with its manifestations, escape, and avoidance.

The Rule of Private Events

From a cultural perspective, purposeful control undeniably works in the successful manipulation of the world. The world outside the skin works according to verbally constructed rules. The problem is that these same rules are different in the world of private experience because private events are not mere objects to be manipulated: they are historical and automatic. The more general track, "If bad events are removed, then bad outcomes can be avoided," is a track that is quite effective in some contexts, but not this one. The following dialogue shows how the issue of the uncontrollability of private experiences is broached.

THERAPIST: OK. I think I understand what you have been doing. Any others that you noticed.

CLIENT: No. That is about it.

THERAPIST: OK. Actually, there are probably a lot of others that will percolate up as we proceed, but it is not important at this point that we know every one. We just need to get a sense of the range of things involved. What I want to do today is to try to get a clearer sense of this set of things—I want to have us get clearer about what digging even is anyway. And I want to give it a name—not to figure it out intellectually, but just to have a way of talking about it in here.

CLIENT: You want us to have a name for the theme.

THERAPIST: Right. I believe that most of what you have been doing is quite logical, sensible, and reasonable, at least according to your mind and my mind. The outcome isn't what you hoped it would be, but it seems to me that you've done pretty much the normal thing. You've really tried hard and fought the good fight. All these digging moves you just listed. Aren't they the kinds of things people do?

CLIENT: Maybe not normal people, but people like me sure do. It's like that support group I go to. It is almost laughable. Every single person in there has the same story. I mean you can tell even before they open their mouths what the story will be.

THERAPIST: Exactly. Because we all show how the system works. Consider this as a possibility. Everyone's story is similar (and similar to yours) because what you are doing is what we are all trained to do. It's just that it doesn't work here. Human language has given us a tremendous advantage as a species because it allows us to break things down into parts, to formulate plans, to construct futures we have never experienced, and to plan action. And it works pretty well. If we look just at the part of our existence that involves what goes on outside the skin, it works great. Look at all the things the rest of creation is dealing with, and you'll see we do pretty well. Just look around this room. Almost everything we see in here wouldn't be here without human language and human rationality. The plastic chair. The lights. The heating duct. Our clothes. That computer. And so on. So we are warm, it won't rain on us, we have light—in regard to the stuff nonhumans are struggling with, we pretty much have it made. You give a dog or a cat all this stuff—warmth, shelter, food, social simulation—and it is about as happy as it knows to be. But without humans, dogs and cats are outside in the cold. So we've solved the problems nonverbal critters face. We are also the only species that commits suicide, and we can be miserable when they would be happy. Really, really important things—important to us as a species competing with other life forms on this planet—have been done with human language. There is an operating rule for things outside the skin that works great: If you don't like something, figure out how to get rid of it and get rid of it. And that rule works fine in most of our life. But consider the possibility—just consider it—that that rule does not work in the world between your ears. That last little bit of human existence is a pretty important part because it is where life satisfaction lies, but it is only a small proportion of our total lives. Yet suppose that same rule worked just terribly in that last few percentage points of life. In your experience, not in your logical mind, look and see whether it's not like this: In the world inside the skin, the rule actually is, If you aren't willing to have it, you've got it.

CLIENT: If I'm not willing to have it, I will . . .

THERAPIST: Just look at it. For example, you've been struggling with anxiety.

CLIENT: Oh, yeah.

THERAPIST: You are not willing to have it.

CLIENT: No way.

THERAPIST: But if it is really, really important not to have anxiety, and then you start to get anxious, that is something to get anxious about.

CLIENT: If I'm not willing to have it, I have it . . .

THERAPIST: Weird, huh? Just to put a name on it, let me say it this way:
In the outside world, our mind's fascination with prediction and
control works great. Figure out how to get rid of something, give
your mind the job, and watch it go! But when it comes to private
events like unpleasant thoughts, feelings, memories, or bodily sensations, the solution isn't deliberate control, the problem is deliberate
control. If you try to avoid or eliminate your own thoughts or feelings, you are in an unworkable position. Unfortunately, our minds
think control is the answer for everything. If you don't like a memory or the prospect of feeling bad, just eliminate the cause and you
don't have to feel it. So your mind tells you to start digging.

CLIENT: You mean, if I don't get so uptight about being anxious, I'll be
less anxious?

THERAPIST: Maybe—but notice, there is a paradox here. Suppose it
really is true that "if you are not willing to have it, you do." What
could you do with such knowledge? If you are willing to have it in
order to get rid of it, then you are not willing to have it and you will
get it again. So you can't trick yourself. You can't dig with what I'm
saying here . . . or at least if you do, nothing positive will happen.

Very often clients pick up on the word *control* in helpful ways;
for instance, "I've always had a problem when I wasn't in control,"
or "My husband says I'm a control freak," or "I'm a pretty controlling person." If that happens, the ACT therapist can harness these
issues to the therapeutic agenda. For example, the therapist can respond, "We are all control freaks—we have minds that just can't let
go of the idea that control is the solution for everything!" This uses
the issue while avoiding assigning the same meaning to "control
issues" that the client may be implicating. For example, the client may
have been told that "the problem that causes my (the client's) suffering is that I try to control everything." This could be just one more
rule that the client may have picked up as a way of explaining the
causes of his or her suffering, and if it is an old rule we can be sure
that it is not powerful enough to be of major help now.

Providing some understanding about how control is programmed
avoids destructive pliance in several ways. First, it is normalizing. The
therapist is saying that the client is not bent, broken, or defective. The
client is merely suffering a normal side effect of language. There is little
in this to defend against. There is also an element of paradox inherent in
the rule "If you're not willing to have it, you've got it." This is a funny

sort of rule, because even though we can understand the rule, it is not clear how to follow it. A degree of confusion is an ally when excessive sense making is a problem.

The *Polygraph Metaphor* is a core intervention in this phase of therapy. It is especially good with anxiety- or mood-disordered clients.

> Suppose I had you hooked up to the best polygraph machine that's ever been built. This is a perfect machine, the most sensitive ever made. When you are all wired up to it, there is no way you can be aroused or anxious without the machine's knowing it. So I tell you that you have a very simple task here: All you have to do is stay relaxed. If you get the least bit anxious, however, I will know it. I know you want to try hard, but I want to give you an extra incentive, so I also have a .44 Magnum, which I will hold to your head. If you just stay relaxed, I won't blow your brains out, but if you get nervous (and I'll know it because you're wired up to this perfect machine), I'm going to have to kill you. So, just relax! . . . What do you think would happen? . . . Guess what you'd get? . . . The tiniest bit of anxiety would be terrifying. You'd naturally be saying, "Oh, my gosh! I'm getting anxious! Here it comes!" BAMM! How could it work otherwise?

This metaphor can be used to draw out several paradoxical aspects of the control and avoidance system as it applies to negative emotions. As the following scripts suggest, modifying the language within the metaphor keeps the impact of the exercise intact while allowing the client's different issues to be addressed.

1. *The contrast between behavior that can be controlled and behavior that is not regulated successfully by verbal rules.* "Think about this. If I told you, 'Vacuum the floor or I'll shoot you,' you'd vacuum the floor. If I said, 'Paint the house or I'll shoot,' you'd be painting. That's how the world outside the skin works. But if I simply say, 'Relax, or I'll shoot you,' not only will it not work, but it's the other way around. The very fact that I would ask you to do this would make you damn nervous."

2. *How this metaphor reflects the client's stance toward unwanted private events.* "Now, you have the perfect polygraph machine already hooked up to you: It's your own nervous system. It is better than any machine humans have ever made. You can't really feel something and not have your nervous system in contact with it, almost by definition. And you've got something pointed at you that is more powerful and more threatening than any gun—your own self-esteem, self-worth, the

workability of your life. So you actually are in a situation very much like this. You're holding the gun to your head and saying, 'Relax!' So guess what you get? BAMM!"

3. *How even seemingly successful attempts to make this situation work really don't.* "So see if this isn't true: What you've done is that you've found that if you take a Valium [or whatever the client is doing: drinking alcohol, avoidance, denial, etc.] for at least a little while, then you can manipulate how you feel. But as soon as it wears off it doesn't work anymore. Instead of seeing the whole game as a hopeless and useless enterprise—which it is—you've been trying to win it, and nearly killing yourself in the process."

Other interventions can be used to show how weak deliberate verbal control is when applied to the world of private events. Depending on what the client is struggling with, it may be helpful to use experiential exercises to develop this point in regard to thoughts, memories, or other domains of psychological events. The *Chocolate Cake Exercise* is particularly effective with clients who are struggling to control obsessive thoughts or ruminations.

> Suppose I tell you right now that I don't want you to think about something. I'm going to tell you very soon. And when I do, don't think it even for a second. Here it comes. Remember, don't think of it. Don't think of . . . warm chocolate cake! You know how it smells when it first comes out of the oven. . . . Don't think of it! The taste of the chocolate icing when you bite into the first warm piece. . . . Don't think of it! As the warm, moist piece crumbles and crumbs fall to the plate. . . . Don't think of it! It's very important; don't think about any of this!

Most clients get the point immediately and may laugh uncomfortably, nod, or smile. Others may respond by insisting that they did not think about anything. As illustrated in the following dialogue, the ACT therapist can use this exercise to further highlight the futility of mental control or thought suppression strategies.

THERAPIST: So could you do it?

CLIENT: Sure.

THERAPIST: And how did you do it?

CLIENT: I just thought about something else.

THERAPIST: OK. And how did you know you did it?

CLIENT: What do you mean?

THERAPIST: The task was not to think of chocolate cake. So what did you think of?

CLIENT: Driving a race car.

THERAPIST: Great. And how did you know that thinking of a race car was doing what I asked? So that you could report success?

CLIENT: Well I was saying, "Great, I'm thinking of a race car . . ." (*pauses*)

THERAPIST: Yes. And continue on. I'm thinking of a race car and I'm not thinking of . . .

CLIENT: Chocolate cake.

THERAPIST: Right. So even when it works, it doesn't.

CLIENT: It's true. I did think of cake, but I pushed it out so fast I almost didn't think of it.

THERAPIST: And isn't this similar to what you have done with your obsessive thoughts?

CLIENT: I try to push them out of my mind.

THERAPIST: But see the problem. All you are doing is adding race cars to chocolate cake. You can't 100% subtract chocolate cake deliberately, because to do it deliberately you have to formulate the rule, and then there you are, because the rule contains it. If you are not willing to have it . . .

CLIENT: You do.

The point can also be made in respect to physical reactions. We might say to the client something like, "Don't salivate when I ask you to imagine biting into a wedge of lemon. Don't salivate as you imagine the taste of the juice on your lips and tongue and teeth." These exercises help the client to make direct contact with the ineffectiveness of conscious purposeful control in these domains.

HOW EMOTIONAL CONTROL IS LEARNED

For the client, one of the most unsettling aspects of having to face the "control doesn't work" issue is the thought that repeatedly applying a seemingly unworkable strategy proves there is something wrong with the client "deep down inside." Most clients have little appreciation for how random social conditioning actually is. Instead of approaching the issue from the perspective of random and accidental learning, the client may begin to see failed control strategies as an indictment of underlying stability.

Experiential exercises are particularly useful for demonstrating how easy it is to condition a irrelevant and nonfunctional private response. Assisting the client to understand how language conditioning occurs is helpful, because it undermines the credibility of focusing on having the proper content as a means to psychological health. There is something absurd about defining one's self-worth on the basis of particular feelings, thoughts, attitudes, and so on, when these reactions are often established through accidental and whimsical circumstances that are totally out of the individual's control. The *What Are the Numbers? Exercise* is an ACT intervention designed to demonstrate the arbitrary nature of personal history.

THERAPIST: Suppose I came up to you and said, "I'm going to give you three numbers to remember. It is very important that you remember them, because several years from now I'm going to tap you on the shoulder and ask 'What are the numbers?' " If you can answer, I'll give you a million dollars. So remember, this is important. You can't forget these things. They're worth a million bucks. OK. Here are the three numbers: Ready? One, . . . two, . . . three. Now—what are the numbers?

CLIENT: One, two, three.

THERAPIST: Good. Now don't forget them. If you do, it'll cost you a lot. What are they?

CLIENT: (*laughs*) Still one, two, three.

THERAPIST: Super. Do you think you'll be able to remember them?

CLIENT: I suppose so. If I really believed you I would.

THERAPIST: Then believe me. A million dollars. What are the numbers?

CLIENT: One, two, three.

THERAPIST: Right. Now if you really did believe me (actually I lied) it's quite likely that you might remember these silly numbers for a long time.

CLIENT: Sure.

THERAPIST: But isn't that ridiculous? I mean, just because some head-shrinker wants to make a point here, you might go around for the rest of your life with "One, two, three." For no reason that has anything to do with you. Just an accident, really. The luck of the draw. You've got me as a therapist, and next thing you know you have numbers rolling around in your head for who knows how long. What are the numbers?

CLIENT: One, two, three.

THERAPIST: Right. And once they are in your head, they aren't leaving. Our nervous system works by addition, not by subtraction. Once stuff goes in, it's in. Check this out. What if I say to you that it's very important that you have the experience that the numbers are not one, two, three. OK? So I'm going to ask you about the numbers, and I want you to answer in a way that has absolutely nothing to do with one, two, three. OK? Now, what are the numbers?

CLIENT: Four, five, six.

THERAPIST: And did you do what I asked you?

CLIENT: I thought, "Four, five, six," and I said them.

THERAPIST: And did that meet the goal I set? Let me ask it this way: How do you know four, five, six is a good answer.

CLIENT: (*chuckles*) Because it isn't one, two, three.

THERAPIST: Exactly! So four, five, six still has to do with one, two, three, and I asked you not to do that. So let's do it again: Think of anything except one, two, three—make sure your answer is absolutely unconnected to one, two, three.

CLIENT: I can't do it.

THERAPIST: Neither can I. The nervous system works only by addition—unless you get a lobotomy or something; four, five, six is just adding to one, two, three; one, two, three is in there, and these numbers aren't leaving. When you're 80 years old, I could walk up to you and say, "What are the numbers?" and you might actually say, "One, two, three" simply because some dope told you to remember them! But it isn't just one, two, three. You've got all kinds of people telling you all kinds of things. Your mind has been programmed by all kinds of experiences. [Add a few relevant to the client, such as "So you think, 'I'm bad,' or you think, 'I don't fit in.' But how do you know that this isn't just another example of one, two, three? Don't you sometimes even notice that these thoughts are in your parent's voice or are connected to things people told you?"] If you are nothing more than your reactions, you are in trouble. Because you didn't choose what they would be, you can't control what shows up, and you have all kinds of reactions that are silly, prejudiced, mean, loathsome, scary, and so on. You'll never be able to win at this game.

Seeing that reactions are programmed undermines both the credibility of mounting a successful struggle against undesirable psychological content (because these reactions are automatic conditioned responses) and the need for this struggle (because they do not mean what they say they mean). "I'm bad" is not inherently any more meaningful than "One, two, three."

Theoretically, this kind of exercise makes more evident the *process* of verbal relations, not just the *results* of verbal relations. The result of that shift is that the stimulus functions of verbal events are not as dominant, and thus the rule-control they exert is lessened. Rarely are we aware of the specific histories that have created various relational networks. If we were, we would probably not take the results of this training quite so seriously.

EXAMINE THE APPARENT SUCCESS OF CONTROL

The ACT therapist must begin to undermine the seemingly overwhelming experience that supports control as an effective psychological strategy. This is best accomplished by connecting the client to the costs of using this change agenda in the wrong places. In so doing, the ACT therapist is essentially establishing a discrimination. There are times when the control agenda works, and there are times when it does not. The following dialogue demonstrates how the ACT therapist undermines confidence in the control agenda.

THERAPIST: If conscious, deliberate, purposeful control does not work very well, you have to wonder why we all use it so much. I can think of four primary reasons. One we have already pointed to: It works very well in most aspects of your life. But there is more to it than that. For one thing, try to recall how often you heard things as a young child like "Stop crying or I'll give you something to cry about," or "Stop crying there is nothing scary in here. Stop it and go to sleep," or "Stop being such a baby about this. You're acting like a two-year old."

CLIENT: Some of those exact things were said to me. That one about "I'll give you something to cry about" was something my mom would do when she was mad. I'd be crying and she'd spank me if I didn't stop, but that made it even harder to stop.

THERAPIST: Right. What do you think was the message from all of that?

CLIENT: Shut up.

THERAPIST: Yeah, that you can and should be able to suppress undesirable emotions at will. Just do it and shut up.

CLIENT: I was never good at it, though.

THERAPIST: Neither was I. Of course, what was actually happening was that Mom was saying, in effect, "I don't like feeling what I feel when you feel what you feel, so you stop feeling what you feel so I don't have to feel what I feel." If people can actually do that, you have to wonder why Mom just didn't do it in the first place instead of asking a child to do what she couldn't do. It's like saying, "I can't just get rid of mine, so you just get rid of yours so I can get rid of mine."

CLIENT: The message was that I was supposed to cool it. It goes back as far as I can remember.

THERAPIST: So you were explicitly taught that you can and should control emotions, worry, and so on, just by deliberately controlling them. And this seems right, because you look at these giants called "grownups" and they don't cry like you do, they don't worry like you do, they don't have fears like you do. To a child it looks as though they can usually control their emotions—except when they explode, and then that just makes it all the more important to control them if that is the alternative.

CLIENT: It's different as an adult.

THERAPIST: Exactly. Now we know that adults can't do it either. Heck, half of the adults we looked up to were drinking Martinis every night, taking tranquilizers, avoiding situations like crazy, and whatever else they were doing to get through the day. But as a kid you didn't know that, so it appeared to you that this message—"Just control it"—was something they knew how to do. They weren't crying like you were.

CLIENT: You are talking about stuff that happened when I was real little.

THERAPIST: Yeah—all the more difficult to root it out. These tracks were laid down when you were just a little kid and a lot of the learning was by example, not simply by a verbal rule here or there. Anyway, even all of that wouldn't keep us hooked if it weren't for one final thing: It even seems to work for us. For example, when you have a negative thought you can't get rid of, what do you do most often?

CLIENT: Pray, exercise, talk to someone.

THERAPIST: And for a while it works, does it not?

CLIENT: For a while.

THERAPIST: Exactly. And then what.

CLIENT: Usually it comes back.

THERAPIST: Right. But the way all biological organisms work is that immediate gain is more important than delayed results. This is one of the most universal laws of psychology. So your mind says, "Hey, this is working," because of the immediate effect, but in the longer term it doesn't work—in fact, it might even make it worse.

CLIENT: Sometime it works. Or it used to. I used to be able to do relaxation exercises if I got a little nervous, and I'd be OK. Now it is like spitting on a forest fire.

THERAPIST: There is a paradox here. Control moves aren't really harmful in the emotional arena (or with thoughts, memories, and so on) as long as it isn't too important to avoid this stuff, and the stuff being avoided isn't very potent. That's why you have a chance to learn something most people never will—they can more or less get away with it. Even there I think it hurts them—what we call normal isn't so grand, you know. What is our divorce rate, for example—50%? But, yeah, relaxation isn't very harmful until it is used as a weapon in a struggle with unwanted feelings. That's your situation, though, isn't it? And in that situation, control seems to work short term, while it makes it worse long term.

As clients begin to get a sense of the unworkability of control in certain areas, they may also begin to get a sense of the alternative—being present. This can seem quite threatening, and clients may offer a wide variety of cognitive and emotional responses that are presented as a hindrance to moving forward. The following is an extended dialogue from an ACT session in which the client raises confusion as a reason to interrupt the therapeutic work. This is a good illustration of how psychological avoidance appears in session, and it provides an example of how to work with it from an ACT perspective.

CLIENT: It's hard to hang onto what we're doing here.

THERAPIST: So, don't try to.

CLIENT: It's hard not to try to (chuckle and sigh).

THERAPIST: So, notice that you have the thought that you want to try to.

CLIENT: OK.

THERAPIST: And is it OK to think that you want to try to hang onto it? That you need to hang onto it?

CLIENT: I would like to say it's OK, but it's really not. I feel like I should hold onto it (sigh).

THERAPIST: OK, but now let's just think about that. We've got this thing "I got to hang onto this." . . . Is it OK to think, "I've got to hang onto this"?

CLIENT: Sure (*sigh and chuckle*). . . . No—I guess I'm afraid that I won't get it back if I can't hang onto something.

THERAPIST: OK, so you have the thought that it won't come back. . . . Is it OK to have those words, "It won't come back?"

CLIENT: If it didn't come back, that wouldn't be OK.

THERAPIST: But you didn't experience that it didn't come back, right?

CLIENT: Right, just the fear.

THERAPIST: The fear, right.

CLIENT: Uh huh.

THERAPIST: And some words in your head called, "But it wouldn't be OK if it didn't come back."

CLIENT: Right.

THERAPIST: Is it OK to experience the fact that you have the words called, "But it wouldn't be OK if it didn't come back"?

CLIENT: Sure, it's . . . it's OK to have that feeling.

THERAPIST: Great. Next thought.

CLIENT: But what if it doesn't come back? (*giggle*) Same thing?

THERAPIST: That's the next thought. What's here to accept is not what it says it is, but what you experience it to be. Now what did you actually experience?

CLIENT: The fear that I'm getting confused and it might not ever come back. I might not ever understand.

THERAPIST: Is that OK?

CLIENT: The fear is OK, um. So right, um, when I blank, when I blank out, I'm stuck behind the words. . . . I couldn't have told you that. There weren't any thoughts there to describe.

THERAPIST: Isn't that the most amazing thing? That's true. The most amazing thing is that when you look at the world from words, you don't actually see the words.

CLIENT: Yeah, there weren't any. I was just confused. . . . It's hard to do, um.

THERAPIST: Don't make an effort at trying to do this right. Just get present.

CLIENT: I get into a place, and my mind is just nothing, zero.

THERAPIST: Go with that.

CLIENT: And that anything we've been talking about here in the last hour is gone, it's not . . .

THERAPIST: Stay with that.

CLIENT: I can't remember anything.

THERAPIST: OK. Good!

CLIENT: Yeah. The thought is that my mind is a blank and I can't remember.

THERAPIST: OK, "My mind is blank" um—Anything else your mind has to share?

CLIENT: I'm confused.

THERAPIST: Go with that, go right this moment with that confusion.

CLIENT: I need to keep my mind working.

THERAPIST: OK. So you're having a thought that you have to keep your mind working. . . . What are we trying to do here?

CLIENT: Just to look at my thoughts.

THERAPIST: Right, and all we are really trying to do is just be here with whichever ones come up without struggling with them. Whatever shows up. No particular thing has to show up. Notice how hard that was. Each one kept inviting you to struggle and run away.

CLIENT: Right.

THERAPIST: What are the numbers?

CLIENT: One, two, three.

A certain degree of fearlessness is required of the therapist in such circumstances. The therapist is asking only that this client, to the best of his ability, notice what thoughts and feelings are showing up. There is no requirement that the thoughts be clear or well formed or remembered. Yet all of these are thrown up by the client as obstacles to meeting the simple request to notice thoughts and feelings.

The therapist repeatedly undermines psychological avoidance and turns the issue from the content of distressing thoughts and feelings to the unwillingness of the client to experience the psychological content that is immediately present. Incidentally, the client (who was depressed and using drugs) was successfully treated and later identified this session as an important turning point.

THE ALTERNATIVE TO CONTROL: WILLINGNESS

The whole point of ACT is stated in its name: Acceptance and Commitment. This is another way of saying, "Get present and move ahead," or "Start from where you are and go where you choose to go." Up to this point, therapy has focused on undermining the literal control agenda that tells clients that they can move ahead only after they first start from somewhere else. It helps to begin to point to the alternative. The therapist should use the word *willingness* at this point in therapy, because *acceptance* is often interpreted by the client to mean "toleration," which is an entirely different thing, or "resignation," which the client sees as defeat. Metaphors such as the *Two Scales Metaphor* are designed to introduce the concept of control and its relationship to psychological distress. The metaphor should be linked to clients' experience with the futility of struggling to control their own particular disturbing states. It is also useful to link the metaphor to more mundane examples. For instance, nearly everyone has had the experience of trying to fall asleep during a bout of insomnia. It is commonly understood that *trying* to fall asleep makes sleep nearly impossible. This helps to undermine the client's confidence in control strategies and depathologizes the struggle over control. The struggling insomniac is not crazy, but simply using the wrong strategy.

TWO SCALES METAPHOR

Imagine there are two scales, like the volume and balance knobs on a stereo. One is right out here in front of us and it is called "Anxiety." [Use labels that fit the client's situation; if anxiety does not, use a label such as "Anger," "Guilt," "Disturbing thoughts," etc. It may also help to move your hand as if it is moving up and down a numerical scale.] It can go from 0 to 10. In the posture you're in, what brought you in here was this: "This anxiety is too high. It's way up here, and I want it down here, and I want you, the therapist, to help me do that, please." In other words, you have been trying to pull the pointer down on this scale (*the therapist can use the other hand to pull down unsuccessfully on the Anxiety hand*). But now there's also another scale. It's been hidden. It is hard to see. This other scale can also go from 0 to 10. (*Move the other hand up and down behind your head so you can't see it.*) What we have been doing is gradually preparing the way so that we can see this other scale. We've been bringing it around to look at it. (*Move the other hand around in front.*) It is really the more important of the two, because it is this one that makes the difference and it is the only one that you can control. This second scale is called "Willingness." It refers to how open you are to experiencing your own experience when you experience it—without trying to manipulate it, avoid it, escape it, change it, and so on. When Anxiety [or Discomfort, Depression, Unpleasant memories, Obsessive thoughts, etc.—use a name that fits the client's struggle] is up here at 10, and you're trying hard to control this anxiety, make it go down, make it go away, then you're unwilling to feel this anxiety. In other words, the Willingness scale is down at 0. But that is a terrible combination. It's like a ratchet or something. You know how a ratchet wrench works? When you have a ratchet set one way, no matter how you turn the handle on the wrench it can only tighten the bolt. It's like that. When Anxiety is high and Willingness is low, the ratchet is set and

(*continued on p. 134*)

(*continued from p. 133*)
Anxiety can't go down. That's because if you are really, really unwilling to have Anxiety, then anxiety is something to be anxious about. It's as if when Anxiety is high and Willingness drops down, the anxiety kind of locks into place. You turn the ratchet and no matter what you do with that tool, it drives it in tighter. So what we need to do in this therapy is to shift our focus from the Anxiety scale to the Willingness scale. You've been trying to control anxiety for a long time, and it just doesn't work. It's not that you weren't clever enough; it simply doesn't work. Instead of doing that, we will turn our focus to the Willingness scale. Unlike the Anxiety scale, which you can't move at will, the Willingness scale is something you can set anywhere. It is not a reaction—not a feeling or a thought—it is a choice. You've had it set low. You came here with it set low; in fact, coming here at all may initially have been a reflection of its low setting. What we need to do is get it set high. If you do this, if you set Willingness high, I can guarantee you what will happen to anxiety. I'll tell you exactly what will happen, and you can hold me to this as a solemn promise. If you stop trying to control anxiety, your anxiety will be low—or it will be high. I promise you! Swear. Hold me to it. And when it is low it will be low, until it's not low, and then it will be high. And when it is high it will be high, until it isn't high anymore. Then it will be low again. I'm not teasing you. There just aren't good words for what it is like to have the Willingness scale set high—these strange words are as close as I can get. I can say one thing for sure, though, and your experience says the same thing—if you want to know for certain where the anxiety scale will be, then there is something you can do. Just set Willingness very, very low, and sooner or later when Anxiety starts up, the ratchet will lock in and you will have plenty of anxiety. It will be very predictable. All in the name of getting it low. If you move the Willingness scale up, then anxiety is free to move. Sometimes it will be low, and sometimes it will be high, and in both cases you will keep out of a useless and traumatic struggle that can lead only in one direction.

At this point the client will not know exactly what willingness is. Even though the therapist has made it clear that it is not a feeling or a thought, the client will look for willingness of exactly this kind: a feeling of willingness or a belief that is helpful. The client will also believe that the therapist is saying to ignore or tolerate discomfort. It is essential that the therapist be on the lookout for and detect these misunderstandings, as demonstrated in the following dialogue.

THERAPIST: Willingness is what I was talking about when I was talking about learning to hit the ball.

CLIENT: I'm not really sure I know what willingness is.

THERAPIST: And you don't need to right now. Mostly, right now, I'm just putting an alternative on the table, but I don't expect you to go out and hit home runs just because of a little talk. It will take some experience of actually doing it. It is not a verbal skill.

CLIENT: I understand in the abstract, but I can't imagine actually being willing to feel panic.

THERAPIST: And that is exactly some of the verbal glue that your mind has given you to keep the willingness scale down at zero. The fantasy has been that if you have willingness down at zero, anxiety will go down. If you demand that it go away, it will. That is what your mind says, and it keeps holding out for that effect. Yet that is not what your experience tells you, is it? That is not how it actually works. It says the exact opposite, right? It is almost as if you are being victimized by your feelings.

CLIENT: I do feel that way. It is almost a family tradition. My mother used to say, "That's what happens to us. We get screwed in the end." She was always playing the victim. I guess I learned it early.

THERAPIST: It wouldn't be so bad, except that this victim stuff doesn't do anything positive. It just makes your feelings your own enemy and makes life unlivable. Because no matter how hard you play victim, your own anxiety doesn't care. Remember I was talking about response-ability. Well, in this metaphor, you do have an ability to respond—it's just only on the Willingness scale, not on the Anxiety scale. If you were in control, you would have set this discomfort at zero, and it wouldn't be here, right? Who wouldn't have? If we had our way we'd all be swimming in treacle and sugar cubes all day long. But suppose life is giving you this choice: You can choose to try to control what you feel and lose control over your life, or let go of control over discomfort and get control over your life. Which do you choose?

CLIENT: I'd rather be in control of my life—I've always thought I couldn't do that unless anxiety went away first.

THERAPIST: Exactly. That is how our minds are trained to think. So what we need to learn is where control works and where it doesn't; never mind what your mind tells, your experience tells you. . . . It doesn't work over here with the Emotional Discomfort and Disturbing Thoughts knob. However, over here on the Willingness knob—who sets this one?

CLIENT: I do.

THERAPIST: Only you. Only you. I can make you feel things—I can't make you stay open or not to what you have. That is up to you. It is the one thing that always is up to you.

THE COST OF UNWILLINGNESS

It can be helpful at this point to connect variations in willingness and control to the sense of trauma that clients experience when they attempt to control or eliminate unpleasant experiences, only to discover that they have been amplified and now are seemingly "out of control." The following monologue demonstrates how the ACT therapist introduces the concepts of clean and dirty discomfort.

"We should try to distinguish between 'clean' and 'dirty' discomfort. The discomfort that life just dishes up—that comes and goes as a result of just living your life—is clean discomfort. Sometimes it will be high, or it will be low, because of your history, the environmental circumstances in which you find yourself, and so forth. The clean discomfort is what you can't get rid of by trying to control it. Dirty discomfort, on the other hand, is emotional discomfort and disturbing thoughts actually created by your effort to control your feelings. As a result of running away, whole new sets of bad feelings have shown up. That may be a big part of why you are here. That extra discomfort—discomfort over discomfort—we can call 'dirty discomfort,' and once willingness is high and control is low, it kind of falls out of the picture and you're left with only the clean kind. You don't know how much discomfort you'll have left in any given situation once only clean discomfort is there. But be very clear, I'm not saying that discomfort will go down. What I am saying is that if you give up on the effort to manipulate your discomfort, then over time it will assume the level that is dictated by your actual history. No more. No less."

Clients will sometimes think the therapist is saying that all discomfort (or depression, etc.) will go down because most of it is dirty. Paradoxically, even if this were true (in a literal, scientific sense, it probably is), it wouldn't help clinically, because if one tried to apply willingness this way, it would be by definition be an act of unwillingness and the dirty discomfort would be created again.

The *Box Full of Stuff Metaphor* helps make the point. It is often particularly effective with clients who are avoiding or denying painful past life experiences.

THERAPIST: Suppose we had this trash can here (*Grab a box or a trash can*). This (*put various small items in the box, some nice and some repulsive*) is the content of your life. All your programming. There's some useful stuff in here. But there are also some old cigarette butts and trash. Now let's say there are some things in here that are really yucky. Like your first divorce [fit the specifics to the client]. That would be like this (*blow your nose into a tissue and put it in the box*). What would come up?

CLIENT: I'd think of something else.

THERAPIST: OK, so that's this (*take an item and put it in the box*). What else would come up?

CLIENT: I hate it.

THERAPIST: OK, so that's this (*take an item and put it in the box*). What else?

CLIENT: I've got to get rid of this.

THERAPIST: OK, so that's this (*take an item and put it in the box. Depending on the client, this sequence can continue for some time*). Do you see what is happening? This box is getting pretty full, and notice that a lot of these items have to do with that first yucky one. Notice that the first piece isn't becoming less important—it's becoming more and more important. Because your programming doesn't work by subtraction, the more you try to subtract an item, the more you add new items about the old. Now it's true, some of this stuff you can shove back in the corners and you can hardly see it anymore, but it's all in there. Stuffing things back in the corners is seemingly a logical thing to do. We all do it. Problem is, because the box is you, at some level the box knows, is in contact with, literally up next to, all the bad stuff you've stuffed in the corners. Now, if the stuff that's in the corners is really bad, it's really important that it not be seen. But that means that anything that is related to it can't be seen, so it too has to go into the corner. So you have to avoid the situations that will cause light to be cast into the corners. Gradually your life is getting more and more squeezed. And note that this doesn't really change your programming—it just adds to it. You're just stuffing another thing back into the corner. There are more and more things you can't do. Can you see the cost? It must distort your life. Now the point is not that you need to deliberately pull all the stuff out of the corner—the point is that healthy living will naturally pull some things out of the corner, and you have the choice either to pull back to avoid it or to let going forward with life open it up.

This exercise serves several functions. First, it describes metaphorically the additive nature of history. We can only add to the contents of the box. Second, we have just added a bit of history. This bit links, one more time, avoidance and futile struggle. Eventually, as the client engages in some of the real-life avoidance strategies that are like those brought up in the exercise, the *Box Full of Stuff Metaphor* may become psychologically present, or thoughts of digging, and along with them that sense of futility. Finally, the *Box Full of Stuff Metaphor* has a deliteralizing effect on the various reactions the client produces in response to the avoided content, by objectifying them and placing them in the box—one after another. No reaction is given any special treatment according to its literal content. The metaphor is an object lesson in the dispassionate observation of reactions. This repertoire will be expanded substantially in subsequent sessions.

THERAPEUTIC DO'S AND DON'TS

ACT with Enthusiasm, Not Zealotry

ACT is a powerful approach with the potential to turn a client's "worldview" upside down. This means that the client needs to be approached with respect, dignity, and a certain caution. Although it is essential to communicate confidence in the client's ability to get unstuck, the client's position must also be appreciated. It is hard to walk away from years of practice with something that doesn't work. The ACT therapist has to model acceptance of "where the client is at." This means to avoid criticizing the client for being stuck, for falling back into old traps, and so on. The objective is to create a win-win situation for the client, not to make the therapist "right" and the client "wrong."

All client relapses back into control strategies are opportunities to observe both the strength and the persistence of those repertoires (What are the numbers?) and to notice the shift in level of distress as they move between willingness and struggle. If a client insists on rejoining an old strategy, the therapist should be supportive of the client's doing that, the only proviso being that the client is encouraged to notice the ebb and flow of distress as the control agenda resurfaces. The ACT therapist has to be willing to let the world be the way it is. We let the client's own experience be the teacher.

Often, when therapy is proceeding slowly, the therapist is tempted to begin lecturing the client, to point out all the reasons that the client should adopt the new alternative posed by the therapist. This is nearly always indicative of an impasse, and the therapist should seek supervision from other ACT therapists.

Avoid Intellectualizing

A common pitfall is to begin discussing ACT concepts in order to convince the client that the ACT alternative is better than the client's coping strategies. Sessions in which this process is in full gear are easy to identify: The therapist is doing nearly all the talking, and the tone of the interchange ranges from pleading to convincing to coercing or blaming the client. The client is occasionally asked for a response, a statement of agreement or understanding, and regardless of what this response is, the therapist plows forward. The therapist may bounce metaphor after metaphor off the client, then spend a lot of time trying to explain what the metaphors mean. Besides excesses in explanation, lapses into highly technical or theoretical talk are also markers that the therapist is straying from the necessarily experiential core of the work.

Nothing in language is going to convince the client nearly as strongly as the client's own contact with workability through direct experience. This is the direct contingency that will control behavior if the insensitivity produced by rules can be reduced. If mere intellectual and rational persuasion were ever going to work, the client would probably not be seeking therapy in the first place.

Co-opted by Language

A variant on this theme is more insidious and probably more destructive. This phase of ACT allows back into therapy some stable verbal concepts. Control is linked to the client's experience, and a few of the contingencies supporting the improper application of control are described. If this is not done lightly, the therapist may begin to encourage discussions of control strategies within the existing language paradigm. This may involve the therapist's going over the client's early learning history and offering causal explanations of how the client became "stuck" on control (e.g., "Children of alcoholics learn that they have to control the way everyone feels in order to feel safe. Your use of control probably allows you allow to feel safe"). Such "explanations" will undermine ACT, because it begins to recast control as an idiosyncrasy the client has to eliminate, presumably through insight and understanding. Beneath this type of discussion is the same old change agenda: Figure out how you got this internal problem, and then eliminate it.

The Multiproblem Client

The more problems a client has, the more likely it is that control-based strategies will be at the heart of the client's emotional distress and dysfunctional behavior. This means that the multiproblem client will cling more ferociously to control and its manifestations as "core" moves. Our clinical experience is that this phase of therapy goes more slowly with the multiproblem client. Therefore, the therapist needs to patiently and persistently work on the concepts of control, emotional avoidance/

escape, workability, and willingness, without feeling pressured to move into subsequent stages.

A major stumbling block in working with the multiproblem client is trying to push the client beyond where he or she is psychologically ready to go. This usually results in some type of confrontation between the therapist and client over the client's motivation or progress, the therapist's competence, or some other equally unrewarding issue. Therapy with this type of client must include the therapist's relinquishing control in certain areas, while being persistent in staying with the client's experience of the workability of control strategies.

PROGRESS TO THE NEXT STAGE

There are two clear indications that a client may be ready to move into the next stage of ACT. The first is the spontaneous occurrence of willingness moves in situations that used to elicit control moves. The therapist gets a clear sense that the client is more aware of thoughts, feelings, or sensations evoked by an event. The client is showing some evidence of stepping back from the moment and not simply fusing with conditioned responses. This is not usually done perfectly or consistently across situations, but it is clearly present and is experienced as being different by the client.

The second indication is that the client reports a spontaneous example or two of "feeling feelings differently" or of feelings being experienced as less compelling. When the client begins to experience feelings, distressing thoughts, memories, or bodily sensations as less compelling, even when they occur at a high level of intensity, it suggests that the client is beginning to alter the control agenda. For more functional clients, this phase may require only part of a session to perhaps two sessions. Some clients may require more if they are less functional and solidly locked into control types of strategies.

PERSONAL WORK FOR THE CLINICIAN: IS CONTROL THE PROBLEM?

In Chapter 4, you were asked to examine the main problem in your life and the strategies you have used to implement a solution, then to look at those strategies and assess how well they have worked, both in the short run and in the long run. You evaluated these strategies from the viewpoint of "what you tend to do" when facing life problems. In this exercise, you will be asked to look at these strategies more closely. Remember to save your work. It will be used again in the next chapter.

1. Consider each strategy and assess whether it is a "control" strategy or an "acceptance" strategy. You may want to mark each strategy with either a C or an A to make this clearer.
2. Look at the distribution of C's and A's. What does this tell you about your approach to the main problem in your life?
3. Take each C strategy you discovered. What is it that you hoped to control, that is, what is being avoided or what is being eliminated?

CLINICAL VIGNETTE

You are three sessions into working with a 45-year-old man, who has been experiencing severe anxiety attacks, mostly while on the job. He is in a very stressful management position that involves dealing with system change and unhappy workers. He recently moved to the area to live with his woman friend and her 16-year-old daughter. This transition has been difficult, and the relationship has been faltering. Recently, he has experienced anxiety attacks at home. He describes his main coping strategies as deep breathing, distracting himself in work, looking for any physical signs of anxiety, and closing his office door or leaving work early if these signs appear. He is also using a tranquilizer as needed. He states, "This is the only way I can get my anxiety down so I can stay at work." He also says, "I can get calmed down for a while, but for only for 2 or 3 hours before it [the anxiety] starts to come again."

> *Question for the clinician:* How would you conceptualize the client's major coping strategies and their assumed goals? How would you discuss these solutions with the client? What would be your goal (s) in doing so? (Form a reply before reading our answer.)
>
> *Our answer:* It is useful to conceptualize these strategies as control oriented, organized around the necessity of bringing anxiety down, which is another way of saying "keeping anxiety controlled." The client's experience is that these control strategies work in the short run, but in the long run they build his anxiety. Ideally, the therapist would address this paradox in the client's current strategies: They appear to work, but, bottom line, they build anxiety. We might ask him if there are other functions his anxiety might be serving, rather than just being a form of traumatic experience. This may open the door for us to ask, "Are there some things in your life that you legitimately have reason to be anxious about, other than about being anxious?" "Is your

anxiety telling you something that you need to hear?" The ACT goal is to drive a wedge between the man's legitimate anxieties (stressful job, recent move, struggling relationship, uncertain future) and his struggle with anxiety (hypervigilance, avoiding work, drug use).

APPENDIX: CLIENT HOMEWORK

Daily Experiences Diary

To maximize the impact of this set of interventions, a useful homework assignment is to have the client look for a few uncomfortable moments that occur during the week and record impressions as asked for in the Daily Experiences Diary. The therapist should reiterate that this homework is not going to change anything; it is an attempt to gather important information about the scope and content of the client's struggle. The most important part of this assignment is help the client see how each coping strategy used to address an uncomfortable experience did or did not incorporate a control and eliminate philosophy. The therapist should positively reinforce any spontaneous examples of coping strategies that involve simple awareness or acceptance without struggle or evaluation. This is not the same as having it so it will go away. Rather, the therapist is looking for examples in which the client is allowing the experience to occur directly without the ordinary control defenses. If any of these appear, the therapist should make note of the circumstances that were associated with spontaneous acts of acceptance.

Willingness Diary (Suffering/Struggle/Workability Ratings)

In this phase, it is useful to collect willingness measures. The therapist may help the client develop a daily rating form to collect information on the presence of the client's dominant negative experiential states (e.g., anxiety, depression, obsessive worry), willingness (sometimes it helps to call it by its inverse name "struggle," especially early on when willingness will seem to mean "wanting"), and the client's perception of the workability of his or her approach to life during that day.

The client is instructed to sit down at the end of each day and provide a global rating on each dimension for that day. The client is also instructed to make notes about any interesting or unusual experiences that seem connected with higher ratings of willingness/struggle and/or workability or, conversely, observations about processes that seem to heighten negative states and suffering. This is a potentially powerful way of raising the client's level of awareness beyond that of a mere participant (or prisoner) in the "struggle" to that of participant observer. Often the client will quickly notice that struggle is negatively

			DAILY EXPERIENCES DIARY		
Day	What was the experience?	What were your feelings while it was happening?	What were your thoughts while it was happening?	What were your bodily sensations while it was happening?	What did you do to handle your feelings, thoughts, or bodily sensations?
Monday					
Tuesday					
Wednesday					
Thursday					
Friday					
Saturday					
Sunday					

correlated with workability, and positively correlated with suffering or upset. This can become a topic in a later session when the homework is examined.

Identifying Programming Exercise

Between-session assignments can be used to clarify the nature of programmed responses. The Identifying Programming Exercise is often used with clients who have problematic childhood histories to clarify how dysfunctional coping strategies are passed on. The results of the exercise should be discussed as demonstrating how pervasive and arbitrary conditioning is as a form of human learning.

Feeling Good Exercise

The Feeling Good Exercise is useful in having clients appreciate the specific language rules that act as self-instructions in psychologically difficult moments. It

DAILY WILLINGNESS DIARY
At the end of each day, rate the following three dimensions about that day:
Upset—(e.g., Anxiety, Depression, Worry)   1–None to 10–Extreme _____
Struggle—How much effort was put into getting this to go away?   1–None to 10–Extreme _____
Workability—If life were like this day, to what degree would doing what you did today of be part of a vital, workable way of living?   1–Not at all workable to 10–Extremely workable _____
Comments:

(*Note:* If the client's struggles are focused on particular psychological events, modify the form under "Upset" to fit the client's particular issues.)

IDENTIFYING PROGRAMMING EXERCISE

We can't go back and rewrite our past. History, like automatic thoughts and feelings, is a domain that calls for acceptance and not control. Attachment to the programming that we have accumulated through our histories, however, can greatly amplify the relevance of history to the present. For example, if your mother told you that you were bad when you got angry, you most likely are carrying around a bit of programming that is telling you the same thing. The fact that you are carrying this around isn't the problem. It's the fact that we tend to lose perspective and become "fused" with these historical programs. Automatically believing what our programming tells us, we lose identification with our selves as the context in which these historical events have all occurred. The historical nature of these experiences doesn't make them any more "true," or the evaluations we base on them any more "right," than any other kind of experience. They are accumulated content, and like all content, may be useful in some ways and not in others. In order to determine their usefulness, however, it is necessary to gain some perspective on them.

Exercise:

1. Think about a significant emotionally difficult event in your childhood. Write it down.
2. Now see whether you can identify some programming that you are carrying about this event. What did you conclude about the way the world worked? What did you conclude about yourself? Have you formulated any other rules based on this experience? Write down as many of these as you can identify.
3. Repeat with at least one other event.
4. Bring to therapy next time.

FEELING GOOD EXERCISE

Instruction: Listed here are a number of beliefs about negative moments in our lives, for example, feeling bad, having unwanted thoughts or memories, unpleasant physical sensations. For each pair of beliefs, check the one that is closest to how you now address these moments in your life.

_____ 1a. Negative experiences will hurt you if you don't do something to get rid of them.

_____ 1b. Negative experiences can't hurt you, even if they feel bad.

_____ 2a. When negative experiences occur, the goal is to do something to get them under control so they hurt less.

_____ 2b. The attempt to control negative experiences creates problems; the goal is to let them be there, and they will change as a natural part of living.

_____ 3a. The way to handle negative experiences is to understand why I'm having them, then use that knowledge to eliminate them.

_____ 3b. The way to handle negative experiences is to notice they're present without necessarily analyzing and judging them.

_____ 4a. The way to be "healthy" is to learn better and better ways to control and eliminate negative moments.

_____ 4b. The way to be "healthy" is to learn to have negative moments and to live effectively.

_____ 5a. The inability to control or eliminate a negative reaction is a sign of weakness.

_____ 5b. Needing to control a negative experience is a problem.

_____ 6a. The appearance of negative experiences is a clear sign of personal problems.

_____ 6b. The appearance of negative experiences is an inevitable part of being alive.

_____ 7a. People who are in control of their lives are generally able to control how they react and feel.

_____ 7b. People who are in control of their lives need not try to control their reactions or feelings.

can help clients articulate their control-related philosophies, inasmuch as the paired items focus the issue more precisely. The therapist should go through the results and may want to predict that these same rule systems are likely to reappear during the course of therapeutic work.

Rules of the Game Exercise

The Rules of the Game Exercise offers another useful way to have clients appreciate the specific language rules that act as self-instructions in psychologically difficult moments. The client is asked to generate favorite life sayings in each of several life theme areas. These phrases are trite because of their near universal use in the language community. Of special interest are general rules that emphasize overcoming life's difficulties through control strategies or through sheer force of will.

RULES OF THE GAME EXERCISE

Each of us uses certain basic rules about the way "life is" to help guide our functioning. Although these rules are largely arbitrary, we tend to view them as absolute truth. Sayings such as, "No pain, no gain," or "Where there's a will there's a way," have a profound impact on how we view ourselves and life itself.

In this exercise, please take some time to "locate" the most basic rules (perhaps in the form of sayings) with which you operate in each of the content areas listed here.

1. Rules about relationships with other people (e.g., trust, loyalty, competition)

2. Rules about feeling bad inside

3. Rules about overcoming life obstacles

4. Rules about "justice" in life

5. Rules about your relationship with yourself

As the exercise is discussed, the therapist can highlight any number of features of life sayings:

1. How black and white the instruction is (e.g., "Least said, least mended").
2. How severe the consequence for noncompliance is (e.g., "Haste makes waste").
3. How the instruction favors "good content" and discourages "bad content" at the community level (e.g., "Smile and world smiles with you, cry and you cry alone").
4. How undesirable content is laundered to make it desirable (e.g., "You're never happy unless you're unhappy").
5. How undesirable content is to be addressed privately through acts of strength and will (e.g., "The Lord helps those who help themselves").

Clean versus Dirty Discomfort Diary

It is often helpful to have the client work on the practical impact of clean versus dirty discomfort in between sessions. The Clean versus Dirty Discomfort Diary again exposes the client to what has been discussed in session and asks the client to take a "high risk" situation from recent life and practice distinguishing clean from dirty reactions. The client first identifies all the clean discomfort inherent in the situation, then begins to identify secondary consequences associated with using control strategies in that situation. Sometimes, if the client is examining a salient but less emotionally charged situation than that being targeted in therapy, the general distinction is easier to learn. For that reason, it is useful to instruct the client not to focus attention on the same events being discussed in therapy, but another event or situation that has already come and gone.

CLEAN VERSUS DIRTY DISCOMFORT DIARY

Instructions: Each time you run into a situation in which you feel "stuck" or in which you are struggling with your thoughts or feelings, please complete each column here.				
Situation	(Clean stuff) My first reactions	Suffering level	(Dirty stuff) What I did about my reactions	New suffering
What happened to start this?	What immediately "showed up" in the way of thoughts, feelings, memories, or physical sensations?	Rate your immediate distress level on a 1–100 scale (1 = no suffering, 100 = extreme suffering).	Did I struggle with things I didn't like? Did I criticize myself? Did I try to shove my reactions back in, or pretend they weren't there?	Rate your new suffering level on the same 1–100 scale.

•6•

Building Acceptance by Defusing Language

Some things happen that you cannot change;
Some things happen you can rearrange
—CHARLES F. HAYES (age 8)

THEORETICAL FOCUS

There is a distinction between *language* as a learned set of derived stimulus relations and *languaging* as the action of deriving these relations. The distinction, however, is shrouded in language itself. Stimulus functions are stimulus functions, and the process through which they appear are not normally relevant nor salient. Consider the process of transferring stimulus functions through nonverbal means in nonverbal organisms. Pavlov's dogs salivate to anything that reliably predicts the imminent provision of food. This effect does not require that the dog be aware that it is drooling now because of classical conditioning, and there would be no great advantage to the dog for becoming aware. Similarly, the regulatory functions of language that establish its value do not depend on simultaneous awareness of the *process* of language.

There is some evidence that humans at one time were much less aware of language process than they are now. For example, it appears as though it was ordinary in the earliest days of written language for humans to hear their thoughts through their ears (Jaynes, 1976). The ancient concerns about others knowing one's name, the prohibition against saying the name of God, and so on, also appear to be related to

148

the relatively more automatic behavior regulatory functions of language in ancient times—as if knowing someone's name would give one special power over that person.

If the distinction between process and product is hard to detect in written and spoken language, it is virtually undetectable without special effort when it is applied to private verbal events such as thinking, feeling, and remembering. Humans spend a great deal of time living in the world structured by derived stimulus relations and little time simply noticing the process. We spend much more time *in* or looking *from* our thoughts than we do simply observing our thoughts. The mystical religious traditions probably constituted the first well-developed effort to loosen the effects of verbal products over human behavior. In our opinion, psychotherapy systems have been too willing to tamper with verbal products and not willing enough to focus on verbal processes per se.

When the derived functions of language dominate, humans fuse with the psychological contents of verbal events. The distinction between thinking and the referent of thought is diminished. As an end result, certain thoughts or feelings (particularly those with provocative or pejorative meanings) become connected to powerful and predictable behavior patterns. The client comes to see his or her verbal constructions of life as a virtual substitute for tangible life itself. For the anxiety-disordered client, for example, *anxiety* almost ceases to be a mere word, so completely has it become part of a set of physiological, emotional, and cognitive events. The word *anxiety* takes on a literal meaning, and the very reading or thinking of the word can bring into the client's immediate experience the entire spectrum of negatively perceived events with which it is related. Through the power of language, *anxiety,* the word, becomes anxiety, the fact.

This failure to make the moment-by-moment distinction between verbal products and verbal processes spreads to a failure to make distinctions between different kinds of verbal activities. Evaluations are treated as distinctions, for example, and a client thinking "My life is terrible" will take "terrible" to be a description of a primary attribute equivalent to "This chair is blue, this window is clear, and this life is terrible." Unlike blue and clear, "terrible" is a secondary attribute—a quality of the person's affective and evaluative response to an event, not a quality of the event. The person may then act as if he or she is actually in a terrible life, not like a person who has just had the thought "My life is terrible," which is what was actually experienced.

As we will discuss in the next chapter, this same process can make it hard for the person to develop a sense of self that is distinct from the literal content of verbal behavior. Humans apply language to self-recognition and definition processes as well, and derive many descriptive attributes: kind, insecure, intelligent, anxious, and so on. In an important sense, self-identity becomes synonymous with the language of self-conceptualization. In this ultimate form of fusion, the person is "poured together" with the product of language in such a way that the very presence of language operations is masked in the system itself. Both the present chapter and the next discuss this important problem with "literality" or verbal fusion.

There is the usual inherent paradox in attempting to weaken the hegemony of literal meaning. Language cannot be weakened merely by describing the problem, because that very description depends on literal meaning for its impact. ACT attempts, instead, to weaken the excessive grip of literal meaning through the use of *deliteralization* (or, synonymously, cognitive defusion). The essence of the ACT deliteralization strategies is to prey on certain loopholes in the way language functions, to teach the client to see thoughts and feelings for what they are (i.e., a verbally entangled process of minding) rather than what they advertise themselves to be (e.g., the world understood; structured reality). The therapist must, with words, change how words function for the client. The therapist must fight fire with fire—and still keep from being burned. This is the inherent paradox that is at the core of almost every aspect of ACT.

Deliteralization involves establishing contexts in which the distinction between derived and direct stimulus functions is more experientially evident, and in which verbal stimuli have multiple effects, only some of which are derived. The actual process of languaging and thought is experienced as it happens. As a result, additional stimulus functions are available as a basis for action because verbal products are no longer experienced solely as rules that order the world. A thought is understood, but it is also heard as a sound, seen as a habit, or dispassionately observed as an automatic verbal relation. Whether a thought (or any other verbal activity) occasions action is best determined by the workability of that action in a given context, not merely by the literal force or coherence of the thought itself. This is the essence of the distinction between contextual treatments such as ACT and more mechanistically based behavior therapies. This chapter will demonstrate how ACT can help loosen equivalence classes (or derived stimulus relations, more generally) and thus help direct stimulus functions to compete with those that are derived.

CLINICAL FOCUS

In this phase of ACT, the therapist focuses on the following issues:

- How the fusion of self, referents, and language processes creates suffering and makes willingness impossible

- The role of literality in creating cognitive fusion
- The limitations of language in developing an understanding of self or personal history
- How evaluative language processes interfere with our capacity to experience directly
- How the language community reinforces troublesome language processes such as reason giving, emotional control, and literal self-narrative
- Learning verbal conventions that separate thought and thinker, emotion and feeler
- Removing barriers to willingness by learning to see private experiences for what they are, not what they advertise themselves to be

A summary of key goals, strategies, and specific interventions used to achieve these goals is presented in Table 6.1.

ATTACKING THE ARROGANCE OF WORDS

ACT begins to attack the client's confidence in language by demonstrating its limits. Language is the one tool in the human toolbox that purports to be good for all jobs. The fact is that language has a very limited capacity to apprehend and decipher personal experience, but we are taught from the moment of first consciousness that language is the tool for developing self-understanding. There are many exercises that experientially reveal the limitations of private verbal ("mental") behavior. Prior to initiating them, it is helpful to discuss the issue of minding with the client in a way that creates a new frame for these experiences. The *Your Mind Is Not Your Friend Intervention* helps highlight the problem of self-referential language and thought.

> You've probably guessed by now that I'm not a big fan of minds. Its not that I don't think minds are useful, it's just that you can't really live your life effectively between your ears. I'm pretty sure minds evolved to give us a more elaborate way of detecting threats to our survival, and they probably helped organize packs of prehumans in ways that led to less killing, stealing, incest, and so forth. One thing minds didn't evolve for was to help prehumans feel good about themselves. You know, its kind of hard to imagine them sitting around a fire, contemplating their belly buttons, hugging and bonding. And if you look at recent studies of natural thought processes, what you consistently see is that a large percentage of all mental content is negative in some way. We have minds that are built to produce negative content in

TABLE 6.1. ACT Goals, Strategies, and Interventions Regarding Deliteralization

Goals	Strategies	Interventions
1. Teach limits of language in apprehending direct experience.	Show client how language lags behind experience. Distinguish representation from function in language.	Your Mind Is Not Your Friend Intervention Explain motor actions Finding a Place to Sit Metaphor
2. Undermine fusion of self and language.	Interfere with the function of problematic language sequences. Teach strategies for cognitive defusion.	Milk, Milk, Milk Exercise Passengers on the Bus Metapor Soldiers in the Parade Exercise Taking Your Mind for a Walk Exercise
3. Undermine evaluation and automatic rule-governed functions of language.	Undermine confidence in reason giving. Alter deceptive verbal conventions. Create understanding of evaluation versus description in language.	Reasons as causes, discussion and homework And/Be Out Convention Bad Cup Metaphor Cubby holing
4. Teach healthy distancing and nonjudgmental awareness.	Promote willingness skills as alternative to struggle.	Tin Can Monster Exercise Physicalizing Exercise Contents on Cards Exercises Practicing Awareness of Your Experience

the name of warning us or keeping us in line with the pack. We will have to address this paradox: Your mind is not your friend, *and* you can't do without it.

The importance of being knowledgeable and right are powerfully and frequently reinforced within human culture. The arbitrariness of human language means that once it is learned, it becomes relatively independent of immediate environmental support. The combination of these two factors leads to the indiscriminate use of language, often without the client's even being aware of it. The *Finding a Place to Sit Metaphor* helps make this point experientially.

THERAPIST: It is as if you needed a place to sit, and so you began describing a chair. Let's say you gave a really detailed description of a chair. It's a grey chair, and it has a metal frame, and it's covered in fabric, and it's a very sturdy chair. OK. Now can you sit in that description?

CLIENT: Well, no.

THERAPIST: Hmmm. Maybe the description wasn't detailed enough. What if I were able to describe the chair all the way down to the atomic level. Then could you sit in the description?

CLIENT: No.

THERAPIST: Here's the thing, and check your own experience: Hasn't your mind been telling you things like "The world is this way, and that way and your problem is this and that, et cetera"? Describe, describe. Evaluate, evaluate, evaluate. And all the while you're getting tired. You need a place to sit. And your mind keeps handing you ever more elaborate descriptions of chairs. Then it says to you, "Have a seat." Descriptions are fine, but what we are looking for here is an experience, not a description of an experience. Minds can't deliver experience, they only blab to us about our experience elsewhere. So we'll let your mind describe away, and in the meantime you and I will look for a place to sit.

Another useful strategy is to appeal to the client's own experience in areas in which words are not only insufficient but even detrimental. Some tasks are very well regulated by rules, such as finding one's way to the grocery store—go to the first stoplight, turn left, and so forth. However, for some other activities this is not at all helpful. Suppose we had a perfect description of swimming. We could describe its mechanics, even the feel of the water moving over the skin, but we would not then know how to swim. The only way to learn to swim is to get in the water.

This awareness can be built on experientially by asking the client to explain motor actions during therapy. For example, if the client picks up a pen, the therapist can ask for an explanation of how this is done. When the explanation is given (e.g., "Reach for it with your hand"), the therapist can see whether this works by telling his or her own hand to reach. Of course, the hand will not hear and will not reach. The behavior was nonverbal first and only later became verbally governed. Yet language itself claims to know how to do virtually everything, from reaching for a pen to developing a relationship. Verbal knowing rests atop nonverbal knowing so completely that an illusion is created that all knowledge is verbal knowledge. If we suddenly had all nonverbal knowledge removed from our repertoires, we would fall to the floor quite helpless.

DELITERALIZING LANGUAGE

Having made an initial assault on the limits of language as a stand-in for actual experience, the therapist has to provide the client with the experience of making contact with language stripped of its symbolic functions. The following *Milk, Milk, Milk Exercise* was first used by Titchener (1916, p. 425) to try to explain his context theory of meaning. It is a playful way to demonstrate that a literal, sequential, analytical context is required for language stimuli to have any literal (i.e., derived) meaning.

THERAPIST: Let's do a little exercise. It's an eyes-open one. I'm going to ask you to say a word. Then you tell me what comes to mind. I want you to say the word "milk." Say it once.

CLIENT: Milk.

THERAPIST: Good. Now what came to mind when you said that?

CLIENT: I have milk at home in the refrigerator.

THERAPIST: OK. What else? What shows up when we say "milk"?

CLIENT: I picture it—white, a glass.

THERAPIST: Good. What else?

CLIENT: I can taste it, sort of.

THERAPIST: Exactly. And can you feel what it might feel like to drink a glass? Cold. Creamy. Coats your mouth. Goes "glug, glug" as you drink it. Right?

CLIENT: Sure.

THERAPIST: OK, so let's see if this fits. What shot through your mind were things about actual milk and your experience with it. All that happened is that we made a strange sound—*milk*—and lots of these things showed up. Notice that there isn't any milk in this room. None at all. But milk was in the room psychologically. You and I were seeing it, tasting it, feeling it—yet only the word was actually here. Now, here is the exercise, if you're willing to try it. The exercise is a little silly, so you might feel a little embarrassed doing it, but I am going to do the exercise with you so we can be silly together. What I am going to ask you to do is to say the word "milk," out loud, rapidly, over and over again, and then notice what happens. Are you willing to try it?

CLIENT: I guess so.

THERAPIST: OK. Let's do it. Say "milk" over and over again. (*Therapist and client say the word for 1 to 2 minutes, with the therapist periodically encouraging the client to keep it going, to keep saying it out loud, or to go faster.*)

THERAPIST: OK, now stop. Where is the milk?

CLIENT: Gone (*laughs*).

THERAPIST: Did you notice what happened to the psychological aspects of milk that were here a few minutes ago?

CLIENT: After about 40 times they disappeared. All I could hear was the sound. It sounded very strange—in fact, I had a funny feeling that I didn't even know what word I was saying for a few moments. It sounded more like a bird sound than a word.

THERAPIST: Right. The creamy, cold, gluggy stuff just goes away. The first time you said it, it was as if milk were actually here, in the room. But all that really happened was that you said a word. The first time you said it, it was really meaningful, it was almost solid. But when you said it again and again and again, you began to lose that meaning and the words began to be just a sound.

CLIENT: That's what happened.

THERAPIST: Well, when you say things to yourself, in addition to any meaning sustained by the relation between those words and other things, isn't it also true that these words are just words? The words are just smoke. There isn't anything solid in them.

This exercise demonstrates quite quickly that although literal meaning dominates in language, it is not hard to establish contexts in which literal meaning quickly weakens and almost disappears. To many "milk" is a very odd sound, considered (as it almost never is) simply as a sound. It has a funny quality to it, reminding people of sounds made by birds or other animals. These direct properties are so glossed over by its functional symbolic properties, that it is often a revelation to hear—just to hear—"milk," perhaps for the first time since early childhood. This does not mean that milk has lost its literal meaning. Clients still have milk and the mammary secretions of cows in an equivalence class, though it may have loosened somewhat. What has happened is that the transfer of stimulus functions through that equivalence class has been greatly weakened.

A client who is struggling with a particular negative thought can be asked to do this exercise with the thought. It is a bit harder to get the effect with a complete sentence, but it can be done, especially if the thought can be put into a few words. For example, shorten a negative self-description to "I'm bad." This sentence can then be stated as rapidly as possible over and over for a couple of minutes until its meaning dissolves. Once this is experienced, the thought now has two functions: It is referential and evaluative, and it is also just a string of auditory events. The ACT therapist can ask the client to practice actually experiencing "I'm bad" as a string of sounds, in addition to whatever literal meaning it has.

The direct stimulus effects of language are not just auditory. Saying a word requires muscle movement and breathing, for example. The same kind of repeated word exercise can be done with the instruction to notice how one's mouth feels, or what one's diaphragm does while speaking the word. With some practice, it is possible to generalize this effect even to spontaneous speech? As we speak, we can also hear the sound, feel the mouth movements, notice the breathing, observe the eye movements, and so on. This sense is initially easier to learn if the speech is slowed deliberately, but with practice it is possible to be simultaneously aware of the literal content of speech, its natural sound, and the odd muscle movements necessary to produce that sound. It is an eerie feeling to do this during normal therapy interactions, because it instantly reveals the humanness and extended behavioral nature of the interactive process (and instantly places therapist and client on the same plane).

Learning to see the direct stimulus functions of symbols does not eliminate their derived functions, of course, nor would we want them to do so. But they *add* to the derived functions and make it easier for us to observe the *process* of language without fusing entirely with its derived stimulus products. We do not readily fuse with the pure sound, mouth movements, or breathing that are actually here when we say "milk." We do readily fuse with the creamy, cold, gluggy white stuff that is not here. That is the grand illusion, the great shroud that covers human language. Other therapy traditions try to get the client to be properly skeptical about the literal truth of derived stimulus relations (i.e., seeing and challenging irrational thoughts). ACT goes after the grand illusion itself and attempts to pull the shroud to one side often enough that its nature is evident.

Objectifying Language That Pushes Us Around

Another way to defuse or deliteralize language is to objectify it. We have a great deal of experience in dealing with objects in our environment.

The natural distance between person and object often disappears when the things we are struggling with are verbal and, thus, derived. By creating metaphors in which these verbal events are themselves objects, it is easier to use common sense in dealing with our problems.

The *Passengers on the Bus Metaphor* is a core ACT intervention aimed at deliteralizing provocative psychological content through objectification.

Suppose there is a bus and you're the driver. On this bus we've got a bunch of passengers. The passengers are thoughts, feelings, bodily states, memories, and other aspects of experience. Some of them are scary, and they're dressed up in black leather jackets and they have switchblade knives. What happens is that you're driving along and the passengers start threatening you, telling you what you have to do, where you have to go. "You've got to turn left," "You've got to go right," and so on. The threat they have over you is that if you don't do what they say, they're going to come up front from the back of the bus.

It's as if you've made deals with these passengers, and the deal is, "You sit in the back of the bus and scrunch down so that I can't see you very often, and I'll do what you say pretty much." Now, what if one day you get tired of that and say, "I don't like this! I'm going to throw those people off the bus!" You stop the bus, and you go back to deal with the mean-looking passengers. But you notice that the very first thing you had to do was stop. Notice now, you're not driving anywhere, you're just dealing with these passengers. And they're very strong. They don't intend to leave, and you wrestle with them, but it just doesn't turn out very successfully.

Eventually, you go back to placating the passengers, trying to get them to sit way in the back again where you can't see them. The problem with this deal is that you do what they ask in exchange for getting them out of your life. Pretty soon they don't even have to tell you, "Turn left"—you know as soon as you get near a left turn that the passengers are going to crawl all over you. In time you may get good enough that you can almost pretend that they're not on the bus at all. You just tell yourself that left is the only direction you want to turn. However, when they eventually do show up, it's with the added power of the deals that you've made with them in the past.

Now the trick about the whole thing is that the power the passengers have over you is 100% based on this: "If you don't do what we say, we're coming up and we're making you look at us." That's it. It's true that when they come up front they look as if they could do a whole lot more. They have knives, chains, and so forth. It looks as though you could be destroyed. The deal you make is to do what they say so they won't come up and stand next to you and make you look at them. The driver (you) has control of the bus, but you trade off the control in these secret deals with the passengers. In other words, by trying to get control, you've actually given up control! Now notice that even though your passengers claim they can destroy you if you don't turn left, it has never actually happened. These passengers can't make you do something against your will.

The therapist can continue to allude to the bus metaphor throughout deliteralization work. Questions such as, "Which passenger is threatening you now?" can help reorient the client who is practicing emotional avoidance in session.

The bus metaphor casts the relationship between a person and thoughts or feelings the way one might cast a social relationship between a person and bullies. This reframe is useful as a motivative augmental in seeking freedom from literal language. Some of our past efforts to gain social independence can be used to stimulate a similar independence from the hegemony of our own verbal systems: our own minds. However limited our social independence is, independence from our minds is usually much less. This makes sense in another way inasmuch as the source of verbal relations, after all, is dominantly social and external in any case (What are the numbers?). The bus metaphor also nicely structures how the illusion of language works and what the cost is in terms of loss of life direction.

Don't Buy Thoughts

The shift from looking at the world *through* literal meaning to a deliteralized look *at* literal meaning is a subtle one. In ACT, a common phrase for literality is "buying a thought," which is distinguished carefully from "having a thought." The use of the word *buying* again turns attention from products of verbal relations to the verbal actions themselves. The problem is not in the content of private events; verbal relations are arbitrarily applicable, and in some sense everything is related to everything, verbally speaking. Rather, the problem is that the client is operating as if the stimulus functions that result are direct. The client buys representations of the world, to such an extent that the process of thinking is itself hidden behind the content of thinking.

Various meditative and "mindfulness" exercises are useful in distinguishing thinking as a process from the stimulus products of thought. The *Soldiers in the Parade Exercise* was invented by the same client who invented the *Tug-of-War with a Monster Metaphor* described in Chapter

4. She used it as a meditative exercise, and many ACT therapists ask clients to do it as homework in that same fashion. The exercise helps distinguish between thoughts observed as thoughts and thoughts bought as beliefs or concepts.

THERAPIST: I'd like us to do an exercise to show how quickly thoughts pull us away from experience when we buy them. All I'm going to ask you to do is to think whatever thoughts you think and to allow them to flow, one thought after another. The purpose of the exercise is to notice when there's a shift from looking *at* your thoughts, to looking *from* your thoughts. You will know that has happened when the parade stops, or you are down in the parade, or the exercise has disappeared.

   I'm going to ask you to imagine that there are little people, soldiers, marching out of your left ear down in front of you in a parade. You are up on the reviewing stand, watching the parade go by. Each soldier is carrying a sign, and each thought you have is a sentence written on one of these signs. Some people have a hard time putting thoughts into words, and they see thoughts as images. If that applies to you, put each image on a sign being carried by a soldier. Certain people don't like the image of soldiers, and there is an alternative image I have used in that case: leaves floating by in a stream. You can pick the one that seems best.

CLIENT: The soldiers seem fine.

THERAPIST: OK. In a minute I am going to ask you to get centered and begin to let your thoughts go by written on placards carried by the soldiers. Now here is the task. The task is simply to watch the parade go by without having it stop and without your jumping down into the parade. You are just supposed to let it flow. It is very unlikely, however, that you will be able to do this without interruption. And this is the key part of this exercise. At some point you will have the sense that the parade has stopped, or that you have lost the point of the exercise, or that you are down in the parade instead of being on the reviewing stand. When that happens, I would like you to back up a few seconds and see whether you can catch what you were doing right before the parade stopped. Then go ahead and put your thoughts on the placards again, until the parade stops a second time, and so on. The main thing is to notice when it stops for any reason and see whether you can catch what happened right before it stopped. OK?

CLIENT: OK.

THERAPIST: One more thing. If the parade never gets going at all and you start thinking, "It's not working" or "I'm not doing it right," then let that thought be written on a placard and send it down into the parade. OK. Now let's get comfortable, close your eyes, and get centered. [Help the client relax for 1 or 2 minutes.] Now allow the parade to begin. You stay up on the reviewing stand and let the parade flow. If it stops or you find yourself in it, note that; see whether you can notice what you were doing right before that happened, get back up on the reviewing stand, and let the parade begin to flow again. OK, let's begin. . . . Whatever you think, just put it on the cards. [For about 2 to 3 minutes, allow the client to work. Don't underdo it time-wise, and use very few words. Try to read the client reaction and other cues, and add a very few comments, as needed such as, "Just let it flow and notice when it stops." Don't dialogue with the client, however. If the client opens his or her eyes, calmly ask that they be closed and the exercise be continued. If the client starts to talk, gently suggest that even that thought be put on a placard, saying something like, "We will talk more about this when the exercise is finished, but for now there is no need to talk with me. Whatever you think you want to say, let that thought be written down and let it march by too."]. OK, now we will let the last few soldiers go by, and we will begin to think about coming back to this room. [Help the client reorient for 1 or 2 minutes.] Welcome back.

CLIENT: Interesting.

THERAPIST: What did you observe?

CLIENT: Well, at first it was easy. I was watching them go by. Then I suddenly noticed that I was lost and had been for about 15 seconds.

THERAPIST: As if you were off the reviewing stand entirely?

CLIENT: Right. The whole exercise had stopped.

THERAPIST: Did you notice what had been happening right before everything stopped?

CLIENT: Well, I was thinking thoughts about how my body was feeling, and these were being written on the cards. And then I started thinking about my work situation and the meeting with the boss I have Friday. I was thinking about how I might be anxious telling him some of the negative things that have been going on, and next thing you know it's a while later and I'm still thinking about it.

THERAPIST: So when the thought first showed up "I'm going to be meeting with the boss next Friday," was that thought written on a placard?

CLIENT: At first it was, for a split second. Then it wasn't.

THERAPIST: Where was it instead?

CLIENT: Nowhere in particular. I was just thinking it.

THERAPIST: Or it was just thinking you. Can we say it that way? At some point you had a thought that hooked you. You bought it and started looking *at* the world *from* that thought. You let it structure the world. So you started actually working out what might happen, what you will do, and so on, and at that point the parade has absolutely stopped. There is now no perspective on it—you can't even see the thought clearly. Instead you are dealing with the meeting with the boss.

CLIENT: It was like that. It was.

THERAPIST: Did you get that thought back on the placard?

CLIENT: Well, at some point I remembered I was supposed to let the thoughts flow, so I wrote the thought out and let a soldier carry it by. Then things went OK for a while, until I started thinking that this whole exercise is kind of silly.

THERAPIST: And did you just notice that thought, or did it think you?

CLIENT: I bought it, I guess.

THERAPIST: What happened to the parade?

CLIENT: It stopped.

THERAPIST: Right. And check and see whether this isn't so. Every time the parade stopped, it was because you bought a thought.

CLIENT: It fits.

THERAPIST: I haven't met anyone who can let the parade go by 100% of the time. That is not realistic. The point is just to get a feel for what it is like to be hooked by your thoughts and what it is like to step back once you're hooked.

It is useful to encourage clients to engage in awareness exercises that can help them practice observing the contents of consciousness. Several exercises that emphasize the noticing of conscious content, rather than struggling with the contents, involve writing the contents on cards and having clients do various things with the cards.

As progress continues in this phase, the client comes to realize that human minds emit a more or less constant stream of evaluative "chatter." Because sense making is so powerfully useful, this verbal repertoire

CONTENTS ON CARDS EXERCISES

It is useful to encourage the client to engage in awareness exercises that can support practice in observing the contents of consciousness. Cards are used to represent disturbing cognitive content. The use of a physical object takes advantage of the natural distance between objects and the people observing them.

Initially, take a stack of 3″ by 5″ cards and write on them the various thoughts or emotions with which the client is struggling. For example, a card might have written on it, "I'm going to have a panic attack if I go to the store," or "I'll never be able to quit drinking," or "I can't stand this loneliness." Several key thoughts can be written on different cards. Then tell the client that the task is to make 100% certain that none of these cards touch his or her lap. Then flip several of the cards toward the client, one at a time, while the client attempts to deflect them away. Next, ask the client to let the cards land wherever they will and merely to watch them as they do. Flip several more cards, one at a time, landing each on the client's lap. The contrast in effort between just noticing the cards as they land, versus batting them away, makes the underlying point. Once the cards have been used this way, you need not actually write each thought on a card; the client can simply be told, "OK, here comes the thought that . . . [describe the content]."

Other exercises with the cards may be helpful, depending on what sort of struggles the client is having with avoided thoughts. For example, a particularly disturbing thought can be written on a card. Hold the card on the palm of your hand and ask the client to push against the card. Tell the client to hold the thought away, then push the card toward the client. After a few seconds, ask the client how much effort this takes. Then hand the card to the client, ask him or her to hold it, and then to notice the difference in effort. Ask the client to notice that in both instances he or she is equally in contact with the card. This provides a physical metaphor, showing how avoidance increases effort without delivering on the promise of reducing contact.

Yet another card exercise has the client carry several cards with disturbing thoughts on them in a pocket. Sometimes this is combined with a walk outside, with the client choosing where to go while also periodically being given difficult cards to carry by the therapist. Again, this physical metaphor shows that negative content can be carried even while the client is engaging in other purposeful, constructive behavior.

has all the environmental support it needs in most circumstances. The ACT therapist objectifies this repertoire, using the language of the mind. Treating the mind almost as if it were a separate entity is a very powerful deliteralization strategy. It helps the person create some healthy distance between the thinker and the thought.

The *Taking Your Mind for a Walk Exercise* can provide a powerful experience of how busy and evaluative minds can be. In the exercise, the therapist goes for a walk with the client, all the while engaging in the sort of evaluative, second-guessing chatter that the client gets from his or

TAKING YOUR MIND FOR A WALK EXERCISE

Before we start today, it important for us to identify everyone who is in the room. By my count, there are four of us: Me, You, Your Mind, and My Mind. Let's just set out to notice how our minds get in the way of our connecting, of being present with each other. When you notice your mind getting in the way, just mention that it's getting in the way. I'll do the same. Let's see how much time we spend fending off our minds. To do this, I want us to do a little exercise. One of us will be a Person, the other will be that person's Mind. We are going outside for a walk, using a special set of rules: The Person may go where he or she chooses; the Mind must follow. The Mind must communicate nearly constantly about anything and everything: describe, analyze, encourage, evaluate, compare, predict, summarize, warn, cajole, criticize, and so on. The Person cannot communicate with the Mind. If the Person tries to talk to the Mind, the Mind should intervene. The Mind must monitor this carefully and stop the Person from minding the Mind if the rule is violated (by saying, "Never mind your Mind!"). The Person should listen to the Mind without minding back and go wherever the Person chooses to go. After at least 5 minutes, and the Mind will monitor this, we will switch roles. The Person becomes the Mind, and the Mind becomes the Person The same rules will apply for another 5 minutes. Then we will split up and walk quietly and individually for 5 minutes, noticing that each of us is still taking a mind for a walk—it is just the familiar Mind that is inside your head. Follow the same rules as before during these 5 minutes: dispassionately let the Mind describe, analyze, encourage, evaluate, compare, predict, summarize, warn, cajole, point out, and so on, without minding back.

her mind on a daily basis. Having all of the client's "mindstuff" come from an external source can precipitate some defusion and allow the client to become aware of the mind's tendency to chatter, often in quite unhelpful ways.

UNDERMINING REASONS AS CAUSES

Thus far we have discussed ACT deliteralization strategies that can be used in a fairly general way. We now turn to strategies for attacking a particularly burdensome class of thoughts: reason giving. Clients often come to a session with elaborate descriptions of things that happened in their lives that have left them somehow broken and unable to move forward. It is helpful to sensitize the client to the pernicious effect of verbal reason giving. It is one thing to deliteralize single words; it is another entirely to step back from well-worn and treasured verbal formulations. This is particularly important for clients who continually use insight into, and understanding of, past history in ways that are self-defeating.

During sessions, clients often lapse into trying to explain the cause of their problems or begin citing personal history as a reason that things can't change. The therapist can undermine this behavior by focusing attention on its functional utility rather than its literal truth. It can be helpful to ask questions like these:

- "And what is that story in the service of?"
- "And does that description of your past help you move ahead?"
- "Is this helpful, or is this what your mind does to you?"
- "Are you proposing a solution, or is this just your way of digging?"
- "Have you said these kinds of things to yourself or to others before? Is this old?"
- "If you've said this before, what do you think will be different now if you say them again?"
- "If God told you that your explanation is 100% correct, how would this help you?"
- "OK, let's all have a vote and vote that you are correct. Now what?"

Often, the client may think up particular explanations for emotional discomfort and disturbing thoughts that may lead to the misinterpretation of internal experiences or external events that are occurring. For example, when we externalize our explanations, we may miss the role of private events such as fear or anger. When we internalize, we may miss the importance of environmental contexts. The following transcript demonstrates how the ACT therapist uses various interventions to undermine the client's confidence in reasons. The dialogue involves a client who is struggling with urges to relapse into drug use.

THERAPIST: So let's do an exercise. Tell me why you used [drugs] last Tuesday.

CLIENT: (*pause*) Well, I was mad about that stuff that happened at work.

THERAPIST: Why else?

CLIENT: Well, I don't know, I suppose I don't have any support group. You know, to talk about this stuff.

THERAPIST: OK, why else? I mean, those sound like really true reasons. Could you give me some fake reasons?

CLIENT: What do you mean?

THERAPIST: You know, make some up. What reasons could you make up?

CLIENT: Someone forced me to do it?

THERAPIST: Why else?

CLIENT: I accidentally took the pills thinking they were aspirin.

THERAPIST: OK. Can you imagine anyone giving these reasons?

CLIENT: Sure.

THERAPIST: Probably several of them in combination. And if you asked several people, Mom, Dad, you know, you'd get a whole list of reasons. And some might even contradict one another. Hmmm. Something is suspicious here, if the reasons are actually causing you to do things.

CLIENT: What do you mean?

THERAPIST: Well, what about the reasons you just used?

CLIENT: Because of work you mean?

THERAPIST: Sure. Right. But has anything bad ever happened at work like that when you didn't use?

CLIENT: Well, yeah.

THERAPIST: But if the reason caused it, why didn't you use then?

CLIENT: Well, there were other reasons not to use.

THERAPIST: And they were somehow stronger than the other reasons, right? But here's the suspicious part: What if I asked whether there were reasons not to use last Tuesday. Could you think of any?

CLIENT: Sure, I mean, of course.

THERAPIST: For instance, if we did that exercise again, you know, good reasons, bad reasons, Mom's reasons, Dad's, smart reasons, goofy reasons, you know; well, could you have given equally long lists for each perspective?

CLIENT: Mmm, well, it might take a while.

THERAPIST: Say we tried it right now. Could you tell me a reason to use? Sure you could, and if I asked for a reason not to, you could come up with that too. And do you suppose that for any reason to use, you couldn't also come up with a reason not to?

CLIENT: Well, sure.

THERAPIST: And I'll bet you've done that too. Sat and thought of lists of reasons why to and not to—and then you either used or you didn't. And where did all the reasons on the opposite side go once you picked a direction? What if it's the case that we just have this infinite storehouse of reasons that we can draw on for whatever we do? Could it be? And could it be that although these things go together a lot, doing and giving reasons for doing, that one doesn't really cause the other? My guess is that you have been trying to generate enough reasons, really good ones, in order to cause yourself to not use. Isn't it really true that you've got some really powerful reasons to stop using? Why else would you be doing this excruciating therapy? You have great reasons. Could you imagine any stronger reasons than getting your kids back?

CLIENT: Well, no.

THERAPIST: So isn't this suspicious? You've believed that you do this and that for *x* and *y* reasons. But here we have just uncovered two pieces of evidence that this isn't how it works. One is that we seem to have an unlimited supply of reasons and, two, you've already got about the most powerful reasons imaginable. Later we'll talk about an alternative, but for now it's important to just notice.

The point in attacking reason giving is not to do away with reasons. Our clients will always have them, and sometimes they are useful. The point is to see them merely as more private content that should be attended to or followed only if it works to do so.

DISRUPTING TROUBLESOME
LANGUAGE PRACTICES

A number of verbal conventions are adopted in ACT that are designed to disrupt well-formed language practices and to simultaneously create some distance between the client and the contents of the client's mind. These verbal conventions replace common ways of speaking that foster problems of various sorts.

A major target of the assault on normal verbal conventions is the client's use of the word *but*. *But* is commonly used to specify exceptions, carrying with it an implicit statement about the organization of psychological events. Consider the statement "I want to go, but I am anxious." This simple statement carries a deep message about the role of feelings in human action. Considered literally, the statement points to a conflict. Two things are present: wanting to go and anxiety. Furthermore, although wanting to go would normally lead to going, anxiety contradicts this effect of wanting to go. Going cannot occur with anxiety.

The etymology of the word *but* reveals this dynamic quite clearly.

The *Oxford English Dictionary* reveals that the word is from the Old English *be-útan* meaning "on the outside, without." In Middle English this became *bouten* and was gradually phonetically weakened to *bŭten, bŭte,* and thus *but.* The Old English word *be-útan* is itself a combination of *be*—meaning something like the modern word *be*—and *útan,* which is a form of *út*—an early form of our modern word *out.* Etymology in this case reveals the dynamic involved quite clearly: *but* literally means "be - out." It is a call for whatever follows the word to go away or else threaten whatever preceded the word. It says that two reactions that do coexist cannot coexist and still be associated with effective action. One or the other must go. The difficulty we experience with clients who have finely tuned "yes, but" language responses nicely demonstrates how paralyzing this posture can be. In ACT, "but" is attacked directly. The therapist should introduce a verbal convention that involves substituting the word *and* for the word *but.*

AND/BE OUT CONVENTION

There is another little verbal convention I'd like us to adopt here. This is one that we can use throughout our work together. It has to do with our use of the word *but.* This is a word that draws us into the struggle with our thoughts and feelings, because it pits one set of thoughts and feelings against another. *But* literally means that what follows the word contradicts what went before the word. It originally came from the words "be out." When we use it we often say, in effect, "This private event *be out* that private event." It's literally a call to fight, so it is no wonder that it pulls us into the war zone. Let's consider some examples. Here is one: "I love my husband, but I get so angry at him." Here is another: "I want to go, but I am too anxious." Notice that although both say "This *be out* that," what the person actually experiences in both cases is two things: this and that. The "be out" part isn't a description of what happened—it is a proscription about how private events should go together. This proscription, however, is exactly what we are trying to back out of. No one experienced that two private events have to be resolved; instead, two private events were experienced. If the word *but* is replaced by the word *and,* it is almost always much more honest. So in our examples, it is much more honest and direct to say, "I love my husband, and I get angry at him," or to say "I want to go, and I am anxious." So the little convention I'd like us to adopt is to say "and" instead of "but" when we talk. If you try it, you'll see that almost always "and" is more true to your experience. "I want to go, and I am anxious." Both things are true, the wanting to go and the feeling of anxiety. Calling attention to what we're saying with the use of this convention will help make you more sensitive to one of the ways that people get pulled into the struggle with their thoughts and feelings. If you really must say the word *but* at some point, then at least we should say it in a way that emphasizes what we are doing. The original form does this well, so if we really have to say "but," we will say it as "be out."

This is a convention that greatly opens up the verbal and psychological perspective within which clients and therapists can work. *And* is a descriptive, not a proscriptive, term and thus can be associated with many courses of action. All possibilities are open. It is safe for the client to notice and report even the most undesirable reactions inasmuch as there is no need for desired reactions to somehow vanquish them. "I love my husband, *but* I get so angry with him" can make anger a very dangerous feeling for someone committed to a marriage. "I love my husband, *and* I get angry with him" carries little such threat and, in fact, implies an acceptance of the experience of anger within the experience of love. "And" is also more experientially true because many thoughts and feelings can occur within an individual, regardless of their literal contradiction. In other words, *but* is a word that makes sense only when what is at issue is the coherence of the resulting relational network. In other words, "but" is entirely about literal meaning. "And" makes sense whenever the process of thinking and feeling itself is at issue, because whatever was observed and noted was, after all, observed.

EVALUATION VERSUS DESCRIPTION

Evaluations present an especially thorny fusion problem. Distinguishing between evaluation and description is critical, because most clients enter therapy with a great deal of literally held self-talk about good and evil, moral and immoral, correct and incorrect, acceptable and unacceptable, and so on. Much of the evaluative self-talk clients bring to therapy is self-referential. "I am broken, defective, bad," and similar such pejorative statements are common.

Held as literal descriptions, these would be unacceptable to anyone. In addition, if these were descriptions of the *essence* of a person, the only way they could change would be if the essence of the person also changed. In other words, the change and control agenda could hardly be abandoned in this area if negative self-evaluations are merely descriptions of a personal essence. Probing will often reveal that clients are responding to their own self-evaluations as if they were descriptions. Our language makes almost no distinction between the primary property of events themselves and secondary properties occasioned by the emotional evaluations and responses we have to these events. This means the client is likely to infuse events with subjective properties that are treated as objective, external properties of the event. The *Bad Cup Metaphor* can be employed to show how evaluations can masquerade as descrip-

BAD CUP METAPHOR

There are things in our language that draw us into needless psychological battles, and it is good to get a sense of how this happens so that we can learn to avoid them. One of the worst tricks language plays on us is in the area of evaluations. For language to work at all, things have to be what we say they are when we're engaging in the kind of talk that is naming and describing. Otherwise, we couldn't talk to each other. If we describe some-thing accurately, the labels can't change until the form of that event changes. If I say, "Here is a cup," I can't then turn around and claim it isn't a cup but instead is a race car, unless I somehow change the cup. For example, I could mash it into raw materials and use it as part of a sports car. But without a change in form, this is a cup (or whatever else we agree to call it)—the label shouldn't change willy-nilly.

Now consider what happens with evaluative talk. Suppose a person says, "This is a good cup," or "This is a beautiful cup." It sounds the same as if that person were saying, "This is a ceramic cup," or "This is an 8-ounce cup." But are they really the same? Suppose all the living creatures on the planet die tomorrow. This cup is still sitting on the table. If it was "a ceramic cup" before everyone died, it is still a ceramic cup. But is it still a good cup or a beautiful cup? Without anyone to have such opinions, the opinions are gone, because good or beautiful was never in the cup, but instead was in the interaction between the person and the cup. But notice how the structure of language hides this difference. It looks the same, as if "good" is the same kind of description as "ceramic." Both seem to add information about the cup. The problem is that if you let *good* be that kind of descriptor, it means that good has to be what the cup is, in the same way that ceramic is. That kind of description can't change until the form of the cup changes. And what if someone else says, "No, that is a terrible cup!" If I say it is good and you say it is bad, there is a disagreement that seemingly has to be resolved. One side has to win, and one side has to lose: both can't be right. On the other hand, if "good" is just an evaluation or a judgment, something you're doing with the cup rather than something that is in the cup, it makes a big difference. Two opposing evaluations can easily coexist. They do not reflect some impossible state of affairs in the world, such as the cup is both ceramic and metallic. Rather, they reflect the simple fact that events can be evaluated as good or bad, depending on the perspec-tive taken. And, of course, it is not unimaginable that one person could take more than one perspective. Neither evaluation needs to win out as the one concrete fact.

tions. This commonsense metaphor highlights a fairly esoteric philo-sophical idea.

Cubby Holing or Calling a Spade a Spade

Baba Ram Dass (the well-known former Harvard psychologist Richard Alpert, a teacher of Eastern philosophy and techniques) describes a tech-nique that his guru used in working with Ram Dass's self-talk. It is a technique that is easy to use in ACT as well. When Baba Ram Dass would tell his oh-so-interesting stories about his own life, emotions, and psychological processes, his mentor seemed to be interested only in labeling the *kind* of talk he was engaging in, not its content. For example, if he showed emotion, his guru would quietly say, "An emotion." If he said something was terrible, his guru would whisper, "An evaluation."

ACT therapists can employ this verbal convention as a kind of continuous back-channel communication about language processes. Descriptions, evaluations, feelings, thoughts, memories, and so on can simply be labeled in an aside, and the conversation can continue. Once this process is well understood, the client can be asked to do the labeling in the natural stream of conversation. These labels can also be worked into the normal conversation itself, rather than as asides. For instance, a client might restate "I'm a bad person" as "I'm a person and I'm having the evaluation that I'm bad." By its very awkwardness this verbal convention helps break badness out of a well-practiced stream of self-talk, and thus it is deliteralized.

WILLINGNESS: THE GOAL OF DELITERALIZATION

The eventual goal of deliteralization is to neutralize language-based processes that interfere with the client's ability to experience disturbing psychological content. By learning to take the stance of a nonjudgmental observer, the client is freed from the incessant demands of unworkable control strategies. Once we have loosened the grip of literal language, the client is ready to practice willingness with unwanted thoughts, emotions, memories, and bodily states, which will be deliberately elicited by the therapist. Willingness exercises are intended to teach the client to give up the struggle with emotional discomfort and disturbing thoughts.

The following willingness exercise is borrowed from the Gestalt tradition. We call this the *Physicalizing Exercise* because it treats an event being struggled with as if it is a physical object. It starts with a disturbing reaction: an emotion, a bodily state, an obsessive thought, an urge to use drugs, or whatever is relevant to the particular case. The therapist asks the client to put it in front of him or her as if it were an object. The characteristics of the object are then explored. This takes advantage of the natural physical distance we assume between observers and objects.

THERAPIST: Now I want you to imagine yourself setting this depression outside of you, putting it 4 or 5 feet in front of you. Later we'll let you take it back, so if it objects to being put outside, let it know that you will soon be taking it back. See whether you can set it out in front of you on the floor in this room, and let me know when you have it out there.

CLIENT: OK. It's out there.

THERAPIST: So if this feeling of depression had a size, how big would it be?

CLIENT: (*pause*) Almost as big as this room.

THERAPIST: And if it had a color, what color would it be?

CLIENT: Dark black.

THERAPIST: And if it had a speed, how fast would it go?

CLIENT: It would be slow and lumbering.

This process continues with questions about power, surface texture, internal consistency, shape, density, weight, flexibility, and any other physical dimensions you choose. Have the client verbalize each response, but do not get into a conversation. After getting a fairly large sample, go back to a few earlier items and see whether anything is changing (e.g., what was big is now small). Especially if the event hasn't changed much, ask the client if he or she has any reactions to this thing that is big, black, slow, and so forth. Often the client will report being angry with it, repulsed by it, will not want it, will be afraid of it, will hate it, or something of that kind. Get the core, strong reaction and then ask the client to move the first object slightly to the side and to put this second reaction out in front, right next to the initial event. Repeat the entire *Physicalizing Exercise* with the second event. Now take a look at the first event. Usually, when the second event is physicalized, the first will be thinner, lighter, less powerful, and so on. Sometimes these attributes can be turned on and off like a switch; whenever the second reaction is taken literally and used as a perspective from which to examine the first reaction, the first becomes more powerful. When the second reaction is deliteralized by being viewed as an object, the first reaction diminishes.

If the items do not change, the therapist can either look for another core reaction that is holding the system in place or simply stop the exercise. The therapist should never suggest that any particular outcome was expected if it did not occur. Just noticing a reaction as an event—without struggling with it—changes its qualities profoundly. This simple experience can change the context of that reaction when it occurs again in real life. It may be the same reaction, but it is seen differently, even if the client still struggles with it. The next willingness exercise is similar to the first, but examines behavioral domains instead of physical attributes. It is called the *Tin Can Monster Exercise* and usually starts with a partic-

ularly painful or difficult feeling, thought, or memory. (In this example
we will use "panic.")

THERAPIST: Facing our problems is like facing a giant monster who is
   made up of tin cans and string. The 30-foot monster is almost
   impossible to face willingly; if we disassemble him, however, into all
   the cans and string and wire and bubble gum that he's made of, each
   of those pieces is easier to deal with one at a time. I'd like us to do a
   little exercise to see whether that isn't the way it works. Start by
   closing your eyes [add the usual coaching necessary to get the client
   centered, focused, and relaxed]. OK. Let's start by recalling something that happened last summer. Anything that happened is fine.
   When you have something, just let me know.

CLIENT: I went to the lake with my family. We are in a boat.

THERAPIST: Now I want you to see everything that was happening then.
   Notice where you are and what is happening. See whether you can
   see, hear, and smell, just as you did back then. Take your time. [The
   therapist can elicit enough verbal responses to make sure that the
   client is following, and can build on these to encourage the client to
   get into the memory.] And now I want you to notice that you were
   there. Notice that there was a person behind those eyes, and
   although many things have happened since last summer, notice also
   that that person is here now. I'm going to call that person the
   "observer you." From that perspective or point of view, I want you
   to get in touch with this feeling of panic that can show up at work.
   Let me know when you have it.

CLIENT: (pause) I have it.

THERAPIST: I want you to watch your body and see what it does. Just
   stay in touch with the feeling and watch your body, and if you
   notice anything, let me know.

CLIENT: I have a tightness in my chest.

THERAPIST: Now I want you to see whether it is possible to drop the
   rope with that tightness in your chest. The goal here is not that you
   like the feeling, but that you're having it just as a specific bodily
   event. See whether you can notice exactly where that feeling of tightness begins and ends. Imagine that the tightness is a colored patch
   on your skin. See whether you can notice the shape it makes. And as
   you do that, drop any sense of defense or struggle with this simple
   bodily sensation. . . . If other feelings crowd in, let them know we
   will get to them later. Let me know when you are a little more open
   to the tightness.

CLIENT: OK.

THERAPIST: Now I want you to set that reaction aside. Bring the feeling of panic back into the center of your consciousness and again watch quietly for what your body does. See whether there is another reaction that shows itself. As you watch, stay with that observer you— the part of you behind your eyes—and watch from there. Let me know when you have one and tell me what it is. [Repeat for two or three bodily reactions. If the client denies having any, stay with it for a while.]

THERAPIST: This time, just go back and get in touch with that feeling of panic that you've felt at work and let me know when you are in touch with it.

CLIENT: Got it.

THERAPIST: OK. Continue to look for things your body does, but this time just look very dispassionately at all the little things that may happen in your body, and we will just touch each and move on. So with each reaction, just acknowledge it, as you would tip your hat to a person on the street. Sort of pat each on the head, and then look for the next one. Each time, see whether you can welcome that bodily sensation, without struggling with it or trying to make it go away. In a sense, see whether you can welcome it, as you would welcome a visitor to your home.

After this sequence is done with bodily sensations, do the same thing with any behavioral domain of interest: things the person feels pulled to do, thoughts, evaluations, emotions, social roles that come to mind, and so on. The more domains that are covered, the better. Stay with one specific set of reactions at a time. If working on the predisposition to run away, for example, don't let the client also work on thoughts, other actions, emotions, and so on. If you are unsure of what the client is doing, have the client verbalize, but do not get into a conversation. Constantly come back, in creative ways, to the issue of letting go. Usually the last domain is memories, because they can be especially powerful emotionally. Here an additional metaphorical component helps:

"OK, for the last part, I want you to imagine you have all the memories of your life in little snapshots in a picture album. First I want you to flip back through the album until you reach that memory last summer. And once again, see whether you can recall that sense of being a person aware of that scene. Do you have it? Good. Now I want you to reconnect with that feeling of panic. When you are

well connected, start flipping back through the picture album. If
you find yourself gazing at a picture, even if it doesn't make sense
that it might be related to panic, tell me what it is you see."

When a memory is contacted, ask the client questions such as "Who
else is in the picture? How old are you? Where are you? What were you
feeling and thinking at the time? What are you doing?" Have the client
answer questions briefly, but do not enter into a conversation.

"I want you to find a place in that memory where something happened that you avoided. See whether you avoided your own experience in some way. And take this opportunity to drain any sense
of trauma from that memory by seeing whether you are willing to
go now where you would not go psychologically then. Whatever
your reactions to the memory, just see whether you can have that
exactly as it is, have exactly what happened to you as it happened.
That doesn't mean you like it, but that you are willing to have it.
[Repeat this with two or three memories.]
    "OK, when you're ready, I want you to close the album and
picture the room as it was here when you shut your eyes and
began the exercise. When you can picture it and are ready come
back, just open your eyes and come back to the present."

This exercise is time-consuming, but it can be very powerful. It
allows for prolonged exposure to feared experiences in a safe context.
The therapist should help the client to notice the "hooks" that decrease
willingness and the quality of the reactions when those experiences were
bought as opposed to when they were not bought. Without extensive
interpretations, the ACT therapist notes all reactions, big and small,
with a sense of interest in the process and nonevaluative openness to the
content. Because the *Tin Can Monster Exercise* is so powerful, its use is
sometimes delayed until the applied willingness phase described in
Chapter 9.

THERAPEUTIC DO'S AND DON'TS

Being Literal about Deliteralization

The greatest single challenge faced by the therapist in this phase of ACT
is to enter the client's language system, to maintain awareness of it as a
language system, and to avoid falling prey to the many invitations to
fuse with the system. Practically speaking, the therapist cannot use
words to convince the client to deliteralize, but at the same time must

show the client how to deliteralize. The hope is that the client's direct experience with deliteralization and willingness will overcome the seeming illogic of these moves. This process is easy to get lost in, and a cardinal sign of getting lost is usually that the therapist begins to overuse logic with the client. Of course, logic is a language-based operation, so it is highly likely that the use of logic will only feed the client's existing verbal system. Although it is necessary to use words to conduct therapy, we generally like to see these words embedded in metaphors and used to support direct experiential exercises.

Metaphor Abuse

The flip side of this problem is equating the use of metaphors with conducting ACT. Although ACT has specific techniques and strategies, the therapist has to be sensitive to the context of each session and to pick and choose what is most likely to work. Cramming five or six metaphors into a session without a context is just as useless as using logic to convince the client of the virtues of willingness. During the early stages of learning ACT, it is quite common to see the therapist using techniques instead of attending to the functions of the client's verbal behavior. At its worst, this results in a complete disconnect. The therapist is rambling on with metaphors and exercises, and the client is not relating to what the therapist is doing. When done properly, ACT focuses on connecting with the client, seeing the client's particular forms of fusion and avoidance, and tailoring metaphors and exercises to destabilize those forms. The therapist may develop new metaphors or exercises based on the client's history, personal struggles, preferences, and so forth.

PROGRESS TO THE NEXT STAGE

If this phase of ACT work is successful, conditioned private reactions are seen as less compelling. Sacred cows such as "urges to drink," "suicidal impulses," "obsessive thoughts" seem a lot less mysterious and romantic when this shift occurs. Generally, there are two distinctive markers that suggest the client is ready to move on to the next stage. First, the client is spontaneously waking up to troublesome reactions. The client may stop in the middle of a therapeutic interaction and say, "I'm making up reasons right now," or "I just noticed I was getting anxious." The client appears to be noticing reactions at the level of an observer, rather than at the level of a person fused to those reactions. Second, the client reports being able to sustain a stance of willingness in the presence of disturbing content that previously would have produced fusion. This is often reported in the way of an outcome to some highly charged situation. The client may state, "I didn't let my anger run away with me," or "I didn't close down when my spouse started berating me." When the client reports that a well-practiced control or avoidance move did not occur, it is generally due to changes in fusion and a weakening of the social/verbal context of control. It means that the special functions of the verbal community in therapy are beginning to play a more important part. Another instance in which this is observed is when the client directly reports being more willing or shows in a problem situation that the focus was more on staying open and defused than in modulating uncomfortable psychological content.

PERSONAL EXERCISE FOR THE CLINICIAN: YOUR VIEWS OF YOURSELF

In the preceding exercise, we asked you to look at types of strategies you have used to solve the main problem in your life. We asked you to evaluate whether these were control- or acceptance-based strategies. In the case of control strategies, we asked you to think about what private experiences (thoughts, emotions, memories, sensations) you may be trying to avoid or eliminate. Now we want to look at how your self-definition may be influencing your "vision" in this situation. Remember to save your work. We will revisit it in the next chapter.

1. Describe yourself. It will help to give multiple responses to each of the following questions.
   a. I am a person who is . . .
   b. The best things about me are that I am . . .
   c. The worst things about me are that I am . . .
2. Which of these "friends" (something you want to have) and "enemies" (something you don't want to have) are you most strongly committed to as "true statements" about who you are?
3. This is called a "releasing" exercise in which you can relinquish attachment to these notions of yourself. Look at your friends and enemies, and release them in pairs (one friend, one enemy). Releasing means that we will see these statement as statements, not as literal descriptions of realities, one way or the other. The order in which you release them should go from the easiest ones to let go of to the hardest ones to let go of. Write these pairs down as you release them.
4. Look at the last pairs you released. If you bought one or the

other side of these pairs, how might that action influence your ability to respond creatively to your main life problem? Is the restriction as great with the friends as with the enemies?

CLINICAL VIGNETTE

You are in the fifth session with a 31-year-old man who has panic attacks. He has developed an avoidance of freeways and bridges because of the fear of having a panic attack in those settings. He is also uncomfortable being in malls and supermarkets unless he is near an exit. His primary method of controlling his panic has been to avoid situations where panic might be possible or to flee from any situation when he notices the early physical symptoms that he associates with panic. The cost of this avoidance has been high. He has essentially stopped his social life because of his troubles with driving and feeling self-conscious around his friends. He has more or less stopped pursuing a relationship with a woman that he has strong feelings for, but who lives in an area that can be accessed only by freeway driving. He has a good job that is near his home. In this session, he states, "I don't think I'll ever get on top of these panic attacks. When my heart starts pounding, it's like a wave of fear goes over me. All I can think of is 'I'm going to die' or 'I feel like I'm losing my mind.' I feel like a wild animal. I almost don't even know what I'm doing until I come down. Its hard for me to imagine accepting these feelings. I think they would probably just get worse that way."

> *Question for the clinician:* Conceptualize the client's dilemma from the ACT viewpoint on cognitive fusion. How would you respond to these statements from that viewpoint? What strategies/interventions would you use to address them, and what would be your goal(s) in doing so? (Answer this before looking at our answer.)
> *Our answer:* The client is confusing (or pouring together) the content of private experiences (catastrophic thoughts, powerful feelings, somatic symptoms) with the context in which those experiences are occurring (i.e., the client is observing and responding to these symptoms). These experiences, if treated literally, leave no option but to panic. Who wouldn't panic if he or she bought a thought called "I'm going to die" or a physical symptom called "Heart pounding, heart attack"? So, the problem here is how to get the client to step back (move his nose off the computer screen) from these experiences and see them as experiences (thoughts,

feelings, sensations), not what they advertise themselves to be (panic, craziness, death). A variety of deliteralization exercises may help. For the fearsome thoughts, we might do the *Milk, Milk, Milk Exercise.* We might use the *Tin Can Monster Exercise* to get the panic in the room and then deconstruct it into its constituent parts. Our goal would be to elevate the client's willingness to let these symptoms show up, without taking them literally. Then these symptoms would follow some type of natural course, not the ratcheting effect into panic that occurs when cognitive fusion is the dominant response.

APPENDIX: CLIENT HOMEWORK

Reasons as Causes

Having the client work on reason giving between sessions provides a valuable task. The goal of the assignment is to have the client notice instances in real life where he or she is in reason-giving mode. The written experiences are then brought in, and the goals are to help the client recognize the "signals" of reason giving and how it affects the client's mood, self-confidence, and so forth.

Practicing Awareness of Your Experience

This homework allows the client to practice both deliteralization (a form of awareness) and willingness (nonjudgmental detachment) between sessions. It is important to emphasize that these are skills that can be learned, much like other skills. Practice doesn't make perfect, it makes permanent. The more a client experiences willingness and the factors that make it go up or down, the more likely it is that spontaneous willingness moves will occur in the client's life. Generally, the client should engage in the exercise at least once daily for 5 to 10 minutes at the least. It is always important to debrief this type of assignment, to

---

REASONS AS CAUSES HOMEWORK

1. List some of the reasons you are most likely to give to yourself or others for areas in your life that are troublesome.
2. Between now and your next session, try to notice several specific instances in which you catch yourself in the reason-giving mode, using reasons like these or others. Write down several examples. Write down how you were feeling in those situations. Then describe how you felt or what you thought when you noticed yourself giving reasons. Bring this in for discussion at your next session. Are the reasons you caught yourself using similar to those listed above?

---

ensure that the client isn't getting hooked into practicing control strategies in the context of willingness.

PRACTICING AWARENESS OF YOUR EXPERIENCE

Often the buzz of mental activity draws us in, and we become thoroughly caught in it. Sometimes this is so thorough that we can become intensely insensitive to our own moment-to-moment experience. The following meditation allows us to practice observing the buzz of mental activity without doing anything about it.

1. Assume a comfortable sitting position. Try to find a position where you are sitting straight and your shoulders are relaxed.
2. Either close your eyes or arrange yourself so that you are looking at something nondistracting, like a blank wall.
3. Center yourself. Bring yourself to this room you are in, to this space and time. Visualize your physical location: on your block, in your house, in your room, and in this chair. Become aware of your body, of the physical position of your arms and legs, of your feet and hands. Notice the feeling of your body pressing against the chair, of the muscles around your eyes and jaw; notice the feelings of your skin.
4. Become aware of your breathing. Follow a breath as it comes in through your nose, travels through your lungs, moves your belly in and out, and leaves in the opposite direction. Ride the waves of your breathing without attempting to alter it: just notice it and pay attention as it happens.
5. Now, do nothing but observe what comes up. Practice awareness. As sensations emerge in your body, just watch them. As feelings emerge in your awareness, just notice them. As thoughts come into your awareness, just watch them. Watch them come, and watch them go. Don't grab at anything, and don't push anything away.
6. If your mind wanders, if you find yourself getting angry or sad or imagining something you want to say to someone and slipping into fantasy, just notice that you have wandered off and bring yourself back in touch. Notice how you get sucked into the content of your thoughts and start to fuse with them; notice your analytical, judgmental mind. Just notice yourself getting sucked in, and bring yourself back again, gently and without judgment. If you have judgments about how well or how poorly you are doing, just notice these too. Your "job" is simply to practice awareness. This means that if your mind wanders 100 times, then your job is to gently bring it back to this moment 100 times, starting with the present moment.
7. Allow yourself to deeply experience the present moment. Be deeply present with yourself. Even if you are having thoughts or feelings that you don't like, try not to push them away. Adopt an attitude of acceptance toward all parts of your experience: treat every experience gently, even if the experience (the thought or feeling) itself is undesirable. Gently be present with yourself.

•7•

Discovering Self, Defusing Self

Form is only emptiness; emptiness only form
—ZEN SAYING

The emergence of *self* and *mind* in Western language is actually a relatively new phenomenon. Many English words that are now routinely used to connote mental or affective states were not originally designed for that purpose. An excellent treatise on this subject is provided by Skinner (1989) in his analysis of the origins of cognitive thought. For example, if someone says, "I am inclined to do that," it sounds as though an emotional or cognitive state is being described. The term *inclination* literally means "a leaning toward," describing a physical property that can lead to directed action (indeed, "I am leaning toward doing that" is a reasonable synonym). Virtually all terms that refer to complex emotional or cognitive states (e.g., *anxiety, depression*) and most that refer even to simple states of this kind (e.g., *want*) are metaphors based originally on descriptions of physical events. This is not surprising because it seems unlikely that language evolved for the purpose of self-description, self-evaluation, or as a means for describing private experiences.

Out of the issues of blood and bone that originally gave language its value for early humans have come other uses. We have learned to describe ever more subtle states of being, states of mind, behavioral predispositions, and so on. This self-reflexive capacity of human thought is a powerful and potentially dangerous tool, and ACT therapists are very attentive to the precise nature of the dangers.

ACT asks a lot of the client. It asks that verbal defenses be reduced. It asks that psychological monsters be faced. No one can be expected to face psychological pain if self-destruction (literally or metaphorically through relational frames) seems to be the likely result. In order to face one's monsters head-on, it is necessary to find a place from which this is possible. The context in which emotional willingness is fully possible is that of an unchanging self that is not threatened by difficult psychological content. It is one of the great paradoxes of ACT that this self is conceptualized to be a side effect of the very language processes that created the problem to begin with.

THE THEORETICAL FOCUS: VARIETIES OF SELF

ACT distinguishes between three major senses of "self" (Hayes & Gregg, in press). More senses surely exist, but we are interested here only in the senses of self that bear on terms such as *self-knowledge* and the like, not the physical self. These three senses are the conceptualized self, ongoing self-awareness, and self as perspective. Although our clients are often very familiar with their conceptualized selves, they are much less familiar with ongoing self awareness and even less in contact with the most immutable aspect of self: a consciousness perspective or locus. ACT attempts to redefine who the client takes him- or herself to be, and for a simple reason: Some senses of the term *self* are more threatened by change than others. Clients often come into therapy prepared to defend self as conceptualized literal content, and this can greatly restrict the kinds of therapeutic changes that are possible.

ACT therapists take the view that human vitality is most likely when the person voluntarily and repeatedly engages in a kind of conceptual suicide, in which the boundaries of the conceptualized self are torn down and whatever experiences are present in the person's history are made room for in his or her psychology. When we emphasize the client's direct experience through an observing self, we build a stable place from which it is possible to work and from which the ongoing process of self-awareness can honestly go on. We restore for clients what they have already been given but have lost as a result of the domination of the literal content of derived stimulus relations—a place to observe the private war without being in the private war.

The Conceptualized Self

We humans do not merely live in the world, we live in the world as we interpret it, construct it, view it, or understand it. In technical terms, derived stimulus relations dominate over other behavioral processes. Clients invariably have formulated their personal characteristics into what Adler called a "private logic." Clients have told stories, formulated their life histories, defined their dominant attributes, evaluated these attributes, compared their attributes to those of others, constructed cause and effect relations between their histories and attributes, and so on. As a result, as simple a phrase as "I am a person who . . . " can generate dozens, or even hundreds, of supposed attributes in most people.

We do not merely speak, however; we (and others) also listen. Furthermore, the social community expects a correspondence between what we say and what we do, and consequences are doled out accordingly. As we learn that we need to behave in a consistent fashion, we begin to behave in a way so as to maintain our own process of self-reflective categorization and evaluation. We try to live up to our own and others' views of ourselves.

There are several sources of this effort to maintain consistency. First, relational networks that are consistent are inherently more self-supportive, because each part of the network can be used to derive other parts that may have weakened. Second, we have a massive history of learning to detect and maintain consistency. The social community calls this "being right," and from an early age being right is a powerful consequence. Third, phrases such as "I am a person who . . . " literally claim to be about issues of being, as if "I am alive" and "I am kind" are the same sorts of statements. These statements specify equivalence classes, and thus "I" comes to be in the same class as these conceptualized attributes, a process sometimes called "attachment." Fourth, when a person identifies with a particular conceptualization, alternatives to that conceptualization can seem almost life threatening. The relational frame here seems to be "Me = conceptualization" and its entailed derivative "Eliminate conceptualization = eliminate me." Through this frame of coordination, we are drawn into protecting our conceptualized self as if it is our physical self. Through these means, self-descriptions serve as powerful formative augmentals for the importance of protecting the conceptualized self.

The conceptualized self can create severe problems. Often consistency can be maintained more easily simply by distorting or reinterpreting events if they are inconsistent with our conceptualized self. If a person believes him- or herself to be kind, for example, there is less room to deal directly and openly with instances of behavior that could more readily be called cruel. In this way, a conceptualized self becomes resistant to change and variation and fosters self-deception.

Ironically, this means that most people come into therapy wanting to *defend* their particular conceptualized self even if it is loathsome.

They view their familiar ideas about themselves—positive and negative—as one would view dear friends. Most clients are initially so thoroughly trapped by this conceptual prison that they do not know and do not believe that they are imprisoned. The conceptual world in which they live is taken to be a given.

At a university several years ago, an animal activist freed a few dozen pigeons used in animal operant research. Although fully able to fly, the birds sat forlornly next to the front door until the caretakers arrived the next morning. Clients who are attached to their conceptualized selves are like that—even experiences that might open the client up are reinterpreted with the use of existing verbal schemes and promptly reintegrated into the original conceptual prison. To escape a prison, it is necessary to see the prison itself.

Mainstream empirical clinical psychology has encouraged an excessive emphasis on changing the conceptualized self, mainly though its extensive focus on modifying the content of private experiences. Certain thoughts are rational, and others are irrational; certain emotions are good, and others are bad; certain beliefs show high self-esteem, whereas others show low self-esteem; and so on. This kind of categorization is quite familiar to our clients. It's what they have been doing all their lives. Rather than help them win this war between polarities—as most therapies seem to do—ACT therapists work to distinguish clients from their conceptualized content, however good or bad that content may be.

Ongoing Self-Awareness

Although defending a conceptualized self is inherently dangerous and distorting, self-awareness is important in therapy and an ally to a healthy and psychologically vital life. This is true primarily because much of our socialization about what to do in life situations is tied to an ongoing process of verbal self-awareness. Emotional talk is perhaps the clearest example. Although conditions such as anger, anxiety, or sadness are quite varied in the histories that give rise to them, they are quite similar in their social implications. A person who is not able to be aware of and utilize ongoing behavioral states cannot address the highly individualized and changing circumstances that daily life presents. For example, suppose a young girl has been sexually abused for many years by her father. Suppose that during this time expressions of emotion associated with this aversive experience were reinterpreted, ignored, or denied. For instance, the perpetrator might have tried to convince the child that she actually was not upset when indeed she was. With such a history, the person's ongoing self-awareness may be distorted or weak because many conventional verbal discriminations would not have been made: The person may literally not know how she felt. In some deep sense, the person would be flying blind emotionally until this deficit is corrected (i.e., in the context of a therapeutic relationship that helps the person develop more normative self-awareness).

Although ACT assumes that it is inherently constraining to tie one's identity to conceptualized content of any kind, it also assumes that a healthy human life requires continuous and flexible verbal self-knowledge. ACT encourages this in two ways. First, it is rare that content itself is taken to be the important issue. If a person is having a thought, that is a thought. If the person is having an evaluation, that is an evaluation. Where it came from, whether it is correct or desirable, and whether the story being told can explain behavior, is a secondary issue. Rather, ACT therapists encourage clients to see what they see as they see it, without objectifying or concretizing this content in order to justify what was felt or seen. This helps remove the social contingencies that encourage a client to lie or to self-deceive. The irony is that when the specific content of self-knowledge is no longer so much at issue, fluid and useful self-knowledge is more likely to be fostered. There are some data showing that lying in young children follows a similar pattern (Ribeiro, 1989).

Second, ACT therapists try to describe what is going on in therapy, in clients or in themselves, directly and uncritically. An ACT therapist usually looks for direct descriptions of content, not for evaluations, judgments, expectations, interpretations, analyses, and the like. Many ACT exercises train clients to contact psychological content and simply describe it, without adding or subtracting anything.

The Observing Self

The final aspect of self—and that which is most often ignored—has been termed the "observing self" (Deikman, 1982). From the ACT perspective, the observing self is a core phenomenon that is taken to be at the heart of human spirituality. The theory of verbal events presented in Chapter 2 helps us understand the behavioral process this type of self involves, so a brief theoretical extension would be helpful (see Hayes, 1984, and Barnes & Roche, 1997, for more detailed treatments).

From a behavioral point of view, self-awareness is responding to one's own responding. Skinner (1974) used the example of seeing. Most nonhuman animals see, but humans also see that they see. "There is a . . . difference between behaving and reporting that one is behaving or reporting the causes of one's behavior. In arranging conditions under which a person describes the public or private world in which he lives, a community generates that very special form of behavior called knowing. . . . Self-knowledge is of social origin" (Skinner, 1974, p. 30).

Supposedly this happens dominantly through language. As we learn to answer such questions as "What happened to you yesterday?" "What did you see?" "What did you eat?" and so on, there emerges a generalized tendency to respond verbally to one's own behavior. This is important to the social/verbal community because it gives indirect social access to events occurring elsewhere. As Skinner says, "It is only when a person's private world becomes important to others that it is made important to him" (Skinner, 1974, p. 31).

In order to have the ability to report events verbally in a sophisticated manner, however, it is necessary to develop a sense of perspective or point of view and to distinguish it from that of others. For example, we may need to learn to report what we ate this morning, but also what someone else ate. We must learn to report what we see, but also to suppose what it is that others may see. This process of learning to take a perspective is amplified by verbal terms such as *here* and *there*, or *now* and *then*, which are defined in relation to a perspective or locus.

When people are asked many, many questions about their history or experience, the only thing that will be consistent is not the *content* of the answer, but the *context* or perspective in which the answer occurs. "I" in some meaningful sense *is* the location that is left when all of the content differences are subtracted. For example, notice what is consistent in answers to the questions "What happened to you yesterday?" "What did you see?" "What did you eat?" We will answer, "I did such and such," "I saw so and so," and "I ate this and that." The "I" that is referred to is not just a physical organism, it is also a locus, place, or perspective.

As this sense of perspective is formed, a fundamental distinction is available between the literal content of a verbal event and the sense of locus from which observations are made. This distinction forms the basis of the matter–spirit distinction that seems to have emerged in virtually all complex human cultures.

The *Oxford English Dictionary* defines *spirit* as an "incorporeal or immaterial being" and as a "being or intelligence distinct from anything physical." In essence, spirituality is defined negatively as that which is not material or physical. The word *matter* comes from a word meaning "timber" or "building materials," and matter is the "stuff of which a thing is made." *Thing* is defined as "that which is or may be an object of perception, thought, or knowledge." The word *object* comes from a word meaning "to throw"; an object is "a thing thrown down to the senses or the mind." We can go no further, because this definition refers us back to *thing*. If we go back and pick up the word *physical* we find we can go no further there either. The word *physical* comes from a word for nature (thus, the science of physics) and is defined as "of or pertaining to the phenomenal world of the senses; matter."

Putting these various definitions together, "spirit" is a private event that cannot be experienced as a thing or object. In our dualistic culture, matter and spirit are in opposition, but a sense of you-as-perspective has the exact properties of "spirit" so defined. A sense of locus or perspective is not "thing-like" for the person experiencing it. It is not possible to have a different perspective than your own. You can imagine what it might be like to hold a different perspective (it may even be important to do so in order to acquire a sense of perspective), but even as you imagine this you see these imaginings from a local perspective. Everywhere you go, there you are. Anything you know verbally, you were there to know it verbally. One can be conscious of the limits of everything except one's own consciousness. This sense of unity is not "thing-like" at all, because it has no directly available edges or distinctions. Conversely all "things" must be evidently finite—they must have experienced edges or limits. It is the edges or limits that allow us to see a thing. If a thing were absolutely everywhere, we could not see it as a thing. For the person experiencing it, you-as-perspective has no stable edges or limits and thus is not fully experienced as a thing.

We are arguing that the distinction between conceptualized content and a sense of "observing self" is the experiential source of the matter–spirit distinction. That distinction is an ancient one, originating long before a scientific perspective dominated in human culture. Rather than rejecting this distinction, the present analysis suggests that it is a very reasonable and sophisticated one.

Spiritual and religious traditions have dealt most with the observing self. Buddhists have the idea of an "uncarved block" that originates at birth. The uncarved block is the simple wholeness of consciousness itself and is the "ground" for the experience of "being." We would argue that a sense of self as locus or context cannot change once it emerges, because it is so basic and fundamental. As organisms we do have a locus, but, paradoxically, awareness of an experiential locus feels transcendent.

It is not very difficult to help a client recognize the essential connection between the person he or she is today and the person he or she was last summer, and the person who was once a teenager and the person who was once 4 years old. People can remember being behind their eyes in earlier days and can contact that sense now. This sense of observing self is critical to acceptance work because it means that there is at least one stable, unchangeable, immutable fact about oneself that has been experienced directly. That kind of stability and constancy makes it less threatening for a client to enter into the pain and travails of life, knowing in some deep way that no matter what comes up, the "I" defined as the observing self will not be at risk.

Consciousness, awareness, and *being* are terms frequently used to describe contact with the observing self. *Pure consciousness* is a reasonable term for it. Etymologically, *con-sciousness* means "with knowing by the mind" (ironically, the *scious* part of the word comes from the same root as *science*). Pure consciousness comes from being with verbal knowing as a locus, not merely as the content of what is known. To borrow a metaphor from Baba Ram Dass, behind the cloud of literal language processes lies a small bit of blue sky. There is no need for humans to blow the clouds away every moment in order to be reassured that there is blue sky. When we look, it is there. It is the blue sky that envelopes and contains the clouds themselves. Similarly, the observing self (you-as-perspective) is always there, even when we forget that it is. When the clouds of verbal chatter can be seen from the point of view of the sky, the clouds are not so threatening. Contact with the observing self inherently contains a sense of personal wholeness, transcendence, and presence.

Self-as-perspective forms the foundation for a primary move in ACT. In the ACT model, suffering occurs because of needless struggles with the world as structured by literal meaning. The trick lies in teaching the client how to be aware of content, to be aware of the awareness of content, and yet not to be preoccupied with content or attached to it as a matter of personal identity. In other words, we have to teach the client how to notice when thoughts and feelings are present from a perspective of self-as-context, without objectifying these events or mistaking them for "self" in this deeper sense.

An aphorism that touches this point is "Life is really quite simple . . . until we start thinking about it." Rather than using therapy as an opportunity to create new layers of language-based tricks in the name of rational living, correcting cognitive distortions, or creating understanding and insight into prior history, the ACT therapist is going to steer a different course altogether. This course is going to diminish the value and role of content-related verbal processes, while experientially contacting the sense of irreversible wholeness that everyone desires.

CLINICAL FOCUS

This phase of therapy introduces several core perspectives:

- The conceptualized self is inherently polarized—good and bad are functionally related.
- Self-awareness is defined through contact with private experiences; such contact is a healthy activity.

- Self-identity is best tied to self-as-context. The client is not defined by private experiences; rather, the client is the conscious vessel that contains private experiences.
- The experience of an observing self is beyond evaluation, does not change, and has no mechanical qualities.
- Contact with the observing self is inherently peaceful and safe from threatening private experiences.
- The observing self is found in experience, not logic.

Table 7.1 presents a summary of the major therapeutic goals of this phase. For each goal, specific strategies are listed, along with ACT exercises and metaphors that can be used to implement the therapeutic strategies.

UNDERMINING ATTACHMENT
TO THE CONCEPTUALIZED SELF

As is true in any phase of ACT, some clients early on are ready to begin tackling the thorny issues related to self and others are not. Many clients who are psychologically minded, or who have prior experience with meditation or other alternative consciousness-raising experiences, are

TABLE 7.1. ACT Goals, Strategies, and Interventions Regarding Self

Goals	Strategies	Interventions
1. Undermine attachment to the conceptualized self.	Show how attachment to both positive and negative self-concepts is at times detrimental.	Mental Polarity Exercise
2. Create awareness of self-as-perspective.	Help distinguish consciousness from content of consciousness.	Chessboard Metaphor Observer Exercise
	Help appreciate the continuity of consciousness versus the changing nature of content.	
3. Contrast the conceptualized self with the observer self.	Undermine importance ascribed to feeling, thinking, and acting in an entirely coherent fashion.	Faking it Pick an Identity Exercise
	Undermine the "discoveries" of self-analysis.	
	Show arbitrariness of content.	

immediately ready to grasp the issue of self and make headway with it. The ACT orientation toward self and suffering also explains why this approach may work with a broad range of clinical and subclinical conditions that clients present in therapy. In a sense, there is a timelessness to the struggle between content and context—it is a struggle thousands of years old. Therapists and clients are in this language stew together, and there is an intense therapeutic bond that occurs because of this fact.

The early work that is designed to undermine an attachment to a conceptualized self can be fairly straightforward. The linkage between self-conceptualization and successful performance is deeply embedded in popular culture. It has also been widely promoted in psychology (e.g., through concepts like self-efficacy). The client often believes that therapy will help eliminate bad and limiting self-beliefs and induce pure and unadulterated self-confidence. The ACT therapist introduces the idea that it may not be the goodness or badness of beliefs that is a problem, but rather the attachment to the belief itself that is creating the problem.

To begin the process, the therapist can provide the client with several examples of the ways in which overattachment to even very positive beliefs can blind a person. For example, those who are too attached to the idea that the world is a place that is full of goodness are more likely to be preyed upon by the unscrupulous. Those who are too committed to the idea that they are good parents may be blind to ways they are actually harming their children. The therapist may ask such a client to examine some relevant personal experiences and try to come up with situations in which excessive attachment to both positive and negative ideas has been detrimental.

One way to do this more experientially is to use the *Mental Polarity Exercise*. The client often does not appreciate the powerful dialectical properties of language and the arbitrary way this characteristic can affect self-conceptualizations. The client's experience in this exercise will be to notice that any positive identity statement automatically draws its opposite, and any negative identity statement automatically draws its opposite. The point is simply that peace of mind is not possible at the level of content, and thus an attachment to private evaluative thought content will always immediately produce a sense of unease and threat.

BUILDING AWARENESS OF THE OBSERVING SELF

Discussing self-conceptualization at an intellectual level is rarely very helpful. ACT helps the client make experiential contact with the observing self. This involves a series of metaphors and exercises designed to loosen the client's grip on the conceptualized self and instead to notice the process of consciousness and sense of perspective.

MENTAL POLARITY EXERCISE

Have the client close his or her eyes and ask the client to think thoughts that are described by the therapist and see what happens. Encourage the client to really try to believe these thoughts 100%. Start with positive thoughts and gradually make them more and more extreme (e.g., start with "I'm a valid person" and progress to "I'm perfect"). Ask the client to notice what the mind does with this input. Then repeat the same process with negative thoughts (e.g., start with "I have flaws as a person" and progress to "I'm 100% worthless. There is nothing about me that has any positive features.") Again, ask the client to notice what happens.

In debriefing, note what came up, which were harder (positive or negative thoughts), and so on. Usually, the more extreme the positive thoughts, the more the client resisted with negative ones, and vice versa. The point can be drawn out that there is no peace of mind at the level of content, because each pole pulls its opposite. Peace of mind has to be found elsewhere.

Parenthetically, it can be worthwhile to tell the client about the etymology of *perfect*. The first part of the word (*per*) comes from a term that means "thoroughly." *Fect* comes from the same root as the word *factory* and means "made." In normal language, wholeness and perfection seem to be issues of evaluation. If to be perfect is to be thoroughly made, perhaps perfection is more a matter of presence or wholeness. The idea "I am missing something" also comes in a moment that is always absolutely whole. No second contains more life than any other second, even the seconds that are filled with thoughts of how incomplete we are. The experience of that very thought can be complete.

The *Chessboard Metaphor*, a central ACT intervention, connects the client to the distinction between content and the observing self.

Imagine a chessboard that goes out infinitely in all directions. It's covered with black pieces and white pieces. They work together in teams, as in chess—the white pieces fight against the black pieces. You can think of your thoughts and feelings and beliefs as these pieces; they sort of hang out together in teams too. For example, "bad" feelings (like anxiety, depression, resentment) hang out with "bad" thoughts and "bad" memories. Same thing with the "good" ones. So it seems that the way the game is played is that we select the side we want to win. We put the "good" pieces (like thoughts that are self-confident, feelings of being in control, etc.) on one side, and the "bad" pieces on the other. Then we get up on the back of the black horse and ride to battle, fighting to win the war against anxiety, depression, thoughts about using drugs, whatever. It's a war game. But there's a logical problem here, and that is that from this posture huge portions of yourself are your own enemy. In other words, if you need to be in this war, there is something wrong with you. And because it appears that you're on the same level as these pieces, they can be as big or even bigger than you are—even though these pieces are in you. So somehow, even though it is not logical, the more you fight the bigger they get. If it is true that "if you are not willing to have it, you've got it," then as you fight these pieces they become more central to your life, more habitual, more dominating, and more linked to every area of living. The logical idea is that you will knock enough of them off the board that you eventually dominate them—except that your experience tells you that the exact opposite happens. Apparently, the white pieces can't be deliberately knocked off the board. So the battle goes on. You feel hopeless, you have a sense that you can't win, and yet you can't stop fighting. If you're on the back of that black horse, fighting is the only choice you have, because the white pieces seem life threatening. Yet living in a war zone is no way to live.

As the client connects to this metaphor, it can be turned to the issue of the self.

THERAPIST: Now let me ask you to think about this carefully. In this metaphor, suppose you aren't the chess pieces. Who are you?

CLIENT: Am I the player?

THERAPIST: That may be what you have been trying to be. Notice, though, that a player has a big investment in how this war turns out. Besides, whom are you playing against? Some other player? Suppose you're not that either.

CLIENT: . . . Am I the board?

THERAPIST: It's useful to look at it that way. Without a board, these pieces have no place to be. The board holds them. For instance, what would happen to your thoughts if you weren't there to be aware that you thought them? The pieces need you. They cannot exist without you—but you contain them, they don't contain you. Notice that if you're the pieces, the game is very important; you've got to win, your life depends on it. But if you're the board, it doesn't matter whether the war stops or not. The game may go on, but it doesn't make any difference to the board. As the board, you can see all the pieces, you can hold them, you are in intimate contact with them; you can watch the war being played out in your consciousness, but it doesn't matter. It takes no effort.

The *Chessboard Metaphor* is often physically acted out in therapy. For example, a piece of cardboard is placed on the floor and various attractive and ugly things are put on top (e.g., cigarette butts, pictures). The client may be asked to notice that the board exerts no effort to hold the pieces, a metaphor for the lack of effort that is needed in willingness, with the physical act of the board holding things as a metaphor for willingness. The client may be asked to notice that at board level only two things can be done: hold the pieces and move them all in some direction. We cannot move specific pieces without abandoning board level. Whereas the board's job is effortless, the pieces are in a total war. Further, the board is in more direct contact with the pieces than the pieces are with each other—so willingness is not about detachment or dissociation. Rather, when the client becomes attached to a thought or struggles with an emotion, other pieces, although scary, are not really being touched at all.

Once the client has been introduced to the metaphor, it is useful to reinvigorate it periodically by simply asking the client, "Are you at the piece level or at the board level right now?" All the arguments, reasons, and so on that the client brings in are examples of pieces, and thus this metaphor can be a useful tool for attaching cognitive fusion. The notion of board level can be used frequently to connote a stance in which the client is looking *at* psychological content, rather than looking *from* psychological content. The point is that thoughts, feelings, sensations, emotions, memories, and so on are pieces: they are not you. This is immediately experientially available, but the fusion with psychological content can overwhelm this awareness. Metaphors such as the *Chessboard Metaphor* help make the issue concrete.

EXPERIENTIAL EXERCISES WITH THE OBSERVING SELF

ACT therapists are sensitive to the fact that discussions about self-concept and consciousness can quickly become unduly intellectual. The metaphor just described points to the issues involved; however, it does not experientially create the distinction between forms of self-awareness. If someone responds, "So, if that's so, what else can I do? How can I stay at board level?" it is best not to answer the question directly. A good response is, "Well, I don't know. We'll see. But right now let's just notice that it is impossible not to struggle with thoughts and feelings if that is who we are." We have to provide the client with an experience of him- or herself as the conscious context for psychological content.

The *Observer Exercise* (a variant of the *Self-identification Exercise* developed by Assagioli, 1971, pp. 211–217) is designed to begin to establish a sense of self that exists in the present and provides a context for cognitive defusion. This is a key exercise in ACT.

OBSERVER EXERCISE

We are going to do an exercise now that is a way to begin to try to experience that place where you are not your programming. There is no way anyone can fail at the exercise; we're just going to be looking at whatever you are feeling or thinking, so whatever comes up is just right. Close your eyes, get settled into your chair, and follow my voice. If you find yourself wandering, just gently come back to the sound of my voice. For a moment now, turn your attention to yourself in this room. Picture the room. Picture yourself in this room and exactly where you are. Now begin to go inside your skin and get in touch with your body. Notice how you are sitting in the chair. See whether you can notice exactly the shape that is made by the parts of your skin that touch the chair. Notice any bodily sensations that are there. As you see each one, just sort of acknowledge that feeling and allow your consciousness to move on (*pause*). Now notice any emotions you are having, and if you have any, just acknowledge them (*pause*). Now get in touch with your thoughts and just quietly watch them for a few moments (*pause*). Now I want you to notice that as you noticed these things, a part of you noticed them. You noticed those sensations . . . those emotions . . . those thoughts. And that part of you we will call the "observer you." There is a person in there, behind those eyes, who is aware of what I am saying right now. And it is the same person you've been your whole life. In some deep sense, this observer you is the you that you call you.

I want you to remember something that happened last summer. Raise your finger when you have an image in mind. Good. Now just look around. Remember all the things that were happening then. Remember the sights . . . the sounds . . . your feelings . . . and as you do that, see whether you can notice that you were there then, noticing what you were noticing. See whether you can catch the person behind your eyes who saw, and heard, and felt. You were there then, and you are here now. I'm not asking you to believe this. I'm not making a logic point. I am just asking you to note the experience of being aware and check and see whether it isn't so that in some deep sense the you that is here now was there then. The person aware of what you are aware of is here now and was there then. See whether you can notice the essential continuity—in some deep sense, at the level of experience, not of belief, you have been you your whole life.

I want you to remember something that happened when you were a teenager. Raise your finger when you have an image in mind. Good. Now just look around. Remember all the things that were happening then. Remember the sights . . . the sounds . . . your feelings . . . take your time. And when you are clear about what was there, see whether you can, just for a second, catch that there was a person behind your eyes then who saw, and heard, and felt all of this. You were there then too, and see whether it isn't true—as an experienced fact, not a belief—that there is an essential continuity between the person aware of what you are aware of now and the person who was aware of what you were aware of as a teenager in that specific situation. You have been you your whole life.

Finally, remember something that happened when you were a fairly young child, say, around age 6 or 7. Raise your finger when you have an image in mind. Good. Now just look around again. See what was happening. See the sights . . . hear the sounds . . . feel your feelings . . . and then

(*continued on p. 194*)

(continued from p. 193)
catch the fact that you were there, seeing, hearing, and feeling. Notice that you were there behind your eyes. You were there then, and you are here now. Check and see whether in some deep sense the you that is here now was there then. The person aware of what you are aware of is here now and was there then.

You have been you your whole life. Everywhere you've been, you've been there noticing. This is what I mean by the "observer you." And from that perspective or point of view, I want you to look at some areas of living. Let's start with your body. Notice how your body is constantly changing. Sometimes it is sick, and sometimes it is well. It may be rested or tired. It may be strong or weak. You were once a tiny baby, but your body grew. You may have even have had parts of your body removed, as in an operation. Your cells have died, and not all the cells in your body now were there when you were a teenager, or even last summer. Your bodily sensations come and go. Even as we have spoken, they have changed. So if all this is changing and yet the you that you call you has been there your whole life, that must mean that although you have a body, as a matter of experience and not of belief, you do not experience yourself to be just your body. So just notice your body now for a few moments, and as you do this, every so often notice that you are the one noticing [give the client time to do this].

Now let's go to another area: your roles. Notice how many roles you have or have had. Sometimes you are in the role of a [fit these to the client; e.g., "mother . . . or a friend . . . or a daughter . . . or a wife . . . sometimes you are a respected worker . . . other times you are a leader . . . or a follower," etc.]. In the world of form you are in some role all the time. If you were to try not to, then you would be playing the role of not playing a role. Even now part of you is playing a role . . . the client role. Yet all the while, notice that you are also present. The part of you you call you is watching and aware of what you are aware of. And in some deep sense, that you does not change. So if your roles are constantly changing, and yet the you that you call you has been there your whole life, it must be that although you have roles, you do not experience yourself to be your roles. Do not believe this. This is not a matter of belief. Just look and notice the distinction between what you are looking at and the you who is looking.

Now let's go to another area: emotions. Notice how your emotions are constantly changing. Sometimes you feel love and sometimes hatred, sometimes calm and then tense, joyful—sorrowful, happy—sad. Even now you may be experiencing emotions—interest, boredom, relaxation. Think of things you have liked and don't like any longer; of fears that you once had that now are resolved. The only thing you can count on with emotions is that they will change. Although a wave of emotion comes, it will pass in time. Yet while these emotions come and go, notice that in some deep sense that "you" does not change. It must be that although you have emotions, you do not experience yourself to be just your emotions. Allow yourself to realize this as an experienced event, not as a belief. In some very important and deep way you experience yourself as a constant. You are you through it all. So just notice your emotions for a moment and as you do, notice also that you are noticing them [allow a brief period of silence].

Now let's turn to a most difficult area. Your own thoughts. Thoughts are difficult because they tend to hook us and pull us out of our role as observer. If that happens, just come back to the sound of my voice. Notice how your thoughts are constantly changing. You used to be ignorant—then you went to school and learned new thought. You have gained new ideas and new knowledge. Sometimes you think about things one way and some-times another. Sometimes your thoughts may make little sense. Sometimes they seemingly come up automatically, from out of nowhere. They are con-stantly changing. Look at your thoughts even since you came in today, and notice how many different thoughts you have had. And yet in some deep way the you that knows what you think is not changing. So that must mean that although you have thoughts, you do not experience yourself to be just your thoughts. Do not believe this. Just notice it. And notice, even as you realize this, that your stream of thoughts will continue. And you may get caught up in them. And yet, in the instant that you realize that, you also realize that a part of you is standing back, watching it all. So now watch your thoughts for a few moments—and as you do, notice also that you are noticing them [allow a brief period of silence].

So, as a matter of experience and not of belief, you are not just your body . . . your roles . . . your emotions . . . your thoughts. These things are the content of your life, whereas you are the arena . . . the context . . . the space in which they unfold. As you see that, notice that the things you've been struggling with and trying to change are not you anyway. No matter how this war goes, you will be there, unchanged. See whether you can take advantage of this connection to let go just a little bit, secure in the knowl-edge that you have been you through it all and that you need not have such an investment in all this psychological content as a measure of your life. Just notice the experiences in all the domains that show up, and as you do, notice that you are still here, being aware of what you are aware of [allow a brief period of silence]. Now again picture yourself in this room. And now picture the room. Picture [describe the room]. And when you are ready to come back into the room, open your eyes.

The exercise is carried out with eyes closed. The therapist induces a state of relaxed focus and gradually directs the client's attention to dif-ferent domains with which people can become overidentified. Each is examined in turn, and at key moments the therapist punctuates the attention on content with the instruction to notice that someone is notic-ing this content. These punctuations can create a brief but powerful psy-chological state in which there is a sense of transcendence and continu-ity: a self that is aware of content but not defined by that content.

After this exercise, the client's experience is examined, but without analysis and interpretation. It is useful to see whether there were any particular qualities of the experience of connecting with the "you." It is not unusual for clients to report a sense of tranquillity or peace. Life experiences invoked in this exercise, many of which are threatening and anxiety promoting, can be received peacefully and tranquilly (i.e., accepted in a posture of psychological willingness) when they are viewed as bits and pieces of self-content and not as defining the self per se.

It is usually worth touching on the active implications of this experience, if only briefly. The therapist can link the client to experiences with the *Chessboard Metaphor;* for example, "There is one other thing that the board, as a board, can do other than hold the pieces. It can take a direction, regardless of what the pieces are doing at the time. It can see what is there, feel what is there, and still say, 'Here we go!' "

Pick an Identity . . . Any Identity

Sometimes clients are very much involved with self-related talk and self-related logic. A client may have an elaborate network of "insights" into how he or she developed into the person he or she is. Usually these insights are integrated into a life story the client develops about why healthy living is not possible because of a faulty childhood, a lack of self-confidence, low self-esteem, and so forth. This type of process may have been detected earlier in deliteralization work. The *Pick an Identity Exercise* illustrates how language "filters" experience. Further, in changing psychological content rapidly and beyond the normal range for a given individual, the consistent context of self-as-perspective begins to be more evident.

> I want you to play a game with me. It's called the *Pick an Identity Exercise.* Your job is to reach into that box over there and pull out one slip of paper at a time. On each slip of paper I have written down an identity statement. Some of these statements are things that you have told me here. Some of the things describe general characteristics of people. Your job is to pick any four slips of paper, and then I want you to try as hard as you can to imagine that you are the person described in those four slips of paper. Some of the slips will have messages on them that you have told yourself, or seem true of you, and you may see some slips of paper that have messages that you have not thought of. Your job is to take both kinds of messages and try as hard as you can to be that person, right here in the room with me, right now. I'm not trying to change what you believe about yourself. So this is not designed to make you stop believing in any of your ideas about who you are. I'm just interested in seeing what it feels like to actually imagine that you can become the person described by the identity statements, OK?

In this exercise the therapist will place emphasis on helping the client actually take on the characteristics described in the language statement on each slip of paper. Ordinarily, clients will easily assimilate statements that are negative and that they have used before. They may have more trouble with statements that are positive or that are foreign. The therapist's job is to help the client construct the reality of being this person. Then the therapist can ask questions like "What does this person think about his or her career, relationships, and family upbringing?" The therapist may also ask questions such as "How does this person feel around others in a social gathering?" "How does this person feel in an intimate situation?" Once this has been done and the therapist is satisfied that the person has really taken on the imaginary identity, the therapist may ask, "And who is noticing all these thoughts and feelings right now?" Then the exercise is repeated, with a new set of identity slips drawn.

The exercise may be repeated three or four times in a session. There is not necessarily a moral to this exercise. If the client makes remarks about feeling different under different identity formations, then the therapist may point out that different self-related content tends to produce different reactions. However, the most important thing is to simply allow the client to experience directly having different identities. The agenda is not to convince the client that there is a better identity than the one that is currently being held. The mere experience of seeing thoughts as a kind of identity that we take on begins to make the point.

Faking It

A very common theme encountered in ACT is the client's belief that he or she is a "fake." Even though the client may be successful in meeting life demands, struggle continues, with thoughts about having fooled people or about the likelihood of being discovered to be less than he or she pretends to be. The "faking it" motif is a fascinating piece of verbal architecture. Here the mind is literally washing over adaptive, successful human behavior and producing misery and dissatisfaction. The following dialogue reveals how the hegemony of self-evaluation can be undermined through an appeal to self-awareness.

CLIENT: Yes, I went to the get-together with friends like we had planned last week. That did not really affect my depression level, though.

THERAPIST: OK. What did you notice about your depression?

CLIENT: Well, one of the first things that happened when my depression started was that I was involved in a very interesting conversation with a couple who live down the street from me. I noticed that they were both laughing at something that I was saying, which was actually designed to be humorous. But, at the same time . . .

THERAPIST: You mean, *and*, at the same time.

CLIENT: Yes. And at the same time, I knew I was there just because it would help me feel less depressed. I figured that I was not really enjoying it, because of the way I felt. I was saying humorous things, but I wasn't feeling funny, if you know what I mean.

THERAPIST: So you were behaving in ways that were endearing you to these neighbors of yours, and at the same time, your mind was reporting back to you on your feeling state and was also giving you some thoughts to chew on.

CLIENT: Well, mostly, I just felt like I was faking it. At some level, I was sure that they could tell that it wasn't me they were dealing with, but somebody I was trying to be.

THERAPIST: Now let me get this straight. What you're saying is that it wasn't the "real you" who was at this party. The real you was depressed and would not be at the party?

CLIENT: No, the real me would have been at the party depressed and withdrawn, and the fake me was the one who was cracking jokes and making other people laugh.

THERAPIST: OK, so what part of you was there that knew that you were faking it?

CLIENT: Well, I don't know, I'm not sure what you're asking.

THERAPIST: It sounds as though your mind is telling you that it knows what you really are, no matter how you're acting. And that is fine. That kind of stuff is what minds do. What I'm asking is, exactly at the moment that your mind was saying that, who was aware of what it was saying?

THERAPEUTIC DO'S AND DON'TS

Reinforcing the Problem

A key dilemma confronting the therapist in this stage of ACT is the tendency to join the client's language system and begin inadvertently reinforcing talk about the conceptualized self, rather than encouraging direct experience of self that can be used to help live a powerful, committed life. This usually shows itself in the development of an excessive amount of logical, rational talk about why the client can't trust his or her thoughts, the lack of self-confidence, and so on. The best way to offset this pitfall is to focus heavily on experiential exercises and metaphorical talk. The client may misinterpret this process as well, assuming that the therapist's message is that if the client appears not to care about holding onto a particular version of the conceptualized self, then happiness will emerge. It is always important to reaffirm for clients that there is no secret formula that delivers happiness in any consistent way. The objective is to be present with what life appropriately gives the client at any given point in time, in respect to any particular experience. Clients often turn back on themselves in their language and begin evaluating "how well they are staying at board level," as if this were something that could be achieved and never lost. In other words, willingness and detachment experiences provide a new opportunity for the mind to negatively evaluate the client. The ACT therapist should be watching for these subtle self-evaluation processes, which function only to provide more negative content for the conceptualized self.

Spirituality as an Experience, Not a Religion

ACT is not a religion, although many ACT interventions have a distinctly spiritual quality. The ACT therapist must be able to operate from a stance in which perspective, not belief, is what is at issue. There are plenty of religious writings in different cultures dealing with the problems of self-conceptualization and the viability of seeking a deeper form of self-meaning. Religion got there first in the attempt to undo some of the damage caused by "eating from the tree of knowledge." Although many of the ACT messages may be consistent with the messages of different religions, the therapist needs to emphasize the concept of workability for the client, not a belief system. If the client achieves spiritual or religious gains in the process, that is "gravy."

It is perfectly acceptable to use religion-based stories or terms that the client already uses to support ACT interventions. For example, acceptance is much like grace in a religious context, and that connection can be used to show how acceptance is a free, unearned, loving choice and not something that is earned by good content (that connection is made easily inasmuch as *grace* comes from the word *gratis*, or free). Similarly, *confidence* comes from the same root word as *faith* and means "self-fidelity" or "self-faithing." It is helpful to support the client in taking actions of "self-faithing" rather than wait for some other feeling to occur than the one that is there already (e.g., waiting for "confident" feelings to emerge instead of fearful feelings—about the least self-faithing thing one can do).

The Multiproblem Client and Self-Obliteration

More seriously dysfunctional clients sometimes engage in a kind of self-fragmentation in an attempt to adapt to overwhelming personal trauma or to chronic negative environmental stress. Many clients labeled as having character disorders are also victims of self-imposed language-based strategies designed to filter the painful consequences of trauma or chronic distress. The destructive effects of trauma lie less in the event per se than in the escape and avoidance maneuvers used to compensate for the event. The most destructive form of emotional avoidance an individual can make is to fragment the self. At the level of language, such clients often have markedly disturbed identity-related issues, which may lead to pronounced anxiety or fearfulness when exposed to the observing self. Chronically dysfunctional clients may also complain of a sense of boredom, emptiness, or a sense of impending doom. The client may communicate a fear that when he or she is asked to be present with psychological content, some form of psychological annihilation will occur. In metaphorical terms, the client fears falling into a dark hole and never returning. Because self-as-perspective is not thing-like, it can appear to be literal nothingness or annihilation. In a sense this is right, because the observing self does annihilate the overattachment to a conceptualized self. ACT therapists often suggest that clients "kill themselves everyday," but it is the conceptualized self, not self-as-perspective, that is continually killed off (only to reemerge and be killed off again).

In ACT, there is no assumption that dysfunctional clients lack an observing self or are incapable of developing a cohesive self-awareness. In multiple personality disorders, for example, there is one person in the room. The client is being dominated by fragmented content about various conceptualized selves and an avoidance of ongoing self-awareness in the service of avoiding disturbing private content. What dysfunctional clients have in common is their indiscriminate use of emotional avoidance strategies. The client would rather "numb out" (e.g., a borderline client) or be someone else (a person with multiple personality disorder) than confront the dilemmas associated with direct private experience. Although some theories of personality disorder would perhaps discourage confronting identity processes directly (because of a presumed defect in personality organization), ACT strongly promotes the use of experiential and metaphorical exercises that undermine the need for avoidance with such clients. These interventions can undermine the use of fragmentation as an emotional avoidance strategy and help the client to build a cohesive sense of self-awareness and the "I."

PROGRESS TO THE NEXT PHASE

As in any stage of ACT, it is important to learn to recognize signs that indicate that the client is ready to move on to the next phase. Ordinarily, work with the observing self is completed when the client reports a sense of looking at, rather than being caught up in, private experiences. Clients will use language that suggests that they see themselves as separate from their minds. This is particularly noteworthy when it occurs spontaneously, which suggests that it is coming out of the client's experience rather than simply mimicking something the therapist has been saying. Another critical sign at this stage is the ability to laugh at oneself in earnest. In Zen Buddhism, this is referred to as the "all-knowing smile." It really reflects the client's sense of amusement at how seductive self-related processes are, but from a point where this can be laughed at as a forgivable element of human nature. If the Zen saying is true, that a great source of human suffering is the tendency to take ourselves too seriously, then taking oneself lightly through the application of humor, irony, and paradox can only be construed as a healthy life sign. Finally, all these developments are more promising if the client is also beginning to use acceptance and willingness strategies spontaneously in daily life.

PERSONAL WORK FOR THE CLINICIAN: IS YOUR SELF GETTING IN THE WAY?

In the preceding chapter, we asked you to take a look at your positive and negative pieces of self-content. We asked you to release your attachment to them, held as literal truth. We asked you to look at those that were the hardest to let go of and to speculate on how they might be entering into your stuckness with your current main problem. Now we will look at these and other "monsters" you may be avoiding in your attempts to solve the problem. Remember to save your work.

1. What emotion does this problem present that is most difficult for you to deal with?
2. What thought(s) does this problem present that is most difficult for you to deal with? (Suggestion: Some of these may be variants of "hard to let go of" self-related thoughts.)
3. What memory or personal history does this problem present that is difficult? (Suggestion: Some pieces of history act as justification for "hard to let go of" self-content.)
4. Is there anything in these private experiences that, considered on their own terms, you cannot have and still live a vital life? If you can't have them or a part of them, just notice you are not having that part.
5. Are you willing to get in contact with these emotions, thoughts, memories right now? If so, practice having them in a new con-

text. For example, if there is a horrible thought, say the thought out loud 50 times as fast as you can. If it's a painful feeling, hold the feeling in your mind and mentally describe its shape, color, texture, temperature, or smell. Try to see it as a feeling and see yourself feeling it. If it's a painful memory, consider holding it in mind and separating out the physical sensations first, then put them "out there," then move on to the emotions and put them out there, then the images, and put them out there.

6. As you consider each of these content areas, notice also that a conscious person is considering them. Review items 1 to 5, but this time see whether you can also be aware of the person "behind the eyes" who is aware of what you are aware of.

CLINICAL VIGNETTE

You are in the fourth session with a 57-year-old married woman who has been a "closet drinker" for years. Her husband is out of town a lot on business. They have had a somewhat distant marital relationship, but they have "stuck it out." Much of the client's drinking occurs when her husband is gone and she is alone at home. Previous sessions have revealed that her main coping strategies are overcleaning her home, reading books, and watching television. When she "gets quiet," she encounters thoughts like "I deserve to be alone," "I'm never going to find peace and happiness in my life," "I am wasting my life, but I don't know what I'd do with it anyway," "I'm a fake and a coward." This is when she starts drinking. During this session, she says, "All my life, I've had the feeling that I would somehow end up being disappointed and unhappy, and now I'm there."

> *Question for the clinician:* How would you conceptualize this client's dilemma from the ACT viewpoint on versions of self-definition and awareness? What types of strategies would you use to address this issue, and what would be your goal(s) in doing so? (Answer this before looking at our answer!)
>
> *Our answer:* We would see these self-statements as pieces of conceptualized content, the least helpful and most rigid form of self-awareness. These pieces, when held as literal truth, have probably contributed to this client's self-fulfilling prophecy. Our strategy would not be to dispute the truth or falseness of these beliefs, but to enlarge the client's experiential contact with a safer version of self-awareness: self-as-context. We might use the *Chessboard Metaphor* here. To do so, we need to get the black pieces of her

conceptualized content in the room too. As with most self-as-content issues, she is not a carrier of only negative self-beliefs, but positive ones as well. The *Chessboard Metaphor* will help her see that both the negatives and positives are just pieces. Our primary goal in this case would be to neutralize her attachment to the white pieces as truth. Another useful strategy here may be the *Observer Exercise* (the you that you call you). By showing the client experientially that her "you" has been ever present in the face of changing beliefs and expectations about her life, we accomplish much the same awareness shift as with the *Chessboard Metaphor*. If she is going to make meaningful moves in her life, she will have to approach her fears, doubts, anxieties, and hopes from board level.

•8•

Valuing

If we don't decide where we're going, we're bound to end
up where we're headed.

—CHINESE SAYING

ACT assumes that each client already possesses everything that is needed
to define a life direction. What has happened is that the ability to see and
follow a direction has been impaired by verbal fusion and experiential
avoidance. Thoughts about the past, emotions, bodily states, and the
like are often very poor guides to action, especially when they are viewed
in the contexts of literality, control, and reason giving. Chosen values
provide a far more stable compass reading. This is true because thoughts
and feelings often lead in contradictory directions, and they invite a
focus on irrelevant process goals (e.g., getting rid of a certain feeling or
having only certain thoughts). Values can motivate behavior even in the
face of tremendous personal adversity. Clients are hurting, yes . . . value-
less, no. Once awakened, valuing can become a powerful part of a vital
life.

As we shall see, valuing is action of a special kind; it is the kind that
cannot be evaluated by the person engaging in it. Language is very useful
in judging and evaluating actions relative to given standards. Logically,
however, we must reach these standards in some other way than by
judging and evaluating. If we evaluate values, by what values do we
evaluate them? In this sense, valuing transcends logical analysis and
rational decision making. Selecting values is more like postulating,
assuming, or operating on the basis of an axiom than it is like figuring
out, planing, deciding, or reasoning. Valuing is a choice, not a judgment.

ACT is at its core a behavioral treatment. Its ultimate goal is to help the client develop and maintain a behavioral trajectory in life that is vital and valued. *All* ACT techniques are eventually subordinated to helping the client live in accord with his or her chosen values. This means that even such key ACT interventions as defusion and acceptance are, in a sense, secondary. For example, although ACT is emotionally evocative, it differs from some emotion-focused approaches in that there is no interest in confronting painful or avoided private experiences for their own sake. Instead, acceptance of negative thoughts, memories, emotions, and other private events is legitimate and honorable only to the extent that it serves ends that are valued by the client. Helping the client identify valued life goals (this chapter) and implement them in the face of emotional obstacles (the next chapter) both directs and dignifies ACT.

THEORETICAL FOCUS

Behavior is generally shaped by its consequences, both direct and derived; otherwise it would degenerate into random acts with very little significance or survival value. All behavior shaped by its consequences is inherently purposeful. Purpose is not a cause of action, but rather a quality of some forms of action. In the behavioral tradition, much of nonverbal behavior is purposeful in this sense: "Operant behavior is the very field of purpose and intention" (Skinner, 1974, p. 55). But although one can say that the rat presses a lever "in order to get" a food pellet, the future we are speaking of when we say such a thing is *the past as the future in the present* (Hayes, 1992). That is, based on a history of change (the "past"), the animal is responding to present events that have preceded change to other events. It is not the literal future to which the nonverbal organism responds—it is the past *as* the future.

Humans have a different kind of purpose available. In humans, behavior is often guided not just by consequences that have been directly experienced in the past, but also by those consequences that are verbally constructed. Humans learn *if . . . then, before . . . after,* and *cause–effect* relational frames. They can apply these relations to any event, and the functions of the current situation may change accordingly. If a kidnapper tells his victim, "After the clock reaches 12:00, I will kill you," each tick of the clock is likely to be aversive even though no one alive has experienced personal death. "Kill you" in this case is a verbal stimulus with attributes related to it. Many of these attributes have acquired functions, and through the transformation of stimulus functions the verbal concept of death has them as well. The *before . . . after* relation relates the passage of time to this verbally constructed consequence—constructed in the sense that it appears to be a consequence by virtue of its participation in a temporal relational frame. Thus, for verbal organisms, purpose involves *the past as a verbally constructed future in the present.* The future that verbal organisms work toward can thus include many events with which the individual has no direct history at all.

Although ACT focuses on undermining self-defeating forms of verbal control, it also tries to build verbal control where such control works. Valuing is one of those areas. Values are *verbally construed global desired life consequences.* The value of values is that they permit actions to be coordinated and directed over long time frames. Very few human actions are shaped by immediate, direct consequences without significant verbal involvement. In the absence of verbal behavior, consequences are effective over only a very short time frame: minutes to hours at most. Verbal behavior allows consequences to be related to actions even when the consequences are quite delayed. Exactly how this occurs is not yet well understood scientifically. One clue, however, is provided by the taste aversion literature.

Taste aversion (also called the "bait shy effect") is a kind of direct conditioning with extremely delayed consequences, as compared with other forms of direct conditioning. If, for example, an animal is given a novel food to taste and is then made sick, the animal will later avoid the novel food, even if the illness followed the eating by as much as 24 hours. Animals are evolutionarily prepared to relate food-relevant consequences to food-relevant behaviors and cues, but the long time delay effect is more than that. One of the best explanations for this phenomenon is the interference hypothesis originally described by Revusky (1971). In essence, he argued that evolution has simplified the problem by limiting the relevant set of events, which solves the time problem, but only if such events tend to occur infrequently. If, however, we arrange for several different tastes to intervene or otherwise increase the relevant set of events, then taste aversion with long delays deteriorates. Said another way, time is a problem, because with more time there is more and more change and thus it is more and more difficult to detect contingent relationships as compared with chance covariation.

Verbal goals solve this problem presented by time, not through biological evolution and infrequency, but through the extreme specificity permitted by relational networks. Suppose someone tells you, "I will go on vacation in a week. If you mow my lawn for me a week after that, I will pay you $30 at the end of next month." If you follow these directions, the receipt of the $30 in the mail will make it more likely that you will later do what this person asks, but it will probably not make it much more likely that you will open envelopes, even though opening an envelope immediately precedes the receipt of the check. The verbal rule specified a situation, an action, a delay, and a consequence. The $30 is thus verbally placed in a very limited set of events, and change within this set happens far too infrequently for time to present much of a problem.

Verbally constructed contingencies are therefore extremely useful when the consequences of actions are remote, subtle, or probablistic. Many, if not most, human situations are like this. The construction of verbal goals and the actions that will produce them are useful because they specify a small set of relevant events and thus allow people to learn and be guided by consequences that are far more remote than the immediate consequences of importance to nonhumans. Further, they allow people to be motivated to produce outcomes that have never occurred, and to turn their abilities to plan these outcomes. In essence, verbally constructed futures serve as formative and motivative augmentals that can then be tracked.

This effect, in turn, has allowed humans to control their own environments to a much greater degree. Verbally constructed futures act much like actually experienced consequences, but they can be far more abstract, delayed, or probablistic. A human will work to eliminate world hunger even though this outcome has never yet occurred. Small steps toward that goal will be powerfully reinforcing because of the formative augmental effect that establishes lack of hunger worldwide as an important verbal consequence.

If verbal consequences and goals are virtually ubiquitous, why are verbal values needed? Values are more abstract and global than concrete verbal goals and thus provide a kind of verbal glue that makes sets of verbal goals more coherent. This, to some degree, allows a person to avoid working at cross-purposes. For example, if being a loving parent is an important value, it may be easier to spend time with the children instead of watching TV, even though there are useful effects that emerge from TV watching.

The other important feature of values, as compared with other verbal goals, is that values cannot be fully satisfied, permanently achieved, or held like an object. This means that they tend to be relevant over very long time frames, in many situations, and are less subject to satiation and change. This produces a useful kind of persistence. For example, the value of "having intimate, trusting relationships" is not a static achievement; it must be continually sought on a day-by-day basis. We never "reach" being a loving person in the way that we can reach Los Angeles. Concrete life outcomes are obtained through behaving lovingly (e.g., marriage), but note that these concrete outcomes are not the same as the value itself. A marriage can be empty or hostile, for example, or even if it is loving, it does not then absolve the person of the need to continue to behave lovingly.

All normal verbal humans have the capacity for values, for this simple reason: Constructing futures is a basic language function that emerges very early in development, certainly by the preschool years. Valuing requires only this ability, combined with a degree of disentanglement from the more elaborate verbal functions of reason giving and justifications. Thus, developing values in adults is more a matter of removing verbal barriers than establishing the construction of verbal futures. Oddly, when values—verbal events—are treated too verbally and intellectually, they cannot function properly.

At the level of "basic language training," the social/verbal community does not actively promote distinctions between evaluation, justification, rationalization, and valuing. Clients thus tend to comingle valuing with justification and explanation, to such an extent that the functional properties of valuing are virtually buried. Valuing thus tends to produce social and internal pressure to "justify" what one is going to do. For example, the client who is abandoning a very successful but personally unfulfilling career will have to explain again and again why he or she is subjecting the spouse and kids to the risks of unemployment and possible relocation. Justification of actions involves fitting them into existing culturally supported verbal networks. As we will explain later, in many ways this is the exact opposite of valuing, however much it may serve the mainstream culture.

A second and more pernicious effect of the conflation of valuing and justification is that some clients, particularly those with chronic multiproblem profiles, will maintain that they have no real life values at all. When asked to write down what they want their lives to be about, these clients will bring in blank pages. Do these clients really not want their lives to mean anything, or are we witnessing the oppressive effects of language?

Clues are provided in the typical background of chronic multiproblem clients. These clients tend to have been raised in chaotic family environments where contingencies were unpredictable, or they have been exposed to childhood or adolescent trauma (e.g., sexual abuse, violence, severe emotional abuse). Under these conditions, constructing verbal futures leads to disappointment or pain and it seems better not to have powerful goals and values. In this sense, the lack of valuing is a defense. Even with a more functional client, it is common to see the client resist stating values and to cry when finally doing so. It hurts to care about something, particularly if previous caring of that kind was suppressed by pain: what we call "traumatic deflection."

Thus, although values are a part of common everyday parlance, getting even the least disturbed client to make direct contact with salient personal ones is no small achievement. What ACT seeks to do is to penetrate the language-based barriers to making direct contact with personal values, with the conviction that value-driven behavior change is more likely to be sustained over time. At the same time, living in accord with one's values lends an inherent sense of purpose and vitality that will make confronting monsters a legitmate and honorable undertaking.

CLINICAL FOCUS

In this phase of ACT the therapist will address the following issues:

- Learning how values create a sense of life meaning and direction
- Learning the distinction between choice and judgment
- Defining the client's valued directions
- Defining how these values suggest specific life goals
- Defining the actions that will be used to accomplish these goals
- Understanding that valuing is defined in part by behavior, not private content
- Understanding the "hooks" that pull the client out of a valued process of living
- Separating values from unfulfilling social and community pressures

Table 8.1 presents a summary of the major goals, strategy areas, and specific interventions that will be used in this phase.

VALUING: A POINT ON THE COMPASS

The ACT therapist makes several distinctions when discussing the issue of values. Among the most important is distinguishing valuing as feeling versus valuing as an action. These two aspects are often thoroughly confused for the client. The example of valuing a loving relationship with one's spouse is instructive. One's feelings of love may wax and wane across time and situations. To behave lovingly (e.g., respectfully, thoughtfully, etc.) only when one has feelings of love, and to behave in opposite ways when the opposite feelings emerge, would be very likely to have problematic effects on a marriage. Yet this is precisely the pickle we are in when values are confused with feelings, because feelings are not fully under voluntary control and tend to come and go.

This is essentially the same issue we discussed earlier in the context of emotional control and emotional reasoning. The cultural context that supports the association between feelings of love and acts of love is the same

TABLE 8.1. ACT Goals, Strategies, and Interventions Regarding Values

Goals	Strategies	Interventions
1. Understand the importance of value-based living.	Introduce the concept of valuing as action. Distinguish choices and judgments.	Argyle Socks Exercise What Do You Want Your Life to Stand For? Exercise Gardening Metaphor
2. Understand the function of goals in producing healthy living.	Introduce outcome as the process by which process becomes the goal. Teach client hazards of being too outcome focused. Show how choice is necessary for commitment.	Skiing Metaphor Path Up the Mountain Metaphor
3. Outline with the client a value-based life direction in major life domains.	Clarify clients' operative life values. Clarify and reduce external influences that may qualify stated values.	Valued direction narrative Values Assessment Rating
4. Outline the actions the client can take to put values into effect.	Identify goals and actions.	Goals, Actions, Barriers exercise
5. Reduce impact of potential barriers on commitment by changing focus to acceptance.	Identify barriers and classify their characteristics. Eliminate barriers the client is ready to abandon. Introduce valuing and willingness as interdependent.	Bubble in the Road Metaphor

cultural context that supports the client with agoraphobia staying home in the presence of high anxiety and the alcoholic's drinking in the presence of strong urges. If the client bases living entirely on the absence of emotional or cognitive obstacles, then valued directions cannot be pursued in a committed fashion, because sooner or later the obstacle will be encountered. As the client walks along the path of life, emotional obstacles inevitably arise and life asks, "Will you have me?" If the answer is "no," the journey must stop. In the area of values, this means that we must learn to value even when we don't feel like it. We must learn to love even when we are angry, to care even when we are exasperated.

A useful way to distinguish feelings and actions is to start with things the client has no strong feelings about. The following dialogue is an example.

THERAPIST: Let's do a silly little exercise called the *Argyle Socks Exercise*. Do you care how many people wear argyle socks?

CLIENT: No, why should I?

THERAPIST: OK. Well, what I want you to do is really, really develop a strong belief that college boys have to wear argyle socks. Really feel it in your gut. Really get behind it!

CLIENT: I can't.

THERAPIST: Well, really try. Feel overwhelmingly strongly about this. Is it working?

CLIENT: No.

THERAPIST: OK. Now I want you to imagine that even though you can't make yourself feel strongly about this, you are going to act in ways that make argyle socks important to college students. Let's think of some ways. For instance, you could picket the dormitories that have low percentages of argyle sock wearers. What else?

CLIENT: I could beat up college students not wearing them.

THERAPIST: Great! What else?

CLIENT: I could give away free argyle socks to college students.

THERAPIST: Super. And notice something. Although these things may be silly actions, you could easily do them.

CLIENT: And would be forever remembered as that stupid guy who wasted his time worrying about argyle socks!

THERAPIST: Yes, and possibly because of your commitment to it, as the person responsible for bringing argyle socks back into fashion. But also notice this: If you behaved in these ways, no one would ever know that you had no strong feeling about argyle socks at all. All they would see is your footprints . . . your actions.

CLIENT: OK.

THERAPIST: Now here is a question. If you did this, would you be following a value that says that argyle socks are important? Would you in fact be "importanting" about argyle socks?

CLIENT: Sure.

THERAPIST: OK. So what stands between you and acting on the basis of things that you really do hold as important? It can't be feelings if they are not critical even when we are dealing with something so trivial.

Here the ACT therapist is focusing on valuing, *the action*. Efforts at conscious control work in the arena of behavior, but are a problem in the arena of private experiences. It makes much more sense to focus on what can be directly regulated (overt behavior) than on events that cannot easily be controlled (private events). By starting with a trivial matter, the client can see that choosing to hold something as important is not an emotional issue. This may make it somewhat easier to talk about more personally relevant material without conflating feelings and values outcomes.

Choice

Values are useful because they help humans select among alternatives. In humans, selecting among alternatives almost always occurs with concurrent reasons. Reasons, as we noted in a previous chapter, are verbal formulations of causes and effects. They are attempts to answer the question "Why?" To have a precise way of speaking about it, we will call the selection among alternatives based on reasons *judgments*. Judgments are explained, justified, linked to, and guided by verbal evaluations involving the weighing of pros and cons.

For valuing to occur, it is critical that values *not* be confused with judgments—values must instead be *choices*. A choice is a selection among alternatives that may be made with reasons (if reasons are there) but not for reasons. Choices are *not* explained, justified, linked to, or guided by verbal evaluations and judgments. To say that choice is not done for reasons does not mean that there are no historical facts that give rise to a particular choice. Rather, it means that the verbal formulations a given person constructs in regard to a choice do not cause the specific choice to be made. Defined this way, animals can choose but they cannot judge. It seems unlikely that humans, merely because they have added verbal behavior, cannot do what an animal can do quite naturally.

ACT attempts to steer clear of the confusion between chosen action and logically derived action. The following demonstrates how the ACT therapist broaches the issue of judgment and choice:

> "To deal with this issue of valuing, we need to make a distinction. I want us to distinguish between choices and judgments. These two are often confused. A judgment we will define as a selection among alternative courses of action made for a reason. A 'reason' is a verbal formulation of cause and effect, or of pros and cons. When I say 'for a reason,' I mean that the action is linked to the reason, guided by the reason, explained by the reason, or justified

by the reason. So, for example, you may decide to invest in a stock because it has a new product that you think will be successful, has good management, and has a strong record of growth. These reasons guide, explain, and justify the purchase of the stock. Choices are something else. We will define a choice as a selection among alternatives that is not made for reasons, although it is usually made in the presence of reasons because we are such verbal creatures that reasons almost always come along for the ride in any circumstance."

To help the client see the distinction between choices and judgments, the clinician can first explain the distinction intellectually in this way and then put two hands out in front, each in a fist as if holding something, and say, "Quick, choose one." The clinician then asks, "Why did you choose that?" Because the choice is trivial, the most common reaction is "For no reason." (If a reason is given, this trivial choice or a variant can be repeated even more quickly so that the client does not have time to generate reasons.) If the client did not choose a particular fist for a reason, the clinician can then ask in some amazement, "Is that possible? Can you just choose things? And you got away with it? The sky did not fall?"

The clinician can then ask the person to do the same thing while thinking of various reasons for picking the left fist or the right one. For example, the person can be encouraged to think "the right one is better" and then simply to choose one or the other. If that hurdle can be passed, the clinician can say that each hand represents a slightly more important alternative faced by the client (e.g., "The left hand is 'I will buy that table' and the right is 'I will not' "), and the client is asked simply to choose one or the other, now *with* reasons (because anything of importance will evoke an analysis of alternatives) but not *for* reasons. In this fashion, the bar can be gradually raised to an area of values, while maintaining the action as one of choice, not judgment.

If the person keeps offering reasons that address *why* the choice is being made, one strategy is to ask why each reason is true. After this question is repeated two or three times, the usual answer is, "I don't know." This response can then occasion an examination of the "reasonableness" of many such judgments. How reasonable can it be to select among alternatives supposedly for reasons when those reasons are barely skin deep? For example, suppose we ask a client why he or she drinks Diet Coke. The answer will usually be something like "Because I like the taste." If we now ask, "Why do you like the taste?" usually the latency to a credible answer will be very long.

In another variant, the client can specifically be asked to make a choice between two alternatives (e.g., types of food). The therapist can then ask, "Why do you choose that?" This is a trick question, of course. If the person answers it literally, reasons are being formulated, and if the action occurred for these reasons, it was a judgment, not a choice. By repeatedly refusing to accept the answer ("But I did not ask your taste buds to choose—I asked you to choose. And besides, you could have noticed that you liked this food while you chose the other, true?"), the client will often tend to more accurate answers such as "Just because" or "For no reason."

This distinction is important in ACT, not merely because it is the only way to learn how values function, but also because ACT focuses on changing the agenda behind clinically significant behavior that often is reasonable but ineffective. In that sense, willingness versus control is a choice, not a judgment.

Choice has other benefits. For example, it helps the client avoid paralysis when reasoned action does not work. Similarly, it helps the therapist avoid getting entangled with the content and logic of the client's life story.

Most of all, however, the distinction is needed so that clients can value, when valuing works, without needing also to engage in justification and explanation, which can draw them back into the same socially conventional approaches that produced their problems to begin with. Ironically, the language of "free choice" is one of the most powerful forms of language available in this area. It allows each client to be "response-able." The only issues left are what one does and what happens as a result.

In ACT, the language of "free choice" is used frequently, not because it is literally true (scientifically, it is not), but because it is pragmatically true. Some behavior is almost impossible to engage in if it is guided by verbal formulations. That does not mean it is random or literally free. From a scientific perspective, such contingency-shaped behavior occurs because of certain historical conditions, and thus choices are sensible, coherent, and historical. These conditions could be called "reasons," but they are reasons for the scientist, not the person. From the point of view of the client, the closest we can get to speaking about such situations honestly is that choices are "free."

Valuing and Purpose Are Everywhere

Valuing as a behavior is always occurring in the client's life. It cannot be avoided, no matter how shut down and benumbed the client is. Why is this so? Because most behavior is purposeful, whether there is an experienced sense of direction or not. The clock of life is always ticking, and it goes in only one direction: from one moment of now to the next. Any behavior that is historical involves a history of such moments. Any behavior that is consciously purposeful involves a verbally constructed future. In a very real way, behaving *is* valuing, even if the client's thought is, "I'm not really in charge of my life. It is in charge of me. I can't do anything different because I'm trapped in my situation." As the following dialogue demonstrates, the ACT therapist attempts to highlight how the client's behavior reflects values, even if the client is unaware of it.

THERAPIST: I think what you are telling me is that you are not aware of the choices you are making each and every day. So it seems to you as though you aren't acting according to some purpose because you are not aware of having such purposes. If that were actually possible, wouldn't it follow that each day your activity would be completely random? You would be walking around bumping into walls, putting your socks on your hands, brushing your teeth with the toilet brush, going to the wrong place of work, and so forth. Let me ask you, is your life actually that random, or does it just feel as though you are not choosing?

CLIENT: Well, I'm not that out of it, so I guess it mostly feels like I'm not in control of what's happening to me. I don't have any way to change things.

THERAPIST: And choosing to believe what your mind is giving you here, that you are trapped, you proceed to behave like a trapped person, right?

CLIENT: Uh huh.

THERAPIST: I'm not asking you whether you believe you are trapped— what I'm asking is, "Are you able to direct your behavior?" And then I want to know: directed toward what?

It is important not to browbeat the client about this, but rather to gently cut through the illusion that choices are not being made and purposes are not being fulfilled.

What Do You Want Your Life to Stand For?

One of the most powerful ACT "horizon setting" exercises is called *What Do You Want Your Life to Stand For?* This dialogue was with an independently wealthy client who was distressed by his aimlessness:

THERAPIST: If you're willing, I'd like us to do an exercise that might have some very interesting and surprising results, or it may simply get you in touch with something you've known all along. Let's just see what happens.

CLIENT: OK, I'm willing to give it a try.

THERAPIST: This is what I call the *What Do Want Your Life to Stand For Exercise.* I want you to close your eyes and relax for a few minutes and put all the other stuff we've been talking about out of your mind. (*Therapist assists client with relaxation for 2 to 3 minutes.*) Now I want you to imagine that through some twist of fate you have died but you are able to attend your funeral in spirit. You are watching and listening to the eulogies offered by your wife, your children, your friends, people you have worked with, and so on. Imagine just being in that situation, and get yourself into the room emotionally (*pause*). OK, now I want you to visualize what you would like these people who were part of your life to remember you for. What would you like your wife to say about you, as a husband? Have her say that. Really be bold here. Let her say exactly what you would most want her to say if you had a totally free choice about what that would be (*pause and allow the client to speak*). Now what would you like your children to remember you for, as a father? Again, don't hold back. If you could have them say anything, what would it be? Even if you have not actually lived up to what you would want, let them say it as you would most want it to be (*pause and allow the client to speak*). Now what would you like your friends to say about you, as a friend? What would you like to be remembered for by your friends? Let them say all these things—and don't withhold anything. Have it be said as you would most want it. And just make a mental note of these things as you hear them spoken. [The therapist may continue with this until it is quite clear that the client has entered into the exercise. Then the therapist helps the client to reorient back to the session; for example, "Just picture what the room will look like when you come back, and when you are ready just open your eyes"].

CLIENT: That was weird . . . trying to imagine being dead but being there. Sometimes in the past I've thought about suddenly dying. Usually I imagine how blown out everyone would be. How tough it would be on Debbie and the kids.

THERAPIST: So projecting yourself to the point of dying feels like pretty serious business.

CLIENT: Yeah, it seems to kind of dwarf all my problems. At the same time, I get really down on myself because it seems like my life is wasting away.

THERAPIST: I'm curious; when you heard the eulogies, what stood out in the way of things you wanted to be remembered for?

CLIENT: When Debbie said I had been a loving, faithful, attentive husband and a father who always provided for his children. Chuck, the guy I've probably known the longest, said I had been there for him when he needed me the most, when he quit drinking. This actually happened 2 years ago.

THERAPIST: Did anyone stand up and say, "I remember Richard. He spent his life trying to prove he was no fluke"?

CLIENT: (*laughs*) No.

THERAPIST: Did anyone say, "Here lies Richard. He made over two million dollars in his career, and because of that he is eternally worthy"?

CLIENT: (*laughs*) No. What are you trying to tell me?

THERAPIST: Nothing really, just noticing that a lot of things you berate yourself about and struggle with have no connection to what you want to be remembered for. It just seems that you've squeezed yourself mercilessly in the name of things you may not even value.

CLIENT: That's pretty scary, if that's true.

THERAPIST: Yes it is, and it's not about what's true. Its about what works and what doesn't.

In a variant of this exercise, the client can be asked to write a short eulogy on an imaginary tombstone. Often this will demonstrate the dissonance between the client's values and current actions.

THERAPIST: When people die, what is left behind is not so much what they had as what they stood for. For example, have you ever heard of Albert Schweitzer?

CLIENT: Sure. A doctor in Africa, right?

THERAPIST: Right. Now why should you know about this guy? He's dead. Probably most of the people he treated are dead. But he stood for something. So in that same way, imagine that you can write anything you want on your tombstone that says what you stood for in your life. What would you want to have there, if it could be absolutely anything? Think about it for a minute.

CLIENT: He participated in life and helped his fellow human beings.

THERAPIST: Cool; now let me ask you, when you look at what your life is currently standing for, is it standing for that? Are you participating in life and helping your fellow humans?

CLIENT: No, and I'm not sure I can.

THERAPIST: I hear you. So you're on the way to an epitaph like "Spent his entire life wondering whether he had what it took to live it . . . and died unsure."

After completing this exercise in session, it is generally useful to have the client complete the values assessment homework assignment (see pp. 224–225). This helps the client "go on record" with the themes that have emerged during the in-session work. These values will be used repeatedly during the rest of ACT, so the therapist should go over the homework with the client to verify that the key visions of the client are recorded.

Choice and Commitment

If an action is based on reasons, and the reasons change, then the decision itself logically must be altered. In some deep sense this means that true commitments are better done as choices than as judgments. Reasons often point to things that a person cannot control directly. This means that judgments are linked to things a person does not control, and thus one's level of commitment can potentially be undermined.

Marriage illustrates this process clearly. Marriage is a commitment, yet half of all marriages end in divorce. How could this be? In part it occurs because people do not know how to make commitments. They try to make them on the basis of judgments, decisions, and reasons, not choices. In so doing they put their commitments greatly at risk. Suppose, for example, that a man marries a woman "because she is beautiful." If his spouse then has a horribly disfiguring accident, that implies that the reason for marriage has left. Even if the man does not want to react in that way, he may have a hard time dealing with what his logical mind feeds him, inasmuch as the original action was based on, linked to, explained by, and justified by this reason and the reason has now changed. This kind of thing happens all that time when people marry and later find that they no longer have the same feelings of love toward their spouses. Marrying because of love is considered quite reasonable in our culture, and love is dominantly thought to be a feeling, not a kind of choice. But feelings of love are extremely unpredictable. We speak of love as if it were an accident; we say that we fall into and fall out of this emotional state, for example. It should not then be a surprise when we fall into and fall out of marriages in much the same way.

If the client can learn to make choices in these areas, things work differently. Consider how much easier it is to keep a marriage vow if marriage is based on a *choice* to marry and if love is considered to be a *choice* to value the other and hold the other as special. These actions are a-reasonable (not unreasonable).

Commitments constitute an area where the resistance to impulse ("insensitivity") that is characteristic of rule-governed behavior is positive. Held as a choice, nothing can happen that justifies and explains abandoning a commitment, because the choice itself does not need to be justified and explained. If any reasons that came along for the ride then change, the choice itself doesn't have to be changed, because the choice was not linked to the reasons. This absence of verbal "cover" is itself a powerful contingency that helps commitments to be kept.

If the client related well to the *Chessboard Metaphor*, the therapist can link the issue of choice back to that metaphor:

> "It's like the *Chessboard Metaphor*. There are only two things the board can do: hold the pieces and move them all. To move the pieces, we have to go from who we are to who we are not, and then try to move them around. A logical decision is a movement of the board actively linked to the pieces. But because we don't control the pieces, movements of that kind are movements we do not control. A choice is moving the board in a direction with the pieces, not for the pieces. Choice is like saying to the pieces, 'We are moving here,' for no other reason than the fact that you choose to do so. To do this, all the pieces must be welcome to come along, and yet not be in charge. So being willing to 'have what you have' is what makes choice possible."

The *Gardening Metaphor* can also be used to highlight how choice allows one to maintain a fixed course in the face of difficult, provocative, or confusing feedback. This metaphor is also useful in directing clients toward committed actions. For example, if a client values a more loving marital relationship, this metaphor may direct the client into a more active role in that area.

OUTCOME IS THE PROCESS THROUGH WHICH PROCESS BECOMES THE OUTCOME

One reason clients get stuck is that they believe attaining goals is the key to happiness and life satisfaction. They try to get what they want in order to be happy. This method of living is oppressive, because it is func-

GARDENING METAPHOR

Imagine that you selected a spot to plant a garden. You worked the soil, planted the seeds, and waited for them to sprout. Meanwhile, you started noticing a spot just across the road, which also looked like a good spot— maybe even a better spot. So you pulled up your vegetables and went across the street and planted another garden there. Then you noticed another spot that looked even better. Values are like a spot where you plant a garden. You can grow some things very quickly, but others require time and dedication. The question is, "Do you want to live on lettuce, or do you want to live on something more substantial—potatoes, beets, and the like?" You can't find out how things work in gardens when you have to pull up stakes again and again. Of course, if you stay in the same spot, you'll start to notice its imperfections. Maybe the ground isn't quite as level as it looked when you started, or perhaps the water has to be carried for quite a distance. Some things you plant may seem to take forever to come up. It is at times like this that your mind will tell you, "You should have planted elsewhere," "This will probably never work," "It was stupid of you to think you could grow anything here," and so on. The choice to garden here allows you to water and weed and hoe, even when these thoughts and feelings show up.

tionally connected to a state of deprivation. Etymologically, the word *want* means "missing." So trying to be happy by achieving goals is living in a world where what is important is constantly missing. The thing that is needed (i.e., having what you want) is not present. Although this may create motivation and directed action, it squeezes out a sense of vitality. If goals and values are confused, this is the typical result.

The trick is to use goals only as a means to engage in a process and to maintain a direction. There is a maxim in ACT to describe this: Outcome is the process through which process becomes the outcome. When the process of living becomes the outcome of interest, we are no longer living in a verbal world of constant deprivation and want in which something else, somewhere else, is always what is needed. When the purpose of life is living, we always have it right here, right now. The *Skiing Metaphor* shows the relationship between outcome and process, as emphasized in ACT.

Suppose you go skiing. You take a lift to the top of a hill, and you are just about to ski down the hill when a man comes along and asks where you are going. "I'm going to the lodge at the bottom," you reply. He says, "I can help you with that," and promptly grabs you, throws you into a helicopter, flies you to the lodge, and then disappears. So you look around kind of dazed, take a lift to the top of the hill, and you are just about to ski down it when that same man grabs you, throws you into a helicopter, and flies you to the lodge. You'd be upset, no? Skiing is not just the goal of getting to the lodge, because any number of activities can accomplish that for us. Skiing is how we are going to get there. Yet notice that getting to the lodge is important because it allows us to do the process of skiing in a direction. If I tried to ski uphill instead of down, it wouldn't work. Valuing down over up is necessary in downhill skiing. There is a way to say this: Outcome is the process through which process can become the outcome. We need goals, but we need to hold them lightly so that the real point of living and having goals can emerge.

Most clients are vulnerable to being too outcome oriented. They constantly monitor how well they are doing, how successful they are as compared with others, and constantly imagine achieving a better state of mind than the one they are currently in. Consequently, many potentially invigorating life initiatives are stopped short because the outcome is not delivered on schedule.

Taking a life direction—having values—does not mean that we can monitor progress along that direction moment by moment. Sometimes we have to keep the faith even when a valued direction takes unexpected turns. The *Path Up the Mountain Metaphor* can be employed to help the client understand the hazards of constantly monitoring immediate progress toward concrete goals, rather than connecting with valuing as a process. Moreover, this metaphor shows that even painful or traumatic phases in life can be integrated into a positive overall path if we learn from them.

VALUES CLARIFICATION: SETTING THE COMPASS HEADING

The process of values clarification provides one of the most intense, intimate clinical experiences in ACT. The therapist is likely to become privy to information about a client that has never been shared with anyone else. This intimacy may then serve as the basis for the hard therapeutic work of implementing value-based behavior change.

In ACT, the values assessment process serves a variety of assessment and intervention purposes. First, the client may become aware of long suppressed values. This process is motivational in the sense that the client may find major discrepancies between valued versus current behaviors. Second, the process of values assessment can help highlight a place in the client's life in which everything is absolutely perfect and pristine.

PATH UP THE MOUNTAIN METAPHOR

Suppose you are taking a hike in the mountains. You know how mountain trails are constructed, especially if the slopes are steep. They wind back and forth; often they have "switchbacks," which make you literally walk back and forth, and sometimes a trail will even drop back to below a level you had reached earlier. If I asked you at a number of points on such a trail to evaluate how well you are accomplishing your goal of reaching the mountaintop, I would hear a different story every time. If you were in switchback mode, you would probably tell me that things weren't going well, that you were never going to reach the top. If you were in a stretch of open territory where you could see the mountaintop and the path leading up to it, you would probably tell me things were going very well. Now imagine that we are across the valley with binoculars, looking at people hiking on this trail. If we were asked how they were doing, we would have a positive progress report every time. We would be able to see that the overall direction of the trail, not what it looks like at a given moment, is the key to progress. We would see that following this crazy, winding trail is exactly what leads to the top.

In a world filled with imperfection, a person's values are perfect. A person's values may not be what someone else thinks they should be, but are always perfect and complete within themselves. Many clients come to us with a sense that deep down, at the most fundamental level, they are somehow terribly flawed. It is difficult to imagine anything more fundamental than a person's values, and it can be tremendously empowering to find that one has a flawless foundation. After reviewing a values narrative with a client, an ACT therapist may ask, "Is there anything at all that is missing from these values? Could they be improved in any way?" If the client can think of a way they could be improved, the improvement is added by this very awareness, as the client obviously already values the component that was missing or needed modification.

ASSESSMENT OF VALUES, GOALS, ACTIONS, AND BARRIERS

In ACT, the values assessment process itself is a relatively structured and straightforward one, entailing the following six steps:

1. Therapist describes values assessment homework exercise to client.
2. Client completes values assessment homework exercise.
3. Therapist and client discuss values in each domain and generate brief values narratives that simplify, focus, and encapsulate the

free-form values statements from the exercise (see the Values Narrative Form). Typically, the main task is to help the client distinguish goals from values and to state his or her values in terms of directions, not merely concrete ends.

4. Therapist distributes the Values Assessment Rating Form.
5. Client rates values narratives.
6. Therapist and client collaborate to generate goals, actions, and barriers related to the client's stated values (see Goals, Actions, Barriers Form).

The values assessment work sheets are reviewed by the therapist and client and then modified in a collaborative fashion. The therapist's job is to clarify the direction inherent in what might be fairly concrete valued ends. The therapist should also be assessing for other factors that are influencing the client's statements about valued ends:

- Values statements controlled by the presence of the therapist, in conjunction with the client's assumptions about what would please the therapist. Relevant consequences are signs of therapist approval and/or the absence of therapist disapproval.
- Values statements controlled by the presence of the culture more generally. Relevant consequences include the absence of cultural sanctions, broad social approval, or prestige.
- Values statements controlled by the stated or assumed values of the client's parents. Relevant consequences are parental approval—actually occurring and/or verbally constructed.

It is difficult to imagine a client who would have values that were not controlled in part by all of the aforementioned variables. The key is whether removal of an influence would significantly affect the potency of the value as a source of life direction. This task cannot be completed in one discussion. The issue of "ownership" of a value is likely to resurface time and again. Some of these issues may be addressed by asking the client to talk about the value while imagining the absence of a relevant social consequence.

To illustrate, consider a client who forwards the value of being well educated. The therapist may ask if the level of valuing (or the value itself) would change if it had to be enacted anonymously: "Imagine that you had the opportunity to further your education, but you could not tell anyone about the degree you achieve. Would you still devote yourself to achieving it?" or "What if Mom and Dad would never know you pursued an education: Would you still value it?" A different tack may also provide some insight into controlling variables. So, for instance, the

VALUES ASSESSMENT HOMEWORK

The following are areas of life that are valued by some people. Not everyone has the same values, and this work sheet is not a test to see whether you have the "correct" values. Describe your values as if no one will ever read this work sheet. As you work, think about each area in terms of the concrete goals you may have and in terms of more general life directions. For instance, you may value getting married as a concrete goal and being a loving spouse as a valued direction. The first example, getting married, is something that could be completed. The second example, being a loving spouse, does not have an end. You could always be more loving, no matter how loving you already were. Work through each of the life domains. Some of the domains overlap. You may have trouble keeping family separate from marriage/intimate relations. Do your best to keep them separate. Your therapist will provide assistance when you discuss this goals and values assessment. Clearly number each of the sections and keep them separate from one another. You may not have any valued goals in certain areas; you may skip those areas and discuss them directly with your therapist. It is also important that you write down what you would value if there were nothing in your way. We are not asking what you think you could realistically get, or what you or others think you deserve. We want to know what you care about, what you would want to work toward, in the best of all situations. While doing the work sheet, pretend that magic happened and that anything is possible.

1. *Marriage/couples/intimate relations.* In this section, write down a description of the person you would like to be in an intimate relationship. Write down the type of relationship you would want to have. Try to focus on your role in that relationship.

2. *Family relations.* In this section, describe the type of brother/sister, son/daughter, father/mother you want to be. Describe the qualities you would want to have in those relationships. Describe how you would treat the other people if you were the ideal you in these various relationships.

3. *Friendships/social relations.* In this section, write down what it means to you to be a good friend. If you were able to be the best friend possible, how would you behave toward your friends? Try to describe an ideal friendship.

4. *Career/employment.* In this section, describe what type of work you would like to do. This can be very specific or very general. (Remember, this is in an ideal world.) After writing about the type of work you would like to do, write about why it appeals to you. Next, discuss what kind of worker you would like to be with respect to your employer and co-workers. What would you want your work relations to be like?

5. *Education/personal growth and development.* If you would like to pursue an education, formally or informally, or to pursue some specialized training, write about that. Write about why this sort of training or education appeals to you.

6. *Recreation/leisure.* Discuss the type of recreational life you would like to have, including hobbies, sports, and leisure activities.

7. *Spirituality.* We are not necessarily referring to organized religion in this section. What we mean by spirituality is whatever that means to you. This may be as simple as communing with nature, or as formal as participa-

tion in an organized religious group. Whatever spirituality means to you is fine. If this is an important area of life, write about what you would want it to be. As with all of the other areas, if this is not an important part of your values, skip to the next section.

8. *Citizenship.* For some people, participating in community affairs is an important part of life. For instance, some people think that it is important to volunteer with homeless or elderly people, lobby governmental policymakers at the federal, state, or local level, participate as a member of a group committed to conserving wildlife, or participate in the service structure of a self-help group, such as Alcoholics Anonymous. If community-oriented activities of this type are important to you, write about the direction you would like to take in these areas. Write about what appeals to you in this area.

9. *Health/physical well-being.* In this section, include your values related to maintaining your physical well-being. Write about health-related issues such as sleep, diet, exercise, smoking, and so forth.

---

therapist may ask, "What if you were to work very hard for a degree, and Mom and Dad knew and were proud, but the day after you received the degree you forgot everything you had learned. Would you still value it to the same degree?" As the client plays with imagined consequences, he or she may be chagrined to find that parental approval is the "straw that stirs the drink." In this case, becoming well educated is not a value at all, but a goal in the service of some other value (i.e., being loved by and loving those who are in my life). Once this value is clarified, it is written down as a desired end. It is not uncommon for some values to change in valence over the course of therapy, or even as a function of the initial assessment.

As noted on the values clarification forms, the client is asked to generate responses in various life domains. Often clients come in with domains left empty. With more dysfunctional clients, all the domains may be empty or may contain very superficial answers. Here, the therapist needs to patiently, and in a nonconfrontational way, discuss each domain. It often helps to go back earlier in the client's life and look for examples of dreams, wishes, or hopes that have disappeared because of negative life events. At other times, the therapist may have to assist the client either in generating the directions inherent in specific life goals or, conversely, in generating specific goals from more global directions. The client may also list ends that are not possible. For example, a woman may say that she wants to regain custody of a child who was given up for adoption 10 years ago. In such instances, the therapist tries to find the underlying value and goals that might be achievable if one were moving in that direction. After discussing and refining the values narratives, the therapist should generate a Values Assessment Rating Form.

VALUES NARRATIVE FORM

Generate a brief narrative for each domain, based on discussion of the client's values assessment homework. If none is applicable, put "None." After generating all narratives, read each to the client and refine. Continue this process, simultaneously watching out for pliance-type answers, until you and the client arrive at a brief statement that the client agrees is consistent with his or her values in a given domain.

Domain	Valued direction narrative
Couples/intimate relationships	
Family relations	
Social relations	
Employment	
Education and training	
Recreation	
Spirituality	
Citizenship	
Health/physical well-being	

VALUES ASSESSMENT RATING FORM

Read and then rate each of the values narratives generated by your therapist and you. Rate how important this value is to you on a scale of 1 (high importance) to 10 (low importance). Rate how successfully you have lived this value during the past month on a scale of 1 (very successfully) to 10 (not at all successfully). Finally, rank these value narratives in order of the importance you place on working on them right now, with 1 as the highest rank, 2 the next highest, and so on.

Domain	Valued direction narrative	Importance	Success	Rank
Couples/intimate relationships				
Family relations				
Social relations				
Employment				
Education and training				
Recreation				
Spirituality				
Citizenship				
Health/physical well-being				

GOALS, ACTIONS, BARRIERS FORM

Given the valued direction listed, work with the client to generate goals (obtainable events) and actions (concrete steps the client can take) that would manifest these values. Using interviews and exercises, identify the psychological events that stand between the client and moving forward in these areas (taking these actions, working toward these goals). If the client presents public events as barriers, reformulate them in terms of goals and place them within their relevant value (the domain may differ from that which originally raised this issue). Then look again at actions and barriers relevant to these goals as well.

Domain	Valued direction	Goals	Actions	Barriers
Couples/intimate relationships				
Family relations				
Social relations				
Employment				
Education and training				
Recreation				
Spirituality				
Citizenship				
Health/physical well-being				

Assessing Goals and Actions

This part of the assessment process asks the client to focus on developing goals and specifying the actions that can be taken to achieve those goals. This is the most applied aspect of the assessment and the most critical, because it directs the therapy. The work on goals, actions, and barriers stands on the foundation of the client's values. Given the direction specified in each life domain, the client is asked to generate specific goals. A goal is defined as a specific achievement, accomplished in the service of a particular value. For example, if the client values contributing to society, we might ask about specific ways in which this value could be put into action, perhaps by getting involved in local organizations. The client then defines actions that would likely achieve the goal. The client may decide to call the Red Cross, to give money to the United Way, or to volunteer at a local soup kitchen. The therapist and client try to generate acts that can take the form of homework. In some cases they may involve single instances. At other times they may involve a commitment to repeated and regular acts. Typical goals and actions may include the following:

1. *Career:* investigating reentering school, applying for a new job, asking for a raise, talking to a career counselor
2. *Leisure:* joining a softball team, attending church, asking someone out on a date, going dancing, having a friend over for dinner, going to an NA meeting
3. *Intimacy:* setting aside special time to spend with a spouse, calling or visiting a child from a former marriage, calling or visiting parents, making amends in severed friendships
4. *Personal growth:* arranging to make payments on back taxes, child support, or bills; learning a foreign language; joining a meditation group

An important aspect of effective goals-action work is to monitor for a close connection between the action, its associated goal, and the associated value. Will this action, if taken, actually produce the goal or lead to it? Is the action feasible and within the client's range of abilities? Does the client understand the temporal relationship between the action and the goal? Some actions are like seeds in the *Gardening Metaphor.* They need to be "put into the ground" and allowed to sprout. Other actions produce immediate results, such as resigning from an unsatisfying job in order to pursue the goal of growing a new career. It is always wise to encourage the client to "accumulate small positives" in the action-goal arena. The impact of little steps taken consistently is generally greater than that of heroic steps done inconsistently. The emphasis is on engaging in actions that feel like "steps in the right direction," that is, actions taken that are experienced as consistent with the client's values and stated goals.

Identifying and Undermining Barriers to Committed Action

Effective behavioral goal setting requires a candid analysis of the barriers the client is likely to encounter that may forestall action. Barriers may involve negative psychological reactions or pressure from outside sources. The client who contemplates resigning from an unfulfilling job will most like encounter thoughts such as, "You're making a big mistake. What if you don't find your dream job, then what'll you do?" Negative anticipatory emotions may also show up, such as fear, anxiety, or shame. External barriers may appear too. The client's spouse may disagree with the decision, may resent the subsequent restrictions in life-style as money becomes tight, or may accuse the client of being selfish rather than self-sacrificing. These external barriers can lead to still more negative private events and more avoidance. The client may also realize that pursuing one course of valued action (e.g., more satisfying and challenging work life) collides with another valued course (e.g., building intimacy in primary relationships). The point is that engaging in valued action nearly always stimulates psychological content in one way or another. Particularly when this content is negative, it can function as a barrier to action. Our clients do not get stuck in life serendipitously. They get stuck because they avoid taking valued actions as a means of avoiding painful emotional barriers.

If previous ACT work has been successful, the client is ready to recognize the barriers for what they are, not what they advertise themselves to be. This part of the values clarification process helps the client identify the barriers to valued action in each domain. As these barriers are discussed, the therapist helps the client to examine several issues:

1. What type of barrier is this? Is it negative private events or an external consequence that conflicts with another value?
2. If this barrier did indeed present itself, is it something you could make room for and still continue to act?
3. What aspect of this barrier is most capable of reducing your willingness to have it without defense?
4. Are any of these barriers just another form of the client's emotional control or emotional avoidance change agenda?

WILLINGNESS TO HAVE BARRIERS AND BARRIERS TO WILLINGNESS

After the client's compass and proposed direction have been set, it is time to reintroduce willingness in a new light: It is a value-based action and is inherently a choice. Independent of some overarching life purpose, why would anyone voluntarily evoke painful personal content or unfavorable personal consequences from the environment? The answer is, no one would. Willingness is dignified by the presence of values, and it makes the embodiment of those values possible.

At this point in therapy, this interdependence is simply touched on and clarified for the client. There is no pressure put on the client to dispense with the "believable" barriers, for those barriers will form the backdrop for the final phase of ACT: committed action. The *Bubble in the Road Metaphor* expresses the linkage between willingness and the ability to take a valued direction.

BUBBLE IN THE ROAD METAPHOR

Imagine that you are a soap bubble. Have you ever seen how a big soap bubble can touch smaller ones and the little ones are simply absorbed into the bigger one? Well, imagine that you are a soap bubble like that and you are moving along a path you have chosen. Suddenly, another bubble appears in front of you and says, "Stop!" You float there for a few moments. When you move to get around, over, or under that bubble, it moves just as quickly to block your path. Now you have only two choices. You can stop moving in your valued direction, or you can touch the other soap bubble and continue on with it inside you. This second move is what we mean by "willingness." Your barriers are largely feelings, thoughts, memories, and the like. They are really inside you, but they seem to be outside. Willingness is not a feeling or a thought—it is an action that answers the question the barrier asks: "Will you have me inside you by choice, or will you not?" In order for you to take a valued direction and stick to it, you must answer yes, but only you can choose that answer.

The ACT therapist weaves these topics together to fit the client's situation: willingness, choice, valuing, actions, and barriers. Living a powerful, vital life is not really possible without willingness to have barriers, a set of valued directions that make dealing with these barriers purposeful, and a choice to act in the face of unpredictable consequences.

THERAPEUTIC DO'S AND DON'TS

Coercive Use of Choice

There is a potentially dark side of the therapeutic intimacy that develops when valuing is on the table. Often, it moves both the therapist and client into the realm of moral judgments. Morals are social conventions about what is good; values are personal choices about desirable ends. To be maximally effective, the ACT therapist must be able to work sincerely with the client. Some clients enter therapy with histories or current problems that are morally repugnant to the therapist, such as battering, addiction, repetitive suicidal behavior, and so on. Values clarification work often exposes these areas, yet the ACT therapist cannot be drawn into the role of "moral detective," using the social influence of therapy to openly or implicitly coerce the client into conforming to broadly held social values. The therapist makes the same move the client is asked to make, namely, to see valuing as essentially a personal exercise.

For example, in working with an alcoholic in the ACT model, there is no assumption that being intoxicated on a daily basis is incompatible with living life in a direction valued by the client. Because the values and direction are the client's to choose, it is actually a legitimate outcome for a client to choose to abuse alcohol. Language, of course, will make it seem as though this choice is the "wrong one" to make, because the interests of society are not served by sanctioning alcoholism. Therapy is a verbal enterprise, and it is therefore inextricably intertwined with social control functions. The therapist must avoid falling into the trap of using choice as a way to blame the client.

The language of "free choice" is a powerful language and can easily be used to coerce the client. This usually occurs when the therapist takes a posture such as, "Well, of course, if you choose to continue drinking, that is your choice. You have to make the choice. I can't do it for you. Just remember that its the choice you made, when it comes time to endure the consequences." Although this posture may be technically correct (it is the client's choice and only the client can live out the consequences), the psychological stance is, "The choice you are making here disappoints me, and you are morally wrong for making it."

On occasion, a client may come to therapy with values that are so divergent from the therapist's that a collaborative working relationship cannot be established. In such cases, the therapist should refer the client elsewhere. In the vast majority of cases, however, client and therapist values are sufficiently similar that a basic schism over valued life directions will not develop.

Confusing Values and Goals

A common problem in this phase of ACT is the therapist's failure to detect goals that are presented as values by the client. For example, the client may say, "I want to be happy." This sounds like a value, but it is not. Being happy is something you can have or not have, like an object. A value is a direction—a quality of action. By definition, values cannot be achieved and maintained in a static state, they must be lived out. When goals are mistakenly taken as values, the inability to achieve a goal seemingly cancels out the value. A practical way to avoid this confusion is to place any goal or value statement produced by the client under the following microscope: "What is this in the service of?" or "What would you be able to do if that was accomplished?" Very often, this exercise will reveal the hidden value that has not been stated. Some "values" are really means to an end, in which case they are not values at all. Experiential avoidance itself is a good example. The means–end relationship is revealed if the therapist asks, "What would avoiding anxiety be in the service of?" or "What would you be able to do if you could avoid anxiety?" The client may answer that it would then be possible to live a more valuable life. The therapist could then ask, "If you weren't anxious, what would you be doing that would tell you that you were living a more valuable life?"

Avoiding anxiety is a pseudovalue, and much of the impact of ACT comes simply from sorting this out and moving more directly to actions linked to values. When the values implicit in current actions are made explicit, the client will often reject them. For example, the client would probably not choose a tombstone that read, "Here lies Fred. He spent his life avoiding anxiety."

The culture is dominated by a focus on object-like outcomes (e.g., goals that are attained). In most cases, the first time the client completes the values exercise it will be an exercise in goal definition, not in values clarification. The therapist's job is to detect this confusion of process and outcome and help the client connect specific behavioral goals to values.

PROGRESS TO THE NEXT PHASE

Conclusion of this phase is marked by the completion of the values, goals, actions, and barriers exercise, and when the identified barriers have been reduced to the "critical few." Another indicator that this phase is over is the client's emerging readiness to engage in action. The client may still report anxiety or uncertainty about handling the "fall-out" from engaging in committed action. At the same time, the client has unequivocally connected to values and has focused on goals and actions that promise to make life better if they are put in motion.

PERSONAL WORK FOR THE CLINICIAN: TAKING A DIRECTION

In the previous two chapters, we asked you to look at the most troublesome thinking, feeling, and personal history aspects of your main problem. You were asked to "make room" for these experiences and to practice seeing them as experiences, rather than as "defining" you. In this exercise you will examine what you want your life to stand for in respect to this problem, and what you may have to be willing to accept along the way. Please save your work; you will need it again in the next chapter.

1. When you think about your life path into the future, what are the most important values you want embodied in your life (e.g., career, intimacy, spirituality, recreation/leisure, friends/family, community belonging, personal growth/challenge)? Try to think of at least one important value in each of these areas.

2. Your main problem can either act as an obstacle to your path or become the forum in which you put your values into action:
   a. How could the problem (or its associated thoughts, feelings, personal history) act as an obstacle to your journey?
   b. How could you use the problem as an opportunity to embody your valued directions in life?

3. What would you have to "make room for" (be willing to have) on your way to transforming this problem into a situation that mirrors your values?

4. Is there anything you would be unwilling to have, even if it meant stepping back from what your values would have you do here?

CLINICAL VIGNETTE

You are in the sixth session with a 48-year-old divorced woman who is the mother of two adult children. She entered treatment because of chronic recurrent depressions that started in her early twenties. As a consequence of these depressions, she was divorced when her children were 11 and 13 years old and, because she believed she was a "bad" mother, relinquished custody of her children to her husband. Her husband developed a severe alcohol problem and was verbally abusive to the children throughout their adolescence. She is disaffected from her children, in part because of her own guilt and in part because they still accuse her of walking out on them. Her current depression seems to have started as a result of a conflict over her birthday party. For different reasons, her two children were unable to attend the party. In doing her "values, choices, goals, and actions" work, she identified rebuilding her relationships with her children as a key goal in the context of her stated value: "Being remembered as a loving, caring, and committed mother." In this session she says, "I don't know how I'm ever going to get them to love me. They have been so badly hurt by my choices, they probably will never forgive me. If I reach out to them and they reject me, I don't know if I could stand the pain."

> *Question for the clinician:* Conceptualize the client's dilemma from the ACT viewpoint on valued action, willingness, choices, controllable outcomes, and emotional barriers. What strategies and/ or interventions would you use, and what would be your goals in doing so? (Complete this part before looking at our answer!)
>
> *Our answer:* The client is struggling with the fact that actions she values taking may not produce the outcomes in others she is seek-

ing. She is confusing the "intention" of being a committed, caring mother (the process) with how her children will end up relating to her (the outcome). There is another unstated, slippery value here as well: "I will not engage in any action that may lead to others hurting or rejecting me." In other words, when her willingness must extend to the point of having to "make room for" the possibility of her children's rejection, she is not willing. So her willingness is conditional, and that is usually problematic. Our strategy here might be to point out the conflict between her stated and unstated values and how one value promotes willingness while the other detracts from it. We might also talk about the issue of choice here. She is free to choose the allegedly safer course (don't do anything that might lead to rejection), taken as a choice. We might wonder out loud whether she made a choice much like that in her divorce. We would employ metaphors that distinguish the action from the outcome to help her grasp the reality that "intending" to be (i.e., standing for) a caring, committed mother is a completely controllable outcome and a valued course of action. Which choice is she going to pick?

•9•

Willingness and Commitment: Putting ACT into Action

Our deepest fear is not that we are inadequate. Our deepest fear is that we are powerful beyond measure. It is our light, not our darkness, that most frightens us. We ask ourselves, "Who am I to be brilliant, gorgeous, talented, fabulous?" Actually, who are you *not* to be? You are a child of God. Your playing small does not serve the world. There is nothing enlightened about shrinking so that other people won't feel insecure around you. We are born to make manifest the glory of God that is within us. It is not just in some of us, it is in every one. And as we let our light shine, we give others permission to do the same. As we are liberated from our fears our presence liberates others.
—NELSON MANDELA

If you always do what you always did, you'll always get what you always got.
—"MOMS" MABLY

THE CLIENT'S QUANDARY AND THE WAY OUT

It is one thing to use the forum of therapy to help a client define a valued direction in life. As many therapists have discovered, it is quite another to get the client to proceed in that direction. Life asks whether the client is willing to pay the price of behavior change. Any change, no matter how unassuming, will trigger intended and unintended consequences,

235

and significant change will almost always elicit a variety of negative private responses in the client. It is in part the avoidance of this class of events (i.e., uncomfortable private experiences) that has led the client into therapy in the first place, and it is only at the point where behavior change is initiated that the client is really faced with the emotional price tag of change. The ACT client has been making room for negative content in the presence of a therapist, but that is quite different from facing the "real thing" in one's life on a daily basis.

This chapter will focus on the "C" of ACT: getting the client to engage in valued actions while making room for their intended or unintended consequences. This phase is entered with the following assumptions: that the unworkable change agenda has been abandoned, that a certain degree of willingness has been created, and that valued directions have been identified. In short, all the ingredients needed to move forward to a valued life are present.

THEORETICAL FOCUS

There are several theoretically important principles that underpin the ACT focus on willingness and commitment. Whereas acceptance often has a somewhat passive quality, willingness and behavioral commitments involve actively engaging in actions that may invite the presence of negatively evaluated thoughts, emotions, and bodily states. Many of the metaphors and exercises described in this chapter are used to call up these avoided private experiences in and out of session.

This phase of ACT also links up in important ways to the values clarification that has preceded it. Not all verbal behavior is problematic. Formulating valued ends and intermediate goals is necessarily a verbal activity. At the same time, behavioral activity that moves a client toward a valued end has an important nonverbal quality. For example, looking at a compass and figuring out which way is North could be considered a verbal event; however, once oriented, stepping northward has an important nonverbal quality. It is only through committed action, and its associated intended and unintended effects, that the client can move from knowing what it is he or she wants from life, to finding out what actually works to achieve those ends.

Put more technically, committed action is the mechanism through which unworkable plys and inaccurate tracks will be undermined, and socially valued but individually meaningless augmentals will be abandoned or significantly reformulated. If the values work described in the preceding chapter has been successful, the client has developed or reestablished augmentals that provide overall verbal purposes where those are most helpful. This sets the stage for a confrontation with unworkable aspects of old rule systems, but old rules and their effect on behavior cannot be detected and changed entirely through verbal means. Only in the context of actual movement toward valued ends will destructive rules systems present themselves fully. Only in the world of actual behavior can new rules that track actual contingencies be tested. Further, there is no way to shape behavior directly without actual contact with contingencies, and a significant goal of ACT is to reduce rule-governed behavior where that form of behavior is not useful. For all of these reasons, ACT without active willingness and commitment is very unlikely to succeed. For more functional clients, the refinements in existing rules may be modest; more dysfunctional clients may be learning what works for the first time.

In this phase of ACT, therapy can resemble a program of systematic exposure and behavior change. What is different from traditional exposure treatment is that the dominant focus is on private events as well as overt situations: emotions, thoughts, bodily sensations, and the like are particularly important. The deliteralization work done earlier allows exposure to thoughts and other private events to occur in a fundamentally different way. In ACT, thoughts are observed as an ongoing behavioral process rather than dealt with referentially or literally. That change seems to permit more direct contact with previously avoided events. The hope is that habituation is enhanced as a result.

During this phase of ACT, clients are likely to formulate rules regarding any emerging unpleasant material that reflect the original problematic rule system. These may come in the form of "Oh, this is terrible, I can't stand this" or possibly in the form of self-plys such as "I must learn to cope with this." The emergence of old rule systems provides in vivo opportunities for the therapist to defuse the client from self-defeating verbal behavior, and to support letting go of that highly routinized verbal repertoire while adopting a more open posture toward direct experience. Cognitive defusion and openness to experience have the side effect of sensitizing the client to natural rather than verbally constructed contingencies, which in turn may allow the client to respond more effectively to environmental demands.

Unlike many other aspects of ACT, commitment is a domain in which the insensitivity produced by rules is actively sought. Many contingencies are delayed, subtle, or probabilistic. Commitment involves the description of valued behavior that one is going to produce and the subsequent production of that behavior under the control of this self-rule. If the behavior is successful in producing valued outcomes, the temporary insensitivity produced by overt commitment will allow those contingencies to be contacted. The work done earlier in ACT to undermine reason giving is particularly helpful in this phase of therapy because it allows no easy verbal escape for self-defeating behavior.

CLINICAL FOCUS

The goal of this phase is to elicit behavior change and then to support the client's commitment to sustaining such change. To achieve this, the therapist will focus on the following therapeutic topics:

- Willingness is the primary condition for committed action.
- Willingness is not wanting, it is an act of choice.
- There is no such thing as being partly willing.
- Willingness does not require heroic steps.
- Committed action inevitably invites unwanted private experiences.
- Commitment is funded by an ongoing process of valuing.
- Barriers can be identified using the FEAR algorithm.
- Committed action can be maintained using the ACT algorithm.
- Pain and trauma can function as barriers to willingness and committed action.
- The victim role can interfere with committed action.
- Forgiveness and self-acceptance can allow commitments to be kept.

Key ACT goals, strategies, and interventions associated with this phase are presented in Table 9.1.

EXPERIENTIAL QUALITIES
OF APPLIED WILLINGNESS

Applying willingness to support action consistent with chosen values is a central goal of ACT. If the client makes powerful contact with a certain issue and begins to struggle, the ACT therapist may ask, "Can you let go of that, right at this moment?" The goal is to increase the client's ability to detect struggle and abandon it, right in the middle of the most difficult moments. There are several manifest qualities of this type of applied willingness that make it a unique form of chosen action.

Willingness Is Not Wanting

The client will sometimes confuse willingness with wanting. It is not uncommon for a client to say in response to the willingness question, "No. I really don't want that." This confusion of willingness and wanting is not helpful. *Want* means "missing" (e.g., "For want of food he

TABLE 9.1. ACT Goals, Strategies, and Interventions Regarding Applied Willingness and Commitment

Goals	Strategies	Interventions
1. To understand qualities of applied willingness and choice.	Show that willingness cannot be limited qualitatively. Show safe ways to limit willingness.	Joe the Bum Metaphor
2. To understand the nature of willingness and commitment and the link between the two.	Show how pain turns into trauma. Show how willingness supports commitment.	Jump Exercise Swamp Metaphor Expanding Balloon Metaphor Take Your Keys with You Metaphor
3. To see how barriers to willingness are formed and are dissolved.	Show how right and wrong affect willingness. Show how forgiveness and self-worth are choices. Show how overt action functions in the implementation of chosen values.	Eye Contact Exercise FEAR and ACT Looking for Mr. Discomfort Exercise High School Sweetheart Metaphor Fish on the hook metaphor Empty Chair Exercise Accepting Self on Faith Exercise Exposure exercises

died") and, yes, no one is missing panic, urges, depression, and so on. That is not the question, however. In the effort to live without willingness, clients are sometimes attached to the idea that if they withhold willingness to have content, the content will go away. Their experience says the exact opposite.

A successful ACT client (one who had had a severe agoraphobia) once said it this way: "I used to hold back willingness as if my life depended on it, because I figured God or someone would rescue me if I held out long enough. It was as if reality or some force should and would care that I was in pain and would come and take it away. Finally, I saw that only one thing could happen if I was unwilling, and that lots of things could happen if I was willing. So now I'm willing as if my life depends on it, because actually my experience tells me that it does." The *Joe the Bum Metaphor* helps make this point experientially.

JOE THE BUM METAPHOR

Imagine that you got a new house and you invited all the neighbors over to a housewarming party. Everyone in the whole neighborhood is invited—you even put up a sign at the supermarket. So all the neighbors show up, the party's going great, and here comes Joe-the-Bum, who lives behind the supermarket in the trash dumpster. He's stinky and smelly, and you think, "Oh no, why did he show up?" But you did say on the sign, "Everyone's welcome." Can you see that it's possible for you to welcome him, and really, fully, do that without liking that he's here? You can welcome him even though you don't think well of him. You don't have to like him. You don't have to like the way he smells, or his life-style, or his clothing. You may be embarrassed about the way he's dipping into the punch or the finger sandwiches. Your opinion of him, your evaluation of him, is absolutely distinct from your willingness to have him as a guest in your home.

You could also decide that even though you said everyone was welcome, in reality Joe is not welcome. But as soon as you do that, the party changes. Now you have to be at the front of the house, guarding the door so he can't come back in. Or if you say, "OK, you're welcome," but you don't really mean it, you only mean that he's welcome as long as he stays in the kitchen and doesn't mingle with the other guests, then you're going to have to be constantly making him do that and your whole party will be about that. Meanwhile, life's going on, the party's going on, and you're off guarding the bum. It's just not life enhancing. It's not much like a party. It's a lot of work. What the metaphor is about, of course, is all the feelings and memories and thoughts that show up that you don't like; they're just more bums at the door. The issue is the posture you take in regard to your own stuff. Are the bums welcome? Can you choose to welcome them in, even though you don't like the fact that they came? If not, what's the party going to be like?

The metaphor reveals two central characteristics of the fantasy that underlies unwillingness: first, that if only invited *and* wanted guests came to the party, life would be grand, and second, that withholding willingness to welcome the unwanted guest will somehow promote peace of mind. The reality is the opposite. In fact, most clients have noticed that when they try hard to stop one reaction from joining the party, other undesirable reactions follow along right behind—what one ACT therapist called "the bum's chums."

Willingness Has an All-or-Nothing Quality

The client may begin to promote the idea that willingness can be achieved via sequential steps. Willingness is not measured by the magnitude of the situation the client tackles; it is a "whole act." As the Zen saying goes, "You cannot jump a canyon in two steps." The *Jump Exercise* makes this point.

Willingness is like jumping. You can jump off lots of things. [Therapist takes a book and places it on the floor and stands on it, then jumps off.] Notice that the quality of jumping is to put yourself in space and then let gravity do the rest. You don't jump in two steps. You can put your toe over the edge and touch the floor, but that's not jumping. [Therapist puts one toe on the floor while standing on the book.] So jumping from this little book is still jumping. And it is the same action as jumping from higher places. [Therapist gets up on a chair and jumps off.] Now this is jumping too, right? Same quality? I put myself out into space, and gravity does the rest. But notice, from here I can't really put my toe down very well. [After getting back up on the chair, the therapist tries awkwardly to touch the floor with a toe.] Now, if I jumped off the top of this building, it would be the same thing. The jump would be identical. Only the context would have changed. But from there it would be impossible to try to step down. There is a Zen saying, "You cannot jump a canyon in two steps." Willingness is like that. You can limit willingness by limiting context or situation. You get to choose the magnitude of your jump. What you can't do is limit the nature of your action and still have it work. Reaching down with your toe is simply not jumping. What we need to do here is learn how to jump: we can start small, but it has to be jumping from the very beginning or we won't be doing anything fundamentally useful. So this is not about learning to be comfortable, or grit-your-teeth exposure, or gradually changing habits. This is about learning how to be willing.

Willingness Is Safely Limited Only by the Size of the Situation

Even with the caveat that heroic steps are not required to apply willingness, any notion of letting "monsters" in the room can be frightening to clients. They do not know what will happen if they let go. Clients see the value of willingness, and yet they want to keep it limited. The agoraphobic client may say, "I'm willing to put up with my heart racing, but if I start to feel dizzy or sick, I'm leaving." There are ways to limit willingness safely, but most of the normal actions taken to limit it are destructive. The client cannot learn willingness by changing its quality, because then the client is not limiting willingness but instead is destroying it. Willingness can safely be limited only by situation. When willingness is limited in a way that changes its qualitative nature, it is no longer willingness. Being half-willing is like being half-pregnant.

RECONNECTING WITH VALUES,
GOALS, AND ACTIONS

The context for discussion about willingness and commitment is the client's values that are attached to a set of desired goals and actions. Willingness will be necessary to help the client "inhale" these barriers and keep moving. At this point, the therapist and client should begin to review the contemplated actions in each of the major life domains. Although it is desirable to have something listed in each domain, this is not essential. What is essential is that the client begins to develop at least one high-priority target. High priority means it is important to the client's values and, because of that, it is highly likely to elicit negative private content—predictions of failure, memories of past failed attempts, fear of emotional consequences, and so forth. As the following monologue demonstrates, it is important for the therapist to keep the focus on willingness, not on barriers.

"There's an issue that underlies the question of willingness, and that issue is, Can you make a commitment and keep to it? Is it possible for you to say, 'It would work for me in my life to do this, and, therefore, I'm doing it' and then to do it? And if you slip, or fail at the attempt, to turn right around and do it again? Is commitment—which is a choice—a real possibility, not only in the area of emotional discomfort and disturbing thoughts, but in other areas of life as well? This is not about someone else's life or standards, this is about you and your standards. We are also not talking about something that will necessarily feel good. In fact, I'm predicting that the first thing you will encounter, if you haven't already, is your own mind blabbing at you, criticizing you, predicting failure, and so on. My question to you is, knowing that all these things will happen and that you may not always live up to your commitment each and every day, are you 100% willing to commit yourself to this? Are you willing to do what would work to enhance your life and to have whatever thoughts, feelings, or memories arise as you do it? What stands in the way of you setting your willingness on high right now?"

Whatever barriers are forwarded should simply be noted by the therapist. These will eventually be revisited during subsequent exposure exercises. The therapist may say, "You have identified some pretty formidable reasons for not being willing to tackle this area. Let me ask you, from your experience, has being unwilling worked to protect you over the long haul from these reactions?"

COMMITTED ACTION AS A PROCESS

It is not unusual for the client to avoid making a commitment because of the fear of failing to keep it. Less functional clients in particular have a long history of failing to keep commitments and an equally long list of reasons for why that is so. Eventually, commitments are avoided as a way to avoid feeling the pain of failure. The following session dialogue with a substance-abusing client highlights the utility of emphasizing the process of committed behavior and deemphasizing the outcome of committed behavior:

THERAPIST: We've been talking a lot about values and what direction you want to head in your life.

CLIENT: Mmmhmmm.

THERAPIST: And one thing that has come through clearly is your sense that getting loaded is inconsistent with where you want to head.

CLIENT: Yeah, well that's for sure.

THERAPIST: And so I'm wondering whether you'd like to make a commitment to not using?

CLIENT: Well, I've tried that. I mean a million times.

THERAPIST: Yes. And what is between you and making that commitment right here and now?

CLIENT: Well, I just . . . I can't . . . I mean I haven't . . . It's just that it wouldn't . . . I mean it wouldn't mean anything. I wouldn't mean it.

THERAPIST: Oh well, I don't want you to make a commitment and not mean it. But is this a commitment that you would like to make—if it was just your choice?

CLIENT: Well, yeah . . . I mean, sure—but . . .

THERAPIST: No, I'd want you to mean it 100%. So what's between you and doing that?

CLIENT: Well, I've done that before, and, well, you know.

THERAPIST: But that's not what I'm asking. What I'm asking is: What's between you and making that commitment right now and 100% meaning it?

CLIENT: But what if I fail?

THERAPIST: How can you fail?

CLIENT: Well, by using.

THERAPIST: Oh, I'm not asking you to commit to an outcome! I'm asking if you can take a stand right now in your life . . . knowing that you will probably screw it up. The commitment is not about that you will never screw up. The commitment is that if you do, when you do, that what you will do then is to pick up and take a direction that you value again.

COMMITTED ACTION INVITES OBSTACLES

Once the client has committed to a valued direction, it is time to act. During this phase the therapist must not only support and help structure the client's "game plan," but also be vigilant for signs that the client is slipping back into avoidance behavior. Many metaphors and exercises are used in this phase to help the client understand that committed action invites obstacles and that moving through these obstacles is necessary for personal growth to occur. The *Eye Contact Exercise* is a core ACT intervention. In an individual session it is done with the therapist and client. In a group session clients can be paired, with the therapist acting as coach.

This exercise ordinarily elicits a host of uncomfortable reactions in

---

EYE CONTACT EXERCISE

During this exercise we will look in each other's eyes for about 3 minutes. It may seem longer when you actually do it, but that's all it takes. What the exercise will consist of—if you're willing to do it—is getting a couple chairs and pulling them close together. The job is to get present with me and maintain eye contact. It is not a stare down. You don't have to say anything, or do anything, or communicate anything—just be present with me. Now, your mind will tell you all sorts of reasons that you can't do that: it will give you body sensations, or perhaps a desire to laugh, or maybe you'll be worrying about how your breath smells, or you'll be bored or distracted. But the purpose of the exercise is simply to notice these things, to experience all the pieces coming up, and to notice how you sort of come and go from being really present, from really experiencing being here with me. [As the client does the exercise, the therapist says things like, "See whether you can stay with the simple reality that there's another person over here, looking at you. See whether you can let go of the sense of wanting to do this 'right.' . . . If you find yourself talking about this, or evaluating it, just notice that you're doing that, and then come back into the room and get in touch with the exercise. . . . I want you to notice the incredible fact that there is another person here, another human being, looking back at you. . . . See whether you can connect with the experience of discomfort in simply being present to another person."]

---

the client (and in therapists that are new to it), and it demonstrates how even a simple committed act can bring up the most painful psychological content. This makes the client appreciate that committed action can be expected to produce barriers and that it is possible to simply have them and move forward.

The exercise is also a potent metaphor for what is called for in important relationships with one's friends, spouse, and family. Excess evaluation, superficiality, and other such defenses can be serious barriers to intimacy. There are few moments as pure and lovely as when two lovers are looking into each other's eyes or a parent is watching a small child at play. Part of what gives those moments an almost transcendent quality is the absence of defense, evaluation, and chatter. The task is simply to behold. We are all capable of it, but sometimes we lose track of that capacity in the day-to-day rush of life.

A MAP FOR THE JOURNEY: FEAR AND ACT

Maintaining committed actions over time can present a particularly thorny problem for some clients. The client with a personal history replete with instances of starting out fast, then running out of gas, is a good example. This type of client gets hooked easily into old avoidance behaviors and lives life in "fits and starts." Chronically depressed clients are typical. Many actions are started, few are maintained. In some instances the symptom pattern may reappear over time, such as substance abuse. At other times new forms of unworkable behavior may appear, such as avoidance of social situations, working 16 hours a day, or starting fights with one's spouse. These unworkable behaviors are typically accompanied by symptoms more traditionally understood: depression, panic attacks, and the like.

In ACT, there are several culprits that contribute to a failure to complete committed actions. The first is that the actions taken are not connected to valued ends by the client. The client is acting on behalf of social values or to receive some type of social approval from family, spouse, therapist, or so forth. In this case, the resistance seen is a kind of counterpliance. A second is literality: the client has been hooked by a barrier to willingness. Often destructive reason giving is used to bolster and uphold these barriers. A third is that the person is taking a step that is too large, without proper practice in making commitments, contacting barriers, defusing and accepting, and maintaining valued actions.

To help orient the client regarding these problems, the client should be taught the FEAR and ACT algorithms. In essence, these are metarules that capture all of ACT in a short formula.

The FEAR algorithm is a self-monitoring procedure designed to help the client pinpoint which type(s) of barriers to willingness have surfaced. FEAR requires the client to look at the following areas:

Fusion with your thoughts
Evaluation of experiences
Avoidance of your experiences
Reason giving for your behavior

This list can be printed on one side of a wallet-sized card. The client is asked to carry it in a wallet or purse or post it in a conspicuous place (e.g., the refrigerator door). When the client is feeling stuck, the algorithm gives some needed guidance about what to look for. On the flip side of the card, the ACT algorithm is presented:

Accept your reactions and be present.
Choose a valued direction.
Take action.

An effective way to practice use of the FEAR and ACT algorithms is to elicit psychological barriers in session. The purpose is to bring up the original reactions by design, deliteralize them, and increase the client's willingness to simply make room for them. If the impact is greater, the therapist and client may go to a setting outside the therapy office that will help stimulate discomfort. For example, a client with agoraphobia can meet with the therapist at a mall. An obsessive–compulsive person can meet with the therapist at home and go though hoarded trash. Alternatively, props (e.g., letters, pictures) that elicit difficult emotions can be brought to the session to enhance direct exposure.

In exposure exercises of this kind, it is helpful to label the purpose in ways that are a bit playful, such as the *Looking for Mr. Discomfort Exercise.* Clients can be asked whether they are ready to look for Mr. Discomfort. If they are unwilling, earlier issues need to be covered again. (e.g., "OK . . . and let's look at the cost of that."). When describing the purpose of exposure exercises, the scene should be set carefully.

In the exposure session, ask the client to look for emotional discomfort and disturbing thoughts. If the client begins to experience discomfort, get a description of what the discomfort is in great detail. Look for specific components: bodily sensations, emotions, memories, thoughts, and so on. For each element, ask the client, "Just see whether you can let go of the struggle with [the disquieting thought, feeling, memory, physical symptom] for just a moment, whether you can be willing to have it, exactly as it is, not as it says it is or as it is threatening to become." If the

---

LOOKING FOR MR. DISCOMFORT EXERCISE

We're going to go out and find Mr. Discomfort, to try to call him forth, talk to him, and find out what's going on in your relationship with him. If Discomfort does not show up, that's OK. Our goal is just to experience being willing to have him there. If he shows up, and at any time you find that you are not willing to stay and see what happens, that's OK, too—and still this is a commitment you've made, so I'd like you to see whether you can stay with it. We're going to go there and maybe do some things that will push your discomfort buttons a bit. However, there will be no tricks, nothing to startle or surprise you; any steps we take I'll suggest first, and you can choose to go along with them or not. Notice that this exercise will not be limited by time; these hot buttons could get pushed any time, so it will not be a matter of getting through this exercise. Clock watching won't apply. If you are just going to endure this, you are digging. We'll quit when the work is done. When Mr. Discomfort shows up, we will try to renegotiate your relationship with him. We're also going to be trying to call up the passengers from the back of the bus, to see whether we can examine and change the nature of the relationship you have with them. We'll be looking at all the dimensions of that relationship, with the goal of helping you let go of the struggle and keeping your hands on the wheel (see *Passengers on the Bus Metaphor* in Chapter 6).

---

client begins to sink into panic, sadness, or some other negative state, suggest that the client direct attention back to the external environment. Ask the client to remain aware of the negative private experiences, but also to notice the other things happening in the external environment.

This type of applied willingness exercise is especially useful when a client is about to retract a commitment because he or she can't "stand it." The client has been hooked into the old change agenda: "If I reduce the valued end, maybe the uncomfortable material will go away or will dissipate to where I can tolerate it." By applying an emotional exposure intervention, the feared private events are deconstructed and will be "seen" differently (i.e., recontextualized) when they show up again in real life.

Journeying and growth metaphors are another powerful means to legitimize obstacles and to make moving through them a valued act. Many clients have long-standing and strongly reinforced avoidance repertoires that can be expected to reappear. As demonstrated in the *Swamp Metaphor*, the client's job is not just to determine a direction, but to reaffirm that direction when obstacles appear. The *Swamp Metaphor* highlights the fact that when we are traveling in a particular direction, the journey can take us across difficult ground. It also communicates that we don't walk into pain because we like pain. We walk through pain in the service of taking a valued direction.

SWAMP METAPHOR

Suppose you are beginning a journey to a beautiful mountain you can clearly see in the distance. No sooner do you start the hike than you walk right into a swamp that extends as far as you can see in all directions. You say to yourself, "Gee, I didn't realize that I was going to have go through a swamp. It's all smelly, and the mud is all mushy in my shoes. It's hard to lift my feet out of the muck and put them forward. I'm wet and tired. Why didn't anybody tell me about this swamp?" When that happens, you have a choice: abandon the journey or enter the swamp. Therapy is like that. Life is like that. We go into the swamp, not because we want to get muddy, but because it stands between us and where we are going.

There is an old saying in strategic therapy that applies here: "Life is one damn thing after another. Our job is to make sure it's not the same damn thing." The necessity of growth and struggle in life is a hard message to hear, and its lack of support from the larger culture no doubt contributes to our fascination with methods of avoidance.

In essence, this phase of ACT asks the client a question: "Given a distinction between a chessboard and the pieces, is the board able to hold those pieces, fully and without defense, as they are and not as they say they are, and move everything in a chosen direction?" A colleague of ours, Victoria Follette, says it this way: "Can you hold and move?"

Think of yourself as the expanding balloon in this *Expanding Balloon Metaphor*. At the edge of the balloon is a zone of growth, where the same question keeps being asked: "Are you big enough to have *this*?" No matter how big you get, there's always more "big" to get, and the same question keeps being asked. When an issue presents itself, you say yes or no. If you say no, you get smaller. If you say yes, you get bigger. If you keep answering yes, it does not necessarily get any easier, because the issue that shows up may seem just as difficult in relative terms. It does become more habitual, however, and your experience provides a reservoir of strength. If a difficult problem arises, you might think you could say, "No, I don't want that problem to be next," but life presents each new issue as your situation evolves, and it may not be possible to choose the sequence of the challenges. Figure 9.1 shows this situation in graphic form. If you hit an issue you refuse to deal with, usually you have to distort your life around that issue until it is faced.

The *Take Your Keys with You Metaphor* is a physical metaphor that presents the relationship between avoidance and action quite

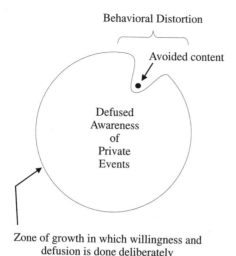

Behavioral Distortion

Avoided content

Defused
Awareness
of
Private
Events

Zone of growth in which willingness and
defusion is done deliberately

FIGURE 9.1. In the balloon metaphor, unwillingness causes distortions of behavior.

clearly. In the metaphor, keys on the client's key ring are said to represent different difficult emotions, memories, thoughts, and reactions. The metaphor highlights two important aspects of these keys. First, picking up the keys and carrying them does not keep the client from going anywhere, and second, the keys can actually open doors that might be locked to us without them. Doing the exercise with the actual keys the client uses also gives the client a physical touchstone, or reminder of his or her goals (where the client is going), the means of going (willingness), and what the client must carry with him or her to move (the client's history and the reactions it may produce). Because we use our keys many times in a day, this metaphor plants a seed that can be contacted frequently outside therapy sessions.

PRIMARY BARRIERS TO COMMITTED ACTION

The client who remains resistant to committed action at this point is often struggling with the effects that significant change will have on a "life story." We use this term loosely to describe personal history as it is constructed by the client, as well as the impact this history has on the conceptualized self. The ostensible purpose of personal history telling is to make sense of what *is* happening as a logical result of what *has* hap-

TAKE YOUR KEYS WITH YOU METAPHOR

Ask whether the client carries keys and whether you can borrow them. Put the keys on the table and say, "OK, suppose these represent the things you've been avoiding. See this key here? That is your anxiety. See this key, that is your anger at your mother." (Continue fitting major issues to the client's keys.) The keys are then placed in front of the client, and the client is asked, "What are you going to do with the keys?" If the client says "Leave them behind," say, "Except that two things happen. First, you find that instead of leaving them behind, you keep coming back to make sure they are left behind, so then you can't go. And second, it is hard to live life without your keys. Some doors won't open without them. So what are you going to do with your keys?" The process continues, waiting for the client to do something. Most clients are a bit uncomfortable about actually picking them up. For one thing, it seems silly (which in itself is another "key"), and for another, the keys are symbols of "bad" things. In that context, actually picking them up is a step forward, and the therapist should keep presenting the keys until they are picked up, without ordering them to be picked up. If the client says, "I would feel silly picking them up," or "What do I need to do?" point to a key and say, "That feeling? That's this one here. So what are you going to do with the keys?" When they are finally picked up, say something like, "OK. Now the question is, where will you go? And notice that there isn't anywhere you can't go with them." Also note that other keys will keep showing up—that is, answering the question affirmatively now does not mean that the same questions won't be asked over and over again by life. The client should also be asked in the natural environment to think about letting go of avoidance of difficult emotions, thoughts, and so on, every time he or she touches, carries, or uses the keys. Suggest that when the keys are used that the client also affirmatively choose to carry his or her experiential "keys."

pened. It is indeed ironic that one of the most threatening moments of all for many clients is when they contact the possibility of actually being different in a positive way, particularly if it threatens the underlying story and may appear to make it wrong. A colleague of ours, Chris McCurry, described it as playing one of two craps games: in one you can win being right about your story, but you have to pay with your own vitality and openness to change; in the other you play for the winnings of vitality and openness to change, but you have to pay with your own self-righteousness.

The threat to one's underlying story may, in the most blatant cases, precipitate rapid relapse, noncompliance, and dropping out of therapy. The ACT therapist must be aware that the real cost of change is experienced at the point of change. However far along a client is in the course of committed action, there is always the possibility that some unintended negative consequence will appear.

Pain, Trauma, and Victimization

Many clients have difficult personal histories containing physical, sexual, and verbal abuse, alcohol- or drug-abusing parents, financial privation, premature or suicidal death of a parent, and so on. These clients have learned that life can be unpredictable and punitive. Such clients may be concerned about the cost of making life-enhancing but potentially painful moves. They may believe that limiting willingness for exposure to painful thoughts, feelings, memories, or sensations will limit their sense of trauma. In fact, the opposite is true. Being willing to experience thoughts and emotions as they are (not as what they say they are) is what makes the difference between an experience that is painful and one that is traumatic. Psychological pain is one thing. It hurts, but it does not in itself do damage. Psychological trauma is pain compounded by an unwillingness to experience the pain. It not only hurts, it damages. By defending against the pain, clients in fact hurt themselves much more, and the effects of their pain may persist.

It is possible to teach the client, from an experiential perspective, the difference between pain and trauma. One way to train the client to make this discrimination is to generate several examples of painful and traumatic events from the client's life. The client is asked to describe these past events in considerable detail; both the original pain and the client's reactions to the actual events (especially the client's control efforts) are "brought into the room." Various domains of response should be carefully inventoried: bodily reactions, emotions, memories, thoughts, and so on. The sense of trauma should be noted. When each reaction comes into awareness, the client is asked to let go of the struggle with this specific reaction. As willingness is applied to these remembered events, the context of the event shifts and there is often an immediate and perceptible reduction in tension. In that shift is the information the client needs to be able to distinguish pain from trauma, because as the client becomes more willing to experience pain, the pain will usually remain but the trauma associated with it will disappear.

It is not uncommon for the client to resist eliciting this material by blocking off the material. When this happens, the therapist should first help the client to notice how burdensome the avoided content feels as it is resisted. The client is asked to just notice any bodily sensations, emotions, or thoughts that are part of the experience of unwillingness. The therapist may ask to client to start by letting go of the struggle with unwillingness, to be willing to be unwilling. If the client is able to make that move, then he or she is gently asked to just notice the difference between struggle and letting go, and to see whether it is possible to let go a little more and to bring up the avoided material.

The client may throw up many obstacles, including a refusal to participate in the exercise at all. All therapists know the experience of the client who sits back and says, "No," or takes the posture, "You can't make me do it." For the ACT therapist, this is just grist for the mill. The client is very familiar, and in a sense comfortable, with this move. The therapist may say something like, "What is showing up seems really intense for you." The client may be asked to notice how the relationship between the client and the therapist feels at that moment. This is not asked as a judgmental question, but as noticing question: "How does it feel to be in this stance, right here, right now, and can you let go of your attachment to that?"

The *High School Sweetheart Metaphor* helps instill an appreciation of how a lack of willingness lets original pain evolve into trauma. Most people know how it feels to lose a first love. This metaphor helps the client make contact with the negative consequences that would follow when one avoids future intimacy in order to be protected from being hurt again.

As the client engages in committed actions, painful emotions may be elicited. The client should understand that a painful situation can be measured this way: "Did it promote your sense of health and wholeness, or did it add to your sense of trauma, damage, and life constriction?" The experience of pain per se is not always a reliable metric, because many forms of growth are painful. Properly done, however, ACT reduces the experience of trauma even when pain is necessarily on the path to a more valued life.

Life Is Not Fair: The Victim Role

A powerful theme, and one that can easily derail the client at this stage, emerges when it becomes clear that living a valued life is possible. This prospect of achieving behavior change simultaneously implies, "You are

---

HIGH SCHOOL SWEETHEART METAPHOR

Recall a time when you were in high school and were in love with someone who rejected you. Can you remember how terrible the pain seemed to be at the time? For some people, this pain leads to lifelong scars, to a pattern of not trusting other people and avoiding opportunities for real intimacy. Look at the pain from your first rejection and ask yourself: How would it have worked if it really was OK just to hurt when you lose something? You have little control over the pain in your life—people will reject you, people will die, bad things will happen. Pain is a part of living none of us can avoid. But what you do have control over is whether the pain turns into trauma. If you are unwilling to hurt, you have to avoid pain. Remember how hard it was for you, as a teenager, to open up after your first real rejection. But if you don't open up, the damage continues and continues.

not broken, you are stuck." As noted earlier, many clients have adopted a life story that, consciously or unconsciously, requires them to remain "broken" in order to prove someone else "wrong." This someone else can be an abusive parent, a family that ignored childhood pleas in regard to sexual abuse by a neighbor, a spouse who suddenly falls in love with another person and leaves. This often makes the client's life little more than an ongoing temper tantrum in which the cry is, "Life's not fair. Look what it's done to me!" The dilemma the client is faced with is, "If I stop being a victim, the wrongdoer will never have to confess and apologize!"

The social/verbal community provides such powerful reinforcement for "being right" that it is somehow satisfying to keep others on the hook even if it is personally destructive. As the following monologue demonstrates, the ACT therapist must identify the functional connection between failing and remaining a victim who demands redress.

> "I want to put an issue on the table, one that you may have some difficulty with, or objections to. That's OK, and if so, I'd like to talk about it. This has to do with how important it is to remain victimized by the wrongs you have experienced in your life. You have a choice between enhancing your life right now, and remaining a victim. If you choose to remain a victim, the only way you can do that is by trading away this opportunity. It is like the legal concept of corpus delicti: If there has been a murder, there should be a dead body. So you nominate yourself to be the dead body to prove that the crime was committed. The question is this: Would you rather keep them (parents, spouse, others) on the hook or live your life? Make no mistake about it, if you get healthy, those you have blamed can sit over there and say, "We raised her right; we were strict and we gave her what she needed to survive. And finally she has come around." If you move ahead, there would no longer be any 'smoking gun' to implicate your parents or anyone else for what they did to you. You will certainly have the thought that your story has been 'wrong.' I don't mean wrong in the sense that these things didn't actually happen; they most certainly did. I do mean wrong in the sense that you can't use your history to retraumatize yourself by acting on the assumption that you are broken because of your history. It is like a fishhook that goes through you and then through others. There may be no way to get yourself off the hook that doesn't seem to let others off."

This type of intervention is always delicate, because the client may feel invalidated by the therapist's refusal to accept the weight of the client's causal argument: "I'm broken because of what has happened to me." The therapist must always assure the client that the events in question are not being disputed. What is being disputed is the necessity of living a self-defeating life in the service of waiting for the recognition and redress that seldom, if ever, comes.

Guilt and Self-Loathing

Progress toward valued ends may slow down when the client believes that keeping a commitment is the only way to atone for past failures. This functionally connects commitment with guilt, and therefore commitment is guilt behavior, even when the client succeeds. The client should understand that life runs in real time; it works by addition, not subtraction. Guilt regarding past failures has no necessary relationship to present commitments. The surest way to undo a commitment is to functionally link it with something that is dead, gone, and can't be changed. Guilt is always connected to "I'm bad" and thus weakens the client's ability to move ahead.

The following transcript from a session with another substance-abusing client demonstrates how the ACT therapist addresses guilt that is interfering with committed action. This client had expressed strong values about his family relations. He viewed himself as the black sheep of his family. His brother, whose love he prized greatly, was going to visit him on the day of the therapy session. The client had recently been released from the hospital with a serious, self-inflicted knife wound, had reentered substance abuse treatment for the ninth time, and had been forced by his financial situation to move his wife and child into a very meager house.

CLIENT: This is my oldest brother, and he is coming to see me, and now I am in this little [house]—last time he saw me I was living down on that 16 acres—had this big house.

THERAPIST: Livin' large.

CLIENT: And now, you know, I mean in this little 600-square-foot little house.

THERAPIST: And a big bandage on your belly.

CLIENT: Big bandage on my belly, so I put on the right clothes so he would not see it; I find myself going through all these things to cover my ass. Went through a panic cleanup at the house so things would look good, putting on this face, you know, ah, and feeling high anxiety, feeling ashamed of myself, I haven't done anything and, you know.

THERAPIST: Lots of passengers showed up.

CLIENT: Yeah, man, everybody, you know; the bus is full, Jack. You know.

THERAPIST: All right, so the question is?

CLIENT: My life could be simple, what's wrong with that, and that's OK. He probably would not care; he'd probably see the simplicity and leave it there. I'm the one going through all these frigging head trips, and if he is or isn't, it really should not matter, but it seems to.

THERAPIST: Well, here are two things . . .

CLIENT: (*laughs*) Yeah.

THERAPIST: . . . as far as your reactions are concerned. One is, do you feel that this is important to you, and the answer to that is yes, and I would suggest that you can no more get rid of that feeling, turn it off and on like a light switch, than you can urges to drink, so my recommendation with that would be . . .

CLIENT: Invite them to the front of the bus.

THERAPIST: By the way, how close are you to your brother?

CLIENT: Very, from what, you know, I hear so many stories from different people, but from what I can see, our family is very close.

THERAPIST: How do you feel about your brother?

CLIENT: I feel very close to him. He is very important to me.

THERAPIST: And you're afraid that if your brother knew that you hadn't been doing real great lately, you know, that you've had some trouble . . .

CLIENT: That it would just be me and the same old, same old, nothing is changed.

THERAPIST: So he'd think less of you?

CLIENT: That he would not think any better of me. 'Cause this has been going on for years.

THERAPIST: I want you to check something out, and that is, you care about being close with your brother, and one of the things that you're doing here is that you're keeping your brother from knowing what is going on with you, so that you can maintain that closeness. See the problem? (*spoken in hushed tones*).

CLIENT: Uh um, yeah, it's like if I had 6 months, and I could say, Hey, I've got 6 months clean and sober—but I've had countless 60 days sober.

THERAPIST: I want you to check out the sort of insidiousness of this, because there is a similar process that I am sure goes on in your own life with you . . . between you and you, between you and your wife, between you and your brother. In order to maintain the illusion of connection, you sever actual connection.

CLIENT: Uh, um.

THERAPIST: Do you follow?

CLIENT: Yeah, I think I understand what you are saying.

THERAPIST: It's like thinking, "Being close to my brother is important to me, so I can't tell him what's going on."

CLIENT: Right, which makes it, which puts you further away.

THERAPIST: Maybe you maintain the illusion of closeness, though.

CLIENT: Yeah.

THERAPIST: But, you know, my guess is that on some level or another you're sort of in touch with . . . and you're sort of carrying this kind of thing where, "I can't let him know what's going on with me." And I wonder, how do you think he would respond if you told him this? And I don't, I'm not suggesting . . . I trust you to do what you need to do, but imagine a scenario like this: What if you were to say something to him like, "You mean really a lot to me, and I know that I haven't done really well, and I kind of am afraid to even let you know that I've had trouble, because you'd think, you know, 'There he goes again,' and I'm afraid to tell you that I'm doing better, because you'd think, 'Oh, there he goes again.'" What if you were to tell him that being close to him means so much to you that what you were inclined to do is to not tell him that you've had some trouble, because you're afraid that he might think less of you?

CLIENT: Uh, um.

THERAPIST: How would he respond to that?

CLIENT: He'd be open armed, I know that. My whole family would. I'm the one that conjures up all this. But when I feel that I've got to approach him, ah, you know, it's like, I can't tell him, how can I tell him? You know, I mean, I'm on food stamps, and, you know, that I, eh, I don't know, I got to paint this bullshit picture, and it is bullshit (laughs).

THERAPIST: I'm wondering what is there between you and taking this opportunity to reaffirm that closeness between you and your brother.

CLIENT: *(pause)* Oh, I don't know.

THERAPIST: As if there were something physical between you and taking this opportunity?

CLIENT: It's probably just coming out and saying it just like you said.

THERAPIST: What would be between you and just saying that?

CLIENT: My fear of disappointing him, I guess.

THERAPIST: And can you bring that one up to the front of the bus and drive?

CLIENT: Yeah, let's do it.

Forgiveness

One of the most elegant forms of willingness is forgiveness. Most clients have a hard time with forgiveness, because it sounds like a change in judgment or evaluation. It sounds like "I used to think you were wrong, but now I've changed my mind." Worse, it may appear to be equivalent to emotional avoidance: excusing, denying, or forgetting old angers and hurts. But the word *forgive* itself suggests a more positive way to approach this difficult topic: We can take it to mean "give that which came before"—literally, *fore-giving*. It means repairing what was lost. *Gift* comes from the Latin *gratis,* or free. In that sense, fore-giving is not earned: it is free.

However, the gift of forgiveness is not a gift to someone else. Giving what went before is most particularly not a gift to the wrongdoer. It is a gift to oneself. If one cannot have the grace that went before a wrongdoing, even if it was valuable, then life's injustices are made permanent. And they are made permanent by the victim's action—not by the actions of a perpetrator. The *Empty Chair Exercise* is a popular therapeutic strategy in Gestalt therapy and other traditions that can be used in ACT to address the issue of forgiveness.

> Have the client sit in one chair, and place an empty chair before him or her. Tell the client to imagine someone sitting in the chair (it may be the client) who needs his or her forgiveness. Ask the client to describe the situation that needs forgiveness, the feelings and thoughts (identified as such) that are associated with the issue, and how he or she has handled these thoughts and feelings in the past. Ask the client if he or she can let go of the struggle with needing vengeance, and to be willing to feel whatever thoughts or feelings are associated with that, as well as those associated with the painful situation. Have the client tell the

"other person" in the chair whatever needs to be said. Also ask the client to verbalize what he or she needs to hear from that other person as part of the forgiveness process.

It is often useful to have the client work on the act of forgiveness and self-acceptance outside the session and independent of any committed action homework. This is often such a pivotal issue for the client that a certain amount of privacy and self-reflection may be beneficial. The *Accepting Yourself on Faith Exercise* is an effective home practice strategy that can be used to process the client's out-of-session self-acceptance work.

ACT AS A BEHAVIOR THERAPY

During the latter portions of this phase, ACT takes on the character of traditional behavior therapy, and virtually any behavior change technique is acceptable. The difference is that behavior change goals, guided exposure, social skills training, modeling, role-playing, couples work, and so on, are integrated with an ACT perspective. Behavior change is a kind of willingness exercise, linked to chosen values. The integration of traditional behavior therapy and ACT in this phase is an important topic, but is well beyond the scope of this book. Fortunately, most ACT therapists seem to have no great difficulty melding the two.

TERMINATION AND RELAPSE PREVENTION

Generally, when valued behavior change has been put into motion and several goals have been accomplished, it is time either to terminate or cut back therapy. Like the expanding balloon, there is no limit to how "big" a client can get, and it is a mistake to suggest that this process must be finished in therapy. Therapy is about getting unstuck. It is not about finishing life. The therapist should make sure that the client exhibits openness to behavior change. It is useful to have the client scale this stance. For example, the therapist may say, "Give me a rating on a 1 to 10 scale of how committed you are to moving forward with your planned actions, even if you have to make room for uncomfortable moments. One equals no commitment at all, and 10 equals complete commitment." Generally, clients should give a rating of 7 or higher at this point of therapy.

Termination essentially involves tapering the frequency of visits over time to allow the client to adjust to the removal of the social support that the therapist has supplied. This can be labeled as a "field experiment" by the ACT therapist. The purpose is not to remove the client's access to therapy. Rather, it is to experiment with longer periods of autonomous functioning, built around periodic "booster sessions" with the therapist. A good tapering plan is to gradually move from weekly to monthly to quarterly booster visits. The purpose of these visits is just to ensure that the client's plan is moving forward and to briefly reinforce key ACT principles. Often, these can be 30-minute visits or less; for some clients, brief telephone contacts will suffice. The more functional a client is, the shorter this tapering phase can be. Clients with long-standing problems, who have benefited from ACT, may need a much slower tapering schedule and will probably benefit from a long-term relapse-prevention approach. This may involve monthly or quarterly visits over several years. The goal of tapering and relapse prevention is to make the transition out of therapy an easy one, while retaining more of an "arms length" relationship with the client. This allows the therapist to periodically monitor how the client is doing and makes it easy for the client to reenter therapy quickly should the need arise.

THERAPEUTIC DO'S AND DON'TS

Even in Relapse, Values Are Permanent

It is not unusual for a client who is backsliding to lapse into defeatism, as if losing focus on a commitment somehow implies that the client has defective values. When clients present this in therapy, the question the therapist asks is, "Which of your values changed during this relapse?" It is important to get the client to answer this very specifically. Usually none of the values has changed. Basic values seldom change; confidence in achieving valued ends can change a lot. The client is no doubt struggling with troublesome thoughts (I'm a failure, I should give up), feelings (shame, anger), and memories (past failures like this), and the most important question is, "So what now?" The ACT therapist may say something like this:

> "Unless your values have changed—'What now?' is the same as 'What before?' If you were to move in the direction you value right now, right at this moment here in therapy, what would you do? If you are committed to heading west, and you find that you have taken a wrong turn and have backtracked 10 miles, is there anything that prevents you from turning the car around and heading west? If you were in a car headed west toward San Francisco, and your mind was telling you that the car will break down, the

road will be closed ahead, or that you will fall asleep at the wheel and get in a wreck, could you continue to drive west? If west is where you want to go, get in the car and start driving."

The Client Owns Committed Action

This phase of ACT involves asking the client to engage in potentially life-altering behavior. Therefore, it is important to make sure the client is fully cognizant of the range of potential consequences of valued actions. The potential problem here is that the therapist's personal agenda for the client may be unduly influencing the client's choices. The client, seeking the therapist's approval, buys into actions without appreciating the gravity of these actions. The ACT therapist has to carefully monitor for this infusion of therapist values. It is sometimes useful to ask, "If I stopped working with you tomorrow for some weird reason and another counselor was sitting here with you, would you be standing by these actions with 100% certainty? Are there some you'd have less certainty about?" The therapist needs to be absolutely clear that what has shown up are the client's values and goals. If there is any doubt whatsoever, it is time to initiate the process of delineating values.

Noncompliance Is Not Failure

A potential trap for the therapist is to view the client's behavior change as a requirement for therapy to be considered a "success." When the client's commitment waivers or the client goes back to old avoidance behaviors, the therapist begins to pressure the client to get the goals and actions accomplished. This is akin to the parenting practice of changing the volume, not the message: If the kid doesn't behave when you say it softly, then say it loudly. Although this may work for some kids, it generally doesn't work too well with clients. In other words, the harder the therapist pushes on the client (an act of therapist unwillingness), the more resistant the client becomes. At its worst, this process can devolve into mutual confrontation, "resistance" interpretations, and even precipitous termination by the client. It is important for the therapist to realize that no matter how carefully the stage is set for the client to choose valued actions, it is a choice only the client can make. Choosing not to go forward with a plan is a legitimate choice, as long as it actually is a choice. The gentlest way to work with a client in such circumstances is to completely validate the client and the dilemma he or she is facing. The therapist might say, "If this were my life and I were seeing the consequences you are seeing, I could well imagine myself choosing not to go forward."

PERSONAL WORK FOR THE CLINICIAN: COMMITTED ACTION

In the preceding chapter, we asked you to look at how you could use your values as a "compass" to help you steer a course through your main problem. We asked you to look for emotional barriers that might entice you to stray from your course. In this chapter, we asked you to look at your willingness to "inhale" those barriers and make this problem work for your values, not against them. You are asked to put your values into action to transform your problem.

1. Pick one value that feels central to you, that you want to put into play in this problem area. Please write it down.
2. Now pick a goal that you would like to achieve, with respect to the problem, that would let you know you are "on track."
3. Now pick an action(s) that will lead you to accomplish that goal.
4. Before you "leave the station," assess whether any obstacles to committed action might be lurking in the shadows.
   a. Is there someone you need to forgive in order to make this move toward greater vitality? Who?
   b. Do you need to forgive yourself for something that you have found hard to swallow? What is it? Are you willing to "fore-give" it?
   c. Is there someone who has wronged you who could escape unpunished if you got healthier? Who? Are you willing to let this happen?
5. Are you willing to make room for any thoughts, feelings, memories, or sensations that arise as a result of your committed actions? (Circle one.)
   Yes (Go forward with your journey and experience it!)
   No (Go back and choose a different valued action, then repeat this exercise.)

CLINICAL VIGNETTE

You are in the seventh session with a 51-year-old married man who has had chronic alcohol abuse problems since his first wife died of cancer at age 38. He has been "on the wagon" many times, the longest period of sobriety being 18 months. During that time he experienced intense anxiety and depression that, in his mind, became so unbearable he "had to" drink. His current wife has been supportive of his attempts to get sober, but is growing weary of his mercurial moods when he isn't drinking and his sullen and withdrawn mood when he is. He believes they are headed for divorce if he doesn't get control of his drinking. He is marginally employed in a job far beneath his skill and education level. He has few friends who are not drinkers. In previous sessions he has disclosed that his primary fear in being sober is slipping back into depression. His primary value was to "be a loving and emotionally available husband," and he picked as an initial action going on a 2-week vacation with his spouse. His stated goal was to do this without using alcohol, as he felt it interfered with his ability to be "present." In this session, after completing the 2-week trip, he says, "This is just like me . . . I can't keep a commitment to anything if it interferes with my drinking. I make it 2 days and, bingo, I'm in the bar laying down boilermakers. My wife sees me snookered and just looks at me like I'm slime. And you know what? She's right! Then, I feel so guilty about ruining our trip, I can't face her, so I avoid talking about it . . . you know, like if I don't mention it, it didn't happen. But I can't hide from the hurt on her face, and I don't know what I'm going to do about it."

> *Question for the clinician:* Conceptualize the client's dilemma from the ACT perspectives on committed action as process versus committed action as outcome, blame versus responsibility, and measuring the size of commitments as a choice. Describe strategies and interventions you might use to address these issues and your goals in doing so. (Answer this before looking at our answer!)
>
> *Our answer:* This type of situation almost never happens with alcoholics, does it? Right. Our conceptualization is that the client is equating the ability to keep a commitment with the ability to make a commitment. In doing so, he misses the important distinction between committed action as a process versus outcome. The outcome of drinking again has overridden the much more important process goal of becoming a "loving and emotionally available husband." His value wasn't, "I want to live life without drinking." It involved doing things in his primary relationship that drinking would undermine.
>
> In this sense, drinking is an obstacle to committed action, not an outcome. The client is also confusing blame and responsibility. He is indeed to blame for his choice to drink, in the sense that it interfered with a valued goal and disappointed his wife. On the other hand, he is still "response-able"; there is nothing that prevents him from choosing the same commitment tomorrow, the next day, and so on. There are many ACT metaphors and exercises we could use. For example, the *Swamp Metaphor*

speaks to the necessity of plowing forward even when the first thing you hit is mud. We might do the *Jump Exercise* to help the client pick a smaller, more feasible but equally committed form of action toward his valued end. The *Eye Contact Exercise* could help him experientially connect with the fact that small commitments can be just as challenging as big ones. We could ask him if any aspect of the value about being a committed and emotionally available husband had changed, based on this outcome. Our primary goal in this situation would be to keep him from "throwing the baby out with the bath water" while helping him refocus and choose to embark again. Choices are always possible, as long as they do not become conceptual prisons.

APPENDIX: CLIENT HOMEWORK

Accepting Yourself on Faith Exercise

THERAPIST: Think of a choice as a postulate or an assumption. An assumption is something we use to do other work—it is where we begin, not what we conclude. Now my question is this: What stands between you and accepting yourself as whole and valid?

CLIENT: I'm not good enough.

THERAPIST: Right. You analyze yourself and find yourself wanting. So you try harder, but then you still feel as though you aren't good enough. And around and round it goes. So what if your acceptability was more like an assumption, not a conclusion? It is more like a faith move: done as a choice, for no reason; before you analyze, not as the product of analysis. If so, you have the choice available right now to "be OK" in a fundamental sense without having to earn it. I'd like to ask you to consider what stands between you and making that assumption, and if you are willing, I'd like you to make such a choice right here, right now. Are you OK or not? Are you acceptable or not? Are you whole, complete, and valid or not? If this is a choice, which do you choose?

[The goal is to help the client see this as a choice and to choose. If it is seen as a choice, few clients will choose self-attack and self-loathing. Usually, any client who does so is tangled up in more self-talk. The therapist may ask the client to stand up and answer the question out loud, as if it were a formal declaration. If the client is able to make a choice that is self-affirming, the therapist should warn the client that this does not mean that one ounce of self-doubt will go away. Such a choice will usually elicit negative "mind talk," in fact, inasmuch as choice is fundamentally threatening to verbal systems based on rationality. When this self-doubt shows up, however, the question is still the same: Are you OK or not? Are you acceptable or not? If the answer is yes (OK, acceptable), then it is OK to be yourself and have self-doubt as experienced content. That content does not mean what it says it means, because the essence of the issue has already been handled by the choice that was made or the assumption or postulate that was embraced.]

•PART III•

Using ACT

In this final part of the book we will examine how ACT approaches some more general clinical issues in the context of a therapeutic relationship. Finally, we return to our original theme—human suffering—and consider some implications of an ACT perspective for the evolution of better ways of dealing with it.

•10•

The Effective ACT
Therapeutic Relationship

The stance of the ACT therapist and the nature of the therapeutic relationship that results is important in producing positive outcomes. ACT, by its very nature, tends to be an intensive, expressive form of psychotherapy. This does not necessarily mean that the sessions are frequent (although ACT has also been conducted successfully in that format), but rather that each session is an emotional and expressive experience for both the client and the therapist.

There is a leveling experience in the relationship between the client and the ACT therapist that emanates from the ACT model itself. The client and the therapist are confronted by many of the same dilemmas in the process of living. The same language traps that capture the client are also those that capture the therapist, both in the therapist's professional role with the client and in the therapist's personal life. Observers of ACT sessions often comment on how strong the connection is between the therapist and client as difficult issues are addressed. ACT purposely capitalizes on the commonality between the client and therapist to help move the client, and by implication, the therapist, forward in their lives.

There are many ways that the therapist can capitalize and build on this genuine bonding, and there are many ways that the therapist can defeat this process through a personal lack of willingness to address issues that the client is being asked to address. In subsequent sections, the most critical of these positive and negative leverage points for the ACT therapist will be examined.

POSITIVE LEVERAGE POINTS IN ACT

It is a sensitivity to the client as viewed from an ACT perspective, not the mechanical application of metaphors, exercises, and concepts, that differentiates effective and ineffective ACT therapists. When therapists are first exposed to ACT, they tend to resonate very strongly to the specific interventions described in previous chapters of this book. They often are attracted to the metaphors, the experiential exercises, the homework assignments, and the iconoclastic feel of challenging the mainstream verbal community. The process of ACT goes well beyond these interventions and strategies, however. For these interventions to function the way they are meant to function, the therapist must be willing to enter into a relationship with the client that is open, accepting, coherent, and consistent with ACT principles.

ACT in a Functional Sense

The defining feature of the effective ACT therapist is the perspective that both encapsulates and informs the work. This is difficult to describe with words, and for a straightforward reason: It is a viewpoint that is characterized by the deliteralization and defusion of language and the therapist's own self-acceptance, willingness, and commitment that emanate from that defusion. Because the issues addressed by ACT have an equally strong impact on the therapist, it is simply not possible for the therapist to be sensitive to the client, as viewed from an ACT perspective, without applying the same perspectives to him- or herself.

For example, suppose an ACT therapist becomes confused in session. The client has said something that has the therapist hooked at the level of literal content. The therapist begins to feel anxious. There is a sense of danger in the room, as if the therapist suddenly feels very much on the spot. The therapist is trying to think what to do next and searches for some ACT-consistent metaphor, exercise, or response.

At that moment, several things could happen, but it would be helpful to first describe the therapist's situation itself from an ACT perspective. The therapist is experiencing some emotions that are not 100% welcome (e.g., confusion, anxiety, fear of looking incompetent). The client's verbalizations are being taken literally. The therapist's own evaluations (e.g., "I'm blowing it") are being taken literally. As a result, the flow and purpose of the session is gone. The therapist is performing for the client—trying to look competent. The two are no longer on the same level field. To go back to the *Chessboard Metaphor,* they are not "board to board" but are relating at "piece level."

Getting hooked like this is not a bad thing. It is not something "good ACT therapists don't do." Indeed, taking such an unrealistic stance is itself an example of getting hooked on a thought (i.e., that this is something "good ACT therapists don't do"). Getting hooked like this is something *all* people do, including people called "clients" and people called "therapists." The issue is not whether the therapist gets caught up on an issue; it will happen. The issue is what happens next. So, for example, the ACT therapist may sit silently for a while, observing his or her evaluations. After some silence, the therapist may say any one of the following, or hundreds of similar things:

- "I'm having some interesting mind chatter about this issue myself—in fact, why don't we just sit here for a minute or two and watch what our minds do in association with this."
- "Boy! Am I getting hooked by this! Does it have you hooked too?"
- "I'm feeling anxious, confused, and incompetent right now. I don't want you to rescue me—I have room for it. I just thought I'd let you know."
- "I feel powerless as I buy my thoughts about this—as though I have to do something, but (and this *is* a 'be-out' kind of thing when I buy those words) I don't know what to do. What shows up for you when you buy these words?"
- "Just to get some perspective on it, why don't we say what you said rapidly, out loud, over and over again, say, 40 times? I'll say it with you, and we can feel slightly silly together. Then we will see what happens. Are you willing?"
- "This thing is heavy. I'd like us to do a little exercise. It will be an eyes-closed kind of thing. We will put that thought out on the table, and I will take you through what your body does, what your emotions do, and what your mind does when it shows up. Are you willing?"

This list could continue indefinitely. Almost any technique imaginable could fit this moment, if the therapist is approaching the moment in an ACT-consistent manner. Conversely, ACT techniques could be employed that are actually inconsistent with the treatment philosophy. For example, the therapist might fight with the anxiety, shove it down, and force out the words "That is just a thought" in a dismissive tone of voice that subtly communicates that the client was wrong to have said what was said. The therapist might perform for the client, or use an ACT metaphor or exercise so as to avoid the discomfort of the moment and to hide behind the role of being a therapist. The therapist might intellectualize, or try to dazzle and confuse the client with ACT psychobabble in order to be "one up."

Used properly, there is a humanizing aspect to the ACT perspective. The therapist sees the client not as a diagnostic label, but as a human being struggling with many of the same life issues as the therapist. In ACT, the effective therapist needs to be willing to step back from the verbal sparring that occurs during psychotherapy, to see words as words, feelings as feelings, and to witness the behavior that is going on in the room from the point of view of an observer. In what follows, we will try to connect certain key ACT concepts to the behavior of the therapist, the client–therapist relationship, and the production of positive leverage in therapy.

Observer Perspective

The ACT therapist develops an almost intuitive suspicion of the process of rationalizing, explaining, and justifying through verbal behavior, instead preferring to take a mindful and experientially open approach to all private events. In ACT training this is referred to as the "observer perspective." The therapist does not adopt such a perspective in relation to the content the client is raising out of defensiveness or condescension. Rather, the therapist is backing up in order to see, the way one might step back from a painting in order to appreciate it. This, of course, closely parallels what the therapist is trying to teach the client to do in the midst of his or her life struggles. It makes intuitive sense that if the therapist is unable to model this ability to take an observer perspective on cognitive and verbal processes, then it is unlikely that this skill will be readily transferred to the client. An especially useful form of modeling occurs when the client can see that the therapist is risking something or allowing personal vulnerability into the room, when avoidance would be an easy alternative.

Wisdom Is Gained by Approach, Not Avoidance

An additional characteristic of the effective ACT therapeutic relationship is the ability to see commitment to values and choices and goals in life as something other than an exercise in developing topographically defined positive outcomes in one's life. Often, the therapist's own personal experience with disheartening personal failures or setbacks in life must be called upon. The ACT therapist approaches obstacles, barriers, and personal setbacks as legitimate forms of growth and experience. Commitment involves getting in contact with these barriers and moving ahead, not by getting over them, not by getting around them, but rather by embracing and moving through or with them.

If the therapist's own life has been characterized by avoiding situations of this type, then it will be much more difficult to model a healthy response. Again and again, the success of therapy boils down to the issue of whether there is a willingness to approach and move through unpleasant obstacles in the name of a valued outcome. Therapists who have learned firsthand that approaching personal obstacles can create a sense of health and vitality are much more likely to be able to impart this knowledge to their clients.

Contradiction and Uncertainty

A defining characteristic of the ACT "field of play" is a willingness to entertain contradictory themes or uncertainties without feeling compelled to use verbal behavior or verbal reasoning to resolve them. The effective ACT therapist must have a great tolerance for paradox, ambiguity, confusion, and irony. Life is full of contradictions, ironies, and things that cannot be entirely explained through deductive reasoning. Indeed, the trap that confronts most people actually comes back to this primary truth: Building a happy life is not always a logical enterprise. If the ACT therapist has touched on this experiential truth in his or her own life, there will be much less of a tendency to help the client begin a process of logical reasoning to determine which contradictions have to be eliminated in order to proceed. In other words, the therapist will experientially connect with the fact that these contradictions exist and that they need not be resolved to move forward. The therapist understands, again nonverbally, that wholeness emerges when contradictory events are allowed to coexist, without the need to resolve them through verbal reasoning.

In the area of uncertainty, the ACT therapist is asking the client to commit to an enterprise that carries significant risks for negative outcomes. It is called "life." The therapist can't guarantee that moving in a new direction will produce any particular outcomes for the client. The ACT therapist does not attempt to "rescue" the client from the fact that there are no guaranteed life outcomes. All that can be guaranteed is that the process is like starting a journey. The destination is important, but so is the journey.

Identification with the Client

Many therapeutic orientations emphasize the need for the therapist to be separate and different from the client (e.g., wiser, more professional, experienced, and balanced, having greater ego strength, and so on). These approaches emphasize that good therapists set good "boundaries," in the belief that the better the therapist instills these boundaries as part of the therapeutic process, the more the client will benefit. This posture can translate into the therapist's taking a "one up" position vis-à-vis the client. The therapist assumes the role of the person who knows how to live a healthy life, and the client assumes the role of the student who needs to learn from the teacher. If this boundary is crossed and the human behind the therapist role is seen, the therapist has failed in some way.

The ACT therapist has an alternative: Both the client and the therapist need to make room for private experiences and do what works in this situation. The successful ACT therapist is clear: "We are in this stew together. We are caught in the same traps. With a small twist of fate, we could be sitting across from each other in opposite roles. Your problems are a special opportunity for you to learn and for me to learn. We are not cut from different cloth, but from the same cloth."

Universality

Taking this position has two dramatic effects on the therapist's behavior and the therapeutic relationship that results. First, problems that the individual client views as unique to his or her own life become much more universal issues. Whereas the client may feel oppressed by the verbal conviction that he or she is alone with this problem, the therapist is able to move to a genuine position of "soft reassurance." Normal reassurance is demeaning. It says, "I am strong and you are weak. I will help you." It is inherently ACT inconsistent. Soft reassurance, on the other hand, is the support that comes when one person is willing to make contact with the other's sense of emotional pain, to validate and normalize it without ducking, despairing, rescuing, buying it, or running away from it. The same emotional, cognitive, and behavioral traps confront not just other people, but the therapist as well. This compassionate and empathetic view of the client's struggle is a fundamental attribute of the effective ACT therapist. This stance cannot be communicated merely through metaphors, experiential exercises, and homework, topographically defined. It cannot be faked. When this stance is taken, then the exercises, metaphors, and other activities of ACT have a power and quality they do not otherwise possess.

Self-Disclosure

A second result of identification with the client is the therapist's willingness to self-disclose when it is helpful. Self-disclosure is an essential aspect of developing a human relationship. This does not mean that the therapist spends more time self-disclosing about his or her life than the client does about his or hers. Rather, self-disclosure flows as a natural and human process. When the client understands that the therapist has torn his or her hair out over some of the same issues the client is struggling with, a strong bond and camaraderie can develop. This camaraderie is reassuring to the client and makes the therapist a much more credible model of acceptance and commitment. At the same time, many of the client's fears about being different or abnormal are allayed when the agent of social control (i.e., the therapist) acknowledges having struggled with similar problems.

Therapeutic Use of Spirituality

Spirituality can be a surprisingly difficult issue for empirical clinicians. Many shy away from the subject entirely, as if it is inherently untrustworthy or beyond the realm of therapeutic work. The ACT therapist who is willing to consider the spiritual side has more room to work and more moves to make to support the client's process of acceptance and change. Many therapists who are exposed to ACT, and who have some prior personal history with Eastern religion or other meditative types of personal growth experiences, comment on the distinct parallels between these types of experiential activities and some of the processes that occur in ACT. In general, therapists who have this type of background find it easier to adopt the ACT perspective.

Spirituality as a mode of intervention is highly valued in ACT. Spirituality does not necessarily imply the use of organized religion or even theistic beliefs, but rather a view of the world that recognizes a transcendent quality to human experience, acknowledges the universal aspects of the human condition, and respects the client's values and choices. Through the deliteralization of language and the adoption of an observer perspective, ACT steps back from a personal struggle and examines it openly and nondefensively. It is an inherently spiritual step in the sense that this kind of perspective taking cannot be justified on the basis of logic, but is based on a direct experience of oneness that comes from the self as context for experiential content.

The ACT therapist should rarely rely on spiritual or religious dogma, however. Indeed, spirituality and religion as such are discussed only if the client brings these issues into the room. Nevertheless, ACT has an inherent and wordless spiritual quality. The ACT therapist needs to get over the initial resistance some have toward raising such issues as "Who are you?" and "What do you want your life to stand for?" If the client wishes to talk about these issues in spiritual or religious terms, there is no reason to resist that process. Most ACT concepts have parallels in the major religious traditions, and so such translation is not difficult. For example, a Christian who understands the concept of an act of faith might be asked to do commitment exercises as "an act of faith."

Radical Respect

One of the most important attributes of an ACT therapist is the ability to remain absolutely neutral in regard to the choices the client is making about how to live his or her life. There is a posture of radical respect in which the basic ability of the individual to seek valued ends is protected.

There is a good deal of implicit social control lodged in therapy. Social control harnessed to the goals of the client is one thing. Social control as a substitute for values and choices is something else. Many therapists who use concepts such as "choice" and "values" subtly direct the client toward outcomes the therapist believes will benefit the client. This often occurs explicitly when therapists are working with clients who are engaging in socially unacceptable behaviors, such as domestic assault, chronic intoxication, and so forth. Often the goal of the therapist with such clients is to eliminate the behavior, regardless of the goals the client may bring to treatment. The clinical use of concepts like "choice" may be used to accomplish these goals. Such an approach is fundamentally at odds with the therapeutic relationship as envisioned in ACT.

In order to focus the client on what works, the ACT therapist has to be willing to occupy a position that focuses on the client's actual experience, not on the therapist's preconceived moral ideas. The effective ACT therapist has to come to the therapeutic interaction with clean hands—otherwise the client and the therapist have an unequal and subtly dishonest relationship. For example, ACT with an agoraphobic client involves no a priori assumption that the client must start getting out of the house. This is not a mind game that the ACT therapist is playing, but a truly compassionate position that comes from life experience and from radical respect for the client.

This experiential truth usually involves understanding that the formula for successful living is unique to each individual. There is no right or wrong way to live one's life. There are only consequences that follow from specific human behaviors. This is a terribly difficult position for new ACT therapists to maintain in the presence of socially undesirable behaviors. It does not mean, however, that the ACT therapist will conspire with the client to say something is working when it is not. For example, if the drug addict is losing a spouse as the result of drug use, and values the relationship with that spouse, the ACT therapist will not pretend that drug addiction has little effect on this valued end. Behind the eyes of even the most decrepit alcoholic lies a human spirit that is trying to make something happen. By acknowledging the vitality of this spirit and emphasizing that life is about making choices, the therapist is able to enter into an honest alliance. If a client values life outcomes that the therapist cannot work with, then the therapist should withdraw from therapy.

Clinical Use of Humor and Irreverence

Because the ACT therapist has fallen into many of same traps as the client, there is an opportunity to capitalize on these shared experiences by taking a somewhat irreverent and ironic view of the client's situation. Irreverence is not condescending to the client. The therapist's irreverence comes from an appreciation of the craziness and verbal entanglements that surround human living.

Many ACT concepts, techniques, and sayings are inherently irreverent. For example, an ACT therapist might say, "The problem here is not that you have problems—it's that they are the same problems. You need some new ones!" If other positive aspects of the ACT therapist's stance are well established, such a comment will not be seen as critical or pejorative. The therapist is poking fun at the system that squeezes down on us all, not just the client's system. By using gallows humor and irony and treating problems somewhat irreverently, the ACT therapist is often able to get the client to question whether problems are being taken too seriously. The likely culprit is fusion with beliefs that life is full of danger, threat, and uncertainty and therefore is to be approached as a very serious proposition.

NEGATIVE LEVERAGE POINTS IN ACT

The ACT model is directive and invasive and involves forming a strong emotional and therapeutic bond with the client. Because of this, the therapist must be mindful of the most common traps that lead to the misuse of ACT strategies.

ACT Is Not an Intellectual Exercise

ACT is a complex set of philosophies, strategies, and techniques. Although the therapy attempts to undermine counterproductive forms of verbal control, most ACT principles and techniques must initially be communicated verbally. The philosophical ideas, basic theoretical research, clever sayings, metaphors, and exercises in ACT have an intellectual appeal for many therapists. It is crucial that this appeal not be converted into seeing ACT as an intellectual exercise with the client. When verbal content is overemphasized, it results in the therapist's engaging in verbal persuasion techniques to get the client to agree that the therapist is right and that the client has been "missing the boat" all along. This is the antithesis of an effective ACT relationship. It essentially reinforces the idea that there is a correct verbal formulation for how to live and that the client has simply adopted the wrong one, as if the client is broken and the therapist is oh, so wise.

It is not the job of the ACT therapist to persuade the client to believe in ACT principles. If an ACT therapist says, "Don't believe a word I'm saying," it has to be sincere (indeed, even this very invocation is not to be believed), and it has to apply to the therapist, not just the client.

When therapists begin intellectualizing ACT, it is manifested in sessions by an excess amount of therapist verbal behavior relative to the purpose of the session, client passivity, and the underuse of nonverbal experiential exercises that could cut through the web of verbal entanglements. The overintellectualized ACT therapist will react with frustration when the client's behavior clearly indicates that he or she is not following what the therapist is trying to say or accomplish. The therapist will fall back on moralizing, lecturing, convincing, and explaining.

This problem is one of the most common issues dealt with in ACT supervision. The therapist's own words will sometimes reveal the true source of the problem. In supervision, therapists will say such things as, "We talked about acceptance," "We discussed the concept of commitment," "I brought up the issue of his avoidance," or "I was trying to show the client that. . . . " ACT is not concerned with the adoption of concepts. It is work in the here and now. Yes, ACT involves issues and it uses words, but only as tools to get in contact with something that is directly and experientially relevant to the client.

The essential point is that if this approach could be readily understood intellectually, no doubt the client would already be using it. The irony is that intellectualizing the ACT perspective, and then idealizing it in therapy, is the single most likely way to prevent the client from developing it in a functional sense. When the client obviously does not understand or feels confused, it is useless and counterproductive for the therapist to rationalize or browbeat the client.

Intellectualization can be a difficult process to correct once it begins in earnest, because the client often tacitly moves into the position of trying to please the therapist by "showing" correct ACT behaviors. Meanwhile, the client's sense of vitality and connection with the therapy drains away. Whereas ACT in its proper application is compassionately confrontational, the intellectualized version of ACT tends to be accusatory and derisive.

The usual correction is to reduce the therapist's verbal domination of session time. As a curative rule of thumb, no more than 20% of the session should involve ACT principles and concepts in a distinctly verbal sense (and even this is a high percentage). Instead, the therapist should use metaphors and exercises, while speaking to real-life events of direct relevance to the client. If a clinician is stuck on intellectualization, he or she should get additional supervision and ask a clinical colleague to watch a session or two. As things get back on track, these guidelines can be withdrawn and therapy can proceed more spontaneously.

Modeling a Lack of Acceptance

Harmful moments in ACT can occur when the therapist is raising issues of acceptance and commitment and at the same time modeling a lack of these behaviors. This occurs most frequently with more disturbed clients, who can frighten or concern therapists with suicidality, self-mutilation, bizarre behaviors, or the like. If the therapist can't accept the client as a human being with real-life, legitimate, honorable dilemmas, then how is the client to accept and move through these dilemmas?

Modeling nonacceptance can occur in several ways during the course of ACT. The therapist can selectively reinforce client thoughts or behaviors that are socially desirable while ignoring or disputing experiences that are negatively evaluated. In other words, the therapist is modeling acceptance of positive events and rejection of negative events—most likely just what the client was already doing before treatment.

A second form of nonacceptance is using the language of choice in a way that is socially coercive. The therapist who is put off by or rejects a client will often fall back on the client's ability to chose in a negative context. In other words, by telling the client, "Well, that's a choice you have to make," the client is really being told, "There is one choice you have to make, and you're not making it."

A third form of nonacceptance occurs when the therapist responds to a negative set of behaviors, cognitions, and feelings by attempting to explore "where you learned that way of thinking." Asking the client where this particular set of thoughts and feelings might be coming from—as if to find out how to remove them—is a sign of trouble. This is to be distinguished from asking the client to describe events that show up in association with the difficult material (including thought about one's history), where the agenda is to see what is there, not to remove it.

This problem is easy to detect through direct observation because of the heavy emphasis placed on history gathering and reason giving.

The solution to this problem is to acknowledge it and let go of it. The therapist should reconsider what personal values are involved in therapy, and from that position go into the next session. Feelings of fear, disgust, or frustration about what is transpiring with a client are not in and of themselves bad. They do not mean what they say they mean. The solution is the same for the therapist as it is for the client. Properly used, this type of difficulty is a good thing, because it means that the therapist can more fully appreciate how hard it is to do what the therapist is asking the client to do. Bringing that into the room can make therapy itself more effective and humane and places the therapeutic relationship on a more egalitarian basis.

Excessive Focus on Emotional Processing

A very common misconception about ACT is that a central goal is to get clients "in touch with their feelings." This ties into a very popular cultural conception regarding the need to release pent-up feelings and past frustrations. A spin-off of this position is to believe that the client's entire psychological distress can be explained as a function of avoiding certain feelings. Therefore, the therapist's first maneuver may be to ask the client what he or she is avoiding in a more or less direct way. The implied assumption here is that if the client gets in touch with what is being avoided, life will automatically assume a positive direction.

Emotional avoidance is a central feature in ACT work with clients, but only insofar as such avoidance blocks the client from taking a committed direction in life. The private events the ACT therapist is interested in are those that surface once the client initiates valued actions. As clients move on the road toward establishing meaning in their lives, negative, avoided feelings, thoughts, and memories will in fact surface. It is these experiences that are the grist for the ACT mill, not an esoteric exercise in getting in touch with feelings because that is inherently healthy.

The therapist may be tempted to jump on the emotional avoidance bandwagon within minutes of starting the first session, because it is so popular in our culture. However, the language accompanying this move often is indistinguishable from the language of other popular psychotherapies that emphasize emotional rediscovery for its own sake. Of all the errors an ACT therapist can make, this one is probably the most seductive, because it is consistent with much of the contemporary literature. Further, it is hard for even experienced therapists to reliably distinguish and undercut this type of emotional wallowing. The solution for this error is to come back to active exercises linked to values and behavior change. If the emotional work is worthwhile, it will be evident at that point.

Countertransference

It is easy for a therapist to become stuck when the therapist and the client stumble on issues that are equally salient for them both. This may occur because the therapist has strong moral beliefs about a certain set of client behaviors (e.g., suicidal behavior) or the client's dilemma closely mirrors a dilemma that the therapist unsuccessfully addressed in his or her own life. The usual errors that result are topic avoidance, advice giving, or excessive reliance on personal experience (e.g., "Don't do what I did").

Even "good" ACT therapists have personal issues and feared psychological content. That is what it means to be human. However, the goal is to acknowledge that personal issues have been engaged that probably won't be beneficial in helping solve the client's dilemma. This is not a personal indictment of the therapist, but a form of self-acceptance for the therapist. In so doing, the ACT therapist models exactly what the client is being asked to do.

THE THERAPEUTIC RELATIONSHIP

In essence, the positive and negative leverage points we have just described define the nature of the therapeutic relationship in ACT. In ACT, therapeutic relationships are strong, open, accepting, mutual, respectful, and loving. Unlike other clinical approaches, ACT does not view the therapeutic relationship per se as an end purpose of therapy. To perceive it thus is, in essence, to hold that clients are missing something that only someone else can provide. Rather, the therapeutic relationship in ACT is important because (1) it is based on a stance toward oneself and others (love, acceptance, respect, openness) that is curative, (2) it allows that stance to be modeled, (3) it creates a social context in which important issues can be evoked (inasmuch as most of the problematic behaviors in an ACT perspective are, at their core, social behaviors), and (4) strong, open, accepting, mutual, respectful, and loving relationships are usually a natural expression of core values in the client and the therapist.

SUMMARY

ACT work is personally challenging. That is the very nature of the work for the client, and it is thus unavoidable for the honest therapist. ACT is also a powerful and intrusive intervention. It raises basic issues of values, meaning, and self-identity. The distinction between ACT topographically defined and ACT functionally defined has to do with the nature and purpose of the therapist's work. When Acceptance and Commitment Therapy is done properly, relationships are intense, personal, and meaningful. The boundaries in a relationship are natural, non-arbitrary, and linked to workability. When developed properly, the relationship itself models the purpose and nature of ACT.

•11•

ACT in Context

Wanting to understand language is like a person made of
salt wanting to explore the undersea depths.
—ZEN SAYING

It is time for a bit of self-reflection and a caution: Don't *believe* a word
in this book. It is one of the burdens of ACT that if the model is correct,
then the model must be held lightly. We mean this both philosophically
and strategically. Philosophically, it does no good to provide an analysis
of how language naturally leads to cognitive fusion and experiential
avoidance, only to turn around and present another "answer" that is to
be held as an "answer." We mean this so radically that we do not even
rule out the possibility that there *is* an answer (that is, even the preceding
sentence is not to be believed). ACT is not a dogma, but it is not a
nondogma either. The confusion and incoherence in this paragraph is
deliberate, not because we are trying to confuse the reader, but because
language is fundamentally incapable of going beyond itself except in the
experiential glimpses provided by paradox and confusion.

Strategically, the ACT model is not to be believed because the
model of treatment development we are following is continuous and
pragmatically oriented. This is an inherently nonlinear process; this
book catches the process of development in flight. As described in Chapter 2, the development model we have followed is a continuous process
of mutual interactions between clinical insights, theoretical work, technical development, basic experimental research, philosophical work,
basic psychopathology research, assessment development, and clinical
outcome research. For good or ill, this feature is a unique characteristic

of ACT. If it is appreciated, however, there is no final analysis of anything. There will be no final truth statement about what ACT is or isn't. ACT and all of its component parts will always be works in progress.

Consider "acceptance," as encompassed in ACT. A considerable body of literature has demonstrated the clinical difficulties produced by experiential avoidance (Hayes et al., 1996), and, conversely, the empirical analyses of acceptance methods are creating excitement in many areas (Hayes, Jacobson, Follette, & Dougher, 1994). We reviewed some of these studies in Chapter 3. Despite all of this interest and even progress in research, "acceptance" is not a thing just because there is a label for it. The thing-like quality of acceptance is yet another trick of human language. We do not suggest throwing out the concept merely because of that—to do so consistently would require that we throw out *all* concepts—but we do suggest that the value of the concept lies in what it buys us pragmatically, however appealing it is to reify the concept itself. We should always remain open to new insights that will accomplish our goals more readily. To have both (getting what it buys us *and* staying open to new things), we need to use the concept *and* to hold it lightly.

We would gladly trade all that we know about acceptance and mindfulness for what we don't know. Experimental measures of acceptance are still relatively crude, the basic psychopathology research on acceptance is in its infancy, and the positive outcomes produced by ACT and other acceptance-based therapies come from packages that include many elements in addition to acceptance.

Even if acceptance stands up over the long term as a useful concept, there may be several kinds of acceptance existing in different domains of human behavior. Acceptance of history, acceptance of consciousness itself, acceptance of specific thoughts, acceptance of feelings, and so on, may be quite different. The ACT model itself suggests that acceptance can involve many different psychological components, including cognitive defusion, choice, abandonment of a control agenda, exposure, and active willingness and commitment. It is not known whether acceptance functions differently with or without any of these elements. There is an aspect to acceptance that seems almost trait-like; other aspects may be quite situationally specific. We do not know how best to establish acceptance or the best conditions under which to use these strategies.

The reader should not take this as an apology for the state of the literature, nor are we implying that acceptance is not a scientifically worthwhile concept, deserving of study in its own right. Our point is more basic. There are many concepts in the empirical clinical literature that are widely researched, widely believed and more poorly understood than proponents would have us believe. Consider an example: "Irrational thoughts cause clinical disorders; more rational thoughts help ameliorate these disorders." You can martial some evidence for the value of rational thoughts or the harm of irrational ones, but the evidence is surprisingly slim when you add in the concept of context. It turns out that the contexts in which irrational and rational thoughts are harmful or helpful, respectively, are at times surprisingly specific (e.g., see Rosenfarb & Hayes, 1984; Hayes & Wolf, 1984; Zettle & Hayes, 1982; for a review see Hayes, Zettle, & Rosenfarb, 1989). For instance, phobic children who are deceived into thinking that the therapist does not know which "rational coping statements" they have been given are no longer helped by those statements. That is, rational coping statements seem to work through pliance and thus stop working if the social context is manipulated so that compliance with a verbal statement can no longer be monitored (see Hayes, Zettle, & Rosenfarb, 1989). Our point is not that irrational cognitions are unimportant, but that even a concept as widely accepted as this must be held lightly so that we are open to new insights.

The same points that we have applied to acceptance apply with equal force to other ACT concepts such as cognitive defusion, deliteralization, and even commitment. Thus, although we invite the reader to take the ACT model seriously, we also advise caution and humility in its application.

One aspect of ACT seems particularly important; it may help link some of the more disparate wings of clinical work. Many clinical traditions, recognizing the situated nature of human action and appreciating the somewhat arbitrary narrative-like quality of any statement about the human condition, have resolved the resulting dialectical discomfort by stepping away from experimental research. In doing so, they have abrogated the responsibility for providing empirical data about efficacy, effectiveness, consumer acceptance, cost, and so forth. Although it is understandable to a degree, this is a form of intellectual nihilism that runs perilously close to being self-serving. In contrast, the ACT model is firmly grounded in the empirical clinical tradition (see Chapter 3 for example), is linked to an active research program, is disconfirmable, and yet is fully respectful of the difficulties inherent in capturing human experience in an experimental bottle.

THE RELEVANCE OF ACT IN THE 21ST CENTURY

As we enter the 21st century, it seems time for human civilization to ask itself the question, "Are we using language or is language using us?" Over the last 5,000 years human progress has been enormous; over the last 100 it has been unfathomable. In almost every physical domain the changes have been positive—we have the technical capabilities to solve many of the basic problems that face us, including food, shelter, and warmth. Yet in almost every behavioral domain recent progress is absent or even negative (Biglan, 1995). For example, the evolution of language has not driven down the prevalence of behavioral disorders; the rates seem to be increasing with each decade. Without belaboring this point, we note a virtual laundry list of social and individual ills that not only have not been improved because of language, but may also be the direct by products of language. Can we passively rely on the normal process of human cultural evolution to create progress in the area of human happiness and pro-social behavior?

We believe that the answer is no. In physical health, biological evolution has eliminated most immediately destructive kinds of structural physical abnormalities. But if we are correct and the landscape of psychological health is dominated by the characteristics of human language, then there are no processes we are aware of that will ensure that psychological health is evolving positively.

There are at least five reasons to be concerned that the process of evolutionary correction will not solve the problem of human misery. First, it has happened too fast to adjust. The most basic forms of human language have existed for only an eye blink of time. Homo sapiens have been on earth for only an evolutionary eye blink—and truly abstract forms of written language, such as those based on an alphabet, are only a few thousand years old. If a list were available, a person with even average intelligence could commit to memory all of his or her ancestors from now until the time before there was written language as we know it. Within such a moment of time, biological evolution has had a very limited opportunity to operate. Humans have barely had time to become acquainted with "The Force," never mind solving its dark side.

Second, verbal behavior pays off biologically. Biological evolution can only operate on competitive disadvantages between genotypes that give rise to differences in the ability to reproduce. Human language, although it may create enormous human misery, can hardly be said to have put us at a competitive disadvantage in our ability to reproduce and survive, either as compared with other animals or as compared within the human family. Abstract verbal abilities are the very essence of intelligent human behavior, as can be seen by factor analyses of virtually any intelligence test. Intelligent behavior, clearly, is a huge competitive advantage in the struggle to produce and to reproduce. Thus, biological evolution will have a hard time weeding out the "dark side" of human language, given its overwhelmingly positive advantages.

Third, verbal behavior pays off for the individual in other areas. Human language does not just give us the ability to criticize ourselves or to imagine that the world will be better when we are gone. It also allows us to reason, plan, and analyze. Many of these activities are powerfully positive in many circumstances. They lead to creativity in the arts and success, not just biologically but also psychologically. The loss of innocence produced by language works for individuals, just not in all areas.

Fourth, verbal behavior pays off culturally. Human cultures can evolve much more rapidly than any other species. Whereas the unit of biological evolution is the gene, the unit of cultural evolution is the cultural practice. A practice is a form of behavior that is passed between individuals and whose prevalence and strength is seen in terms of processes that apply to social propagation and maintenance at the level of the group. Although human language is a psychological adjustment for an individual, it is also a practice at the level of culture.

Even if human misery were 100% due to the side effects of human language, human language would be hard, if not impossible, to eliminate from human culture. This is because symbolic activity enormously increases the ability to pass cultural practices from individual to individual and is thus inherently advantageous at the level of cultural practices. The Japanese snow monkeys that wash sweet potatoes are engaging in a nonverbal cultural practice, but it has to be passed on directly to each generation. We, the present authors, may be long dead, yet a person reading this very book in the future may be influenced by the cultural practices and ways of speaking that have influenced us. Thus, cultures with language—especially written language—can become stronger, more coherent, and longer-lasting as compared with cultures without it. This is so much the case that we at times use the word *culture* to refer exclusively to language-involved practices.

The implication is sobering: Language need not be psychologically positive to survive and prosper, because it is a robust cultural phenomenon. Language is like a virus—almost a different life form that has humans as a host. With each statement and each phrase, we pass on the virus, unable to function without encouraging its spread. The monks see the problem and try silence, chanting, koans, mantras, and prayers, but they too remain infected. Like mitochondria in cells, language in some ways looks like a foreign entity, and yet like cells themselves, we have become dependent on the invader for our existence. Our point is that even if human verbal abilities do in fact lead to the pervasiveness of human suffering, these same abilities carry such great advantages biologically and culturally that it is inconceivable—short of perhaps total nuclear war—that the dark side of language will be weeded out of life on earth anytime soon.

Finally, cultural practices can propagate at the level of the group even if they are horribly destructive to the individual. For the sake of simplicity, let us take the example of suicide. Person X jumps from a tall building. At the level of psychology (the level of the individual organism behaving in a historical and current situational context), all functioning ceases. At the level of biology, all functioning ceases. But as a cultural practice, it is known that a dramatic suicide temporarily increases the likelihood of suicide within the area exposed to knowledge about the suicide. If this is true of suicide, is seems more dramatically true of normal human misery. Suppose a work environment has become unpleasant. Often co-workers will spend a great deal of time talking about how bad things are, how the boss is unfair, and so on. The misery expands and individuals are hurt, but the propagation continues.

The way in which our culture is becoming more and more competitive and achievement oriented may be another example of a cultural good that is harmful to individuals. Most of the readers of this book are high achievers, people who have sought out schooling and have tried to learn how to help people. Yet we know that our dear readers will be as likely as others to die of stress-related illness, to divorce, to become depressed, to suffer from overwhelming anxiety, or to commit suicide. What is true at the level of the individual life is true also at the level of the culture at large. We have no assurance at all that the practices that are producing faster and faster lives, with more and more technology, communication, work, mobility, and stress, and less and less time with our children, human connection, quiet, sharing, or reflection, are in fact leading to happiness for the individuals involved, even though they surely produce more products, goods, services, and knowledge and thus make the culture more competitive. This looks like a behavioral system that is out of control, not one that is evolving positively.

For all these reasons, the assumption of healthy normality need not apply to psychological health. It may be possible to have processes at the psychological level that are at times highly destructive but still useful enough to be developed and maintained at the cultural level. Human symbolic activity, we argue, is a good example of just such a process.

It is not that we need to go backward, nor even that we can. Rather, we need to learn to integrate these human products, abilities, and experiences into a totality that is productive and supportive both for the culture and for the individuals that have, after all, created it.

The only process we can see that has a chance to direct psychological health in a more positive way comprises the deliberate actions of suffering human beings and those who work with them. Therapists in particular are looked to by modern civilization to consider and address such problems. If our thesis is correct, however, merely ameliorating dysfunctional behavior is not enough. For example, suppose a person is impotent and a therapist uses a paradoxical intervention, prohibiting sexual intercourse (à la Masters and Johnson). This intervention cleverly short-circuits the language-based problem (trying to become aroused through threatening self-rules and applying deliberate control where it does not belong). But if it works, it does nothing to help that same person with a similar language-based problem. It would be like finding a blind man caught in a bear trap in his living room, releasing him from the trap, and then leaving it in place to catch him again next time.

If we can understand how language creates the entanglements that make human psychological health and happiness so elusive, then it is our job to try to establish and support cultural practices inside psychotherapy and out that ameliorate these destructive processes in a socially broader way. Acceptance and cognitive defusion, we believe, may be two such practices.

With our children, our clients, and ourselves we need to learn how to prevent disorders, how to support growth, and how to repair things when they are broken, in a way that has broad and long-term beneficial effects. This could be devilishly difficult, because even accurate insights quickly become dogmas to be believed—and there we are again, entangled in language.

Psychotherapy has often had the perverse effect of actually undermining existing traditions that may promote psychological health. Some spiritual and religious traditions, for example, are among the best-documented sources of physical and psychological health (Larson, 1998), particularly the more experiential, accepting, and mystical practices such as meditation and prayer. This is not surprising, because these cultural traditions were among the first to emerge after human language really began to evolve into the elaborate symbolic system we have today. Yet psychotherapists often attack spiritual and religious traditions as if they were inherently toxic to an individual's autonomy and psychological health.

The reasons for this skepticism are understandable. It is known that rigid and punitive religious systems are toxic to human health (Larson, 1998). There are dramatic examples of harmful social control and dogma in religion (e.g., cult suicide, ethnic cleansing). Often, clients who seek out psychotherapy are likely to be among those who have been harmed. But we need to be less arrogant and more open to aspects of human culture that are helpful.

In this larger context, ACT is one small effort to solve the psychological problems language has created. That is "the work" we have before us, and it is perhaps the most important psychological task we face as a species. If we as psychotherapists take on this burden, we need to look again at the many honorable traditions (religious, spiritual, mystical, therapeutic) that have attempted to address human suffering and try to filter out what works from what does not. The self-help sections of bookstores are crammed with books on how to increase life satisfaction. There clearly is a crying need, and it is one that the more scientific wing of empirical clinical work has simply not yet taken seriously. Even if therapists are interested only in psychopathology per se, the core argument we have presented is that such work takes on a different cast when it is placed in the larger context of human suffering.

ACT is unique not so much in its goals or even its methods, but in the systematic link between goals, methods, and a scientific analysis of verbal behavior. Even if ACT per se proves unimportant, it is our hope that this combination will—at least in some small way—advance the work that our species faces. That work may take many years, perhaps even centuries, but it took much longer than that to develop our verbal abilities as a species.

Humans have eaten from the tree of knowledge, and they have been ashamed ever since. We cannot go back to ignorant innocence, nor would we want to, but perhaps we can do a better job of putting on and taking off specific aspects of human language as they best serve our purposes. As a scientific and human matter, it is vitally important that we learn how.

References

Addis, M. E., & Jacobson, N. S. (1996). Reasons for depression and the process and outcome of cognitive-behavioral psychotherapies. *Journal of Consulting and Clinical Psychology, 64,* 1417–1424.

Ascher, L. M. (Ed.). (1989). *Therapeutic paradoxic.* New York: Guilford Press.

Assagioli, R. (1971). *The act of will.* New York: Viking.

Baer, D. M., Peterson, R. F., & Sherman, J. A. (1967). The development of imitation by reinforcing behavioral similarity to a model. *Journal of the Experimental Analysis of Behavior, 43,* 553–566.

Bancroft, J., Skrimshire, A., & Simkins, S. (1976). The reasons people give for taking overdoses. *British Journal of Psychiatry, 128,* 538–548.

Barkley, R. A. (1997). Behavioral inhibition, sustained attention, and executive functions: Constructing a unifying theory of ADHD. *Psychological Bulletin, 121,* 65–94.

Barnes, D., Hegarty, N., & Smeets, P. M. (1997). Relating equivalence relations to equivalence relations: A relational framing model of complex human functioning. *Analysis of Verbal Behavior, 14,* 57–83.

Barnes, D., & Roche, B. (1997). A behavior analytic approach to behavioral reflexivity. *Psychological Record, 47,* 543–572.

Barrett, D. M., Deitz, S. M., Gaydos, G. R., & Quinn, P. C. (1987). The effects of programmed contingencies and social conditions on response stereotypy with human subjects. *Psychological Record, 37,* 489–505.

Baumeister, R. F. (1990). Suicide as escape from self. *Psychological Review, 97,* 90–113.

Beck, A. T., Rush, A. J. Shaw, B. F., & Emery, G. (1979) *Cognitive therapy of depression.* New York: Guilford Press.

Biglan, A. (1995). *Changing cultural practices: A contextualist framework for intervention research.* Reno, NV: Context Press.

Biglan, A., & Hayes, S. C. (1996). Should the behavioral sciences become more pragmatic? The case for functional contextualism in research on human behavior. *Applied and Preventive Psychology: Current Scientific Perspectives, 5,* 47–57.

Biglan, A., Lewin, L., & Hops, H. (1990). A contextual approach to the problem of aversive practices in families. In G. Patterson (Ed.), *Depression and aggression: Two facets of family interactions* (pp. 103–129). New York: Erlbaum.

Bond, F. W., & Bunce, D. (in press). Mediators of change in emotion-focused and problem-focused worksite stress management interventions. *Journal of Occupational Health Psychology.*

Bush, K. M., Sidman, M., & deRose, T. (1989). Contextual control of emergent equivalence relations. *Journal of the Experimental Analysis of Behavior, 51,* 29–45.

Catania, A. C., Shimoff, E., & Matthews, B. A. (1989). An experimental analysis of rule-governed behavior. In S. C. Hayes (Ed.), *Rule-governed behavior: Cognition, contingencies, and instructional control* (pp. 119–150). New York: Plenum.

Chagnon, N. A. (1983). *Yanomamö: The fierce people.* New York: Holt, Rinehart, & Winston.

Chiles, J., & Strosahl, K. (1995). *The suicidal patient: Principles of assessment, treatment and case management.* Washington, DC: American Psychiatric Press.

Cioffi, D., & Holloway, J. (1993). Delayed costs of suppressed pain. *Journal of Personality and Social Psychology, 64,* 274–282.

Clark, D. M., Ball, S., & Pape, D. (1991). An experimental investigation of thought suppression. *Behaviour Reasearch and Therapy, 29,* 253–257.

Craske, M. G., Miller, P. P., Rotunda, R., & Barlow, D. H. (1990). A descriptive report of features of initial unexpected panic attacks in minimal and extensive avoiders. *Behaviour Research and Therapy, 28,* 395–400.

Dawes, R. M. (1994). *House of cards: Psychology and psychotherapy built on myth.* New York: Free Press.

DeGenova, M. K., Patton, D. M., Jurich, J. A., & MacDermid, S. M. (1994). Ways of coping among HIV-infected individuals. *Journal of Social Psychology, 134,* 655–663.

DeGrandpre, R. J., Bickel, W. K., & Higgins, S. T. (1992). Emergent equivalence relations between interoceptive (drug) and exteroceptive (visual) stimuli. *Journal of the Experimental Analysis of Behavior, 58,* 9–18.

Deikman, A. J. (1982). *The observing self: Mysticism and psychotherapy.* Boston: Beacon Press.

Dougher, M. J., Augustson, E., Markham, M. R., & Greenway, D. E. (1994). The transfer of respondent eliciting and extinction functions through stimulus equivalence classes. *Journal of the Experimental Analysis of Behavior, 62,* 331–351.

Dymond, S., & Barnes, D. (1995). A transformation of self-discrimination response functions in accordance with the arbitrarily applicable relations of sameness, more-than, and less-than. *Journal of the Experimental Analysis of Behavior, 64,* 163–184.

Dymond, S., & Barnes, D. (1996). A transformation of self-discrimination response functions in accordance with the arbitrarily applicable relations of sameness and opposition. *Psychological Record, 46,* 271–300.

Endler, N. S., & Parker, J. D. A. (1990). The multidimensional assessment of coping: A critical evaluation. *Journal of Personality and Social Psychology, 58,* 844–854.

Foa, E. B., Steketee, G., & Young, M. C. (1984). Agoraphobia: Phenomenological aspects, associated characteristics, and theoretical considerations. *Clinical Psychology Review, 4,* 431–457.

Folkman, S., & Lazarus, R. S. (1988). *Ways of Coping Questionnaire.* Palo Alto, CA: Consulting Psychologists Press.

Follette, W. C. (1995). Correcting methodological weaknesses in the knowledge base used to derive practice standards. In S. C. Hayes, V. M. Follette, R. M. Dawes, & K. E. Grady (Eds.), *Scientific standards of psychological practice: Issues and recommendations* (pp. 229–247). Reno, NV: Context Press.

Frazer, J. G. (1911). *The golden bough: A study in magic and religion* (Vol. 3). London: Macmillan.

Galizio, M. (1979). Contingency-shaped and rule-governed behavior: Instructional control of human loss avoidance. *Journal of the Experimental Analysis of Behavior, 31,* 53–70.

Gatch, M. B., & Osborne, J. G. (1989). Transfer of contextual stimulus function via equivalence class development. *Journal of the Experimental Analysis of Behavior, 51,* 369–378.

Geiser, D. S. (1992). *A comparison of acceptance-focused and control-focused psychological treatments in a chronic pain treatment center.* Unpublished dissertation, University of Nevada, Reno, NV.

Gewirtz, J. J., & Stengle, K. G. (1968). Learning of generalized imitation as the basis for identification. *Psychological Review, 75,* 374–397.

Gold, D. B., & Wegner, D. M. (1995). Origins of ruminative thought: Trauma, incompleteness, nondisclosure, and suppression. *Journal of Applied Social Psychology, 25,* 1245–1261.

Greenberg, L. (1994). Acceptance in experiential therapy. In S. C. Hayes, N. S. Jacobson, V. M. Follette, & M. J. Dougher (Eds.), *Acceptance and change: Content and context in psychotherapy* (pp. 53–67). Reno, NV: Context Press.

Greenberg, L. S. (1983). Toward a task analysis of conflict resolution in Gestalt therapy. *Psychotherapy: Theory, Research and Practice, 20,* 190–201.

Greenberg, L. S., & Dompierre, L. M. (1981). Specific effects of Gestalt two-chair dialogue on intrapsychic conflict in counseling. *Journal of Counseling Psychology. 28,* 288–294.

Greenberg, L. S., & Johnson, S. M. (1988). *Emotionally focused therapy for couples.* New York: Guilford Press.

Greenberg, L. S., & Safran, J. D. (1989). Emotion in psychotherapy. *American Psychologist, 44,* 19–29.

Greenberg, L. S., & Webster, M. C. (1982). Resolving decisional conflict by Gestalt two-chair dialogue: Relating process to outcome. *Journal of Counseling Psychology, 29,* 468–477.

Hayes, S. C. (1984). Making sense of spirituality. *Behaviorism, 12,* 99–110.

Hayes, S. C. (1987). A contextual approach to therapeutic change. In N. Jacobson (Ed.), *Psychotherapists in clinical practice: Cognitive and behavioral perspectives* (pp. 327–387). New York: Guilford Press.

Hayes, S. C. (1989). Nonhumans have not yet shown stimulus equivalence. *Journal of the Experimental Analysis of Behavior, 51,* 385–392.

Hayes, S. C. (1991). A relational control theory of stimulus equivalence. In L. J. Hayes & P. N. Chase (Eds.), *Dialogues on verbal behavior* (pp. 19–40). Reno, NV: Context Press.

Hayes, S. C. (1992). Verbal relations, time, and suicide. In S. C. Hayes & L. J. Hayes (Eds.), *Understanding verbal relations* (pp. 109–118). Reno, NV: Context Press.

Hayes, S. C. (1993). Goals and the varieties of scientific contextualism. In S. C. Hayes, L. J. Hayes, T. R. Sarbin, & H. W. Reese (Eds.), *The varieties of scientific contextualism* (pp. 11–27). Reno, NV: Context Press.

Hayes, S. C., & Barnes, D. (1997). Analyzing derived stimulus relations requires more than the concept of stimulus class. *Journal of the Experimental Analysis of Behavior, 68,* 235–270.

Hayes, S. C., Bissett, R., Korn, Z., Zettle, R. D., Rosenfarb, I., Cooper, L., & Grundt, A. (1999). The impact of acceptance versus control rationales on pain tolerance. *Psychological Record, 49,* 33–47.

Hayes, S. C., & Brownstein, A. J. (1986a). Mentalism, behavior–behavior relations, and a behavior analytic view of the purposes of science. *Behavior Analyst, 9,* 175–190.

Hayes, S. C., & Brownstein, A. J. (1986b). Mentalism, private events, and scientific explanation: A defense of B. F. Skinner's view. In S. Modgil & C. Modgil (Eds.), *B. F. Skinner: Consensus and controversy* (pp. 207–218). Sussex, England: Falmer Press.

Hayes, S. C., Brownstein, A. J., Haas, J. R., & Greenway, D. E. (1986). Instructions, multiple schedules, and extinction: Distinguishing rule-governed from schedule controlled behavior. *Journal of the Experimental Analysis of Behavior, 46,* 137–147.

Hayes, S. C., Brownstein, A. J., Zettle, R. D., Rosenfarb, I., & Korn, Z. (1986). Rule-governed behavior and sensitivity to changing consequences of responding. *Journal of the Experimental Analysis of Behavior, 45,* 237–256.

Hayes, S. C., Devany, J. M., Kohlenberg, B. S., Brownstein, A. J., & Shelby, J. (1987). Stimulus equivalence and the symbolic control of behavior. *Mexican Journal of Behavior Analysis, 13,* 361–374.

Hayes, S. C., Gifford, E. V., & Hayes, L. J. (1998). Una apróximacion relacional a los eventos verbales (A relational approach to verbal events). Trans. by T. E. Pena-Correal & N. Sanchez. In R. Ardila, W. López, A. M. Pérez-Acosta, R. Quiñones, & F. Reyes F. (Eds.), *Manual de análisis experimental del comportamiento* (pp. 499–517). Madrid, Spain: Biblioteca Nueva.

Hayes, S. C., & Gregg, J. (in press). Functional contextualism and the self. In C. Muran (Ed.), *Self-relations in the psychotherapy process.* Washington, DC: American Psychological Association.

Hayes, S. C., & Hayes, L. J. (1989). The verbal action of the listener as a basis for rule-governance. In S. C. Hayes (Ed.), *Rule-governed behavior: Cognition, contingencies, and instructional control* (pp. 153–190). New York: Plenum.

Hayes, S. C., & Hayes, L. J. (1992). Verbal relations and the evolution of behavior analysis. *American Psychologist, 47,* 1383–1395.

Hayes, S. C., Hayes, L. J., & Reese, H. W. (1988). Finding the philosophical core: A review of Stephen C. Pepper's *World Hypotheses. Journal of the Experimental Analysis of Behavior, 50,* 97–111.

Hayes, S. C., Hayes, L. J., Reese, H. W., & Sarbin, T. R. (Eds.). (1993). *Varieties of scientific contextualism.* Reno, NV: Context Press.

Hayes, S. C., Jacobson, N. S., Follette, V. M., & Dougher, M. J. (Eds.). (1994). *Acceptance and change: Content and context in psychotherapy.* Reno, NV: Context Press.

Hayes, S. C., & Ju, W. (1997). The applied implications of rule-governed behavior. In W. O'Donohue (Ed.), *Learning and behavior therapy* (pp. 374–391). New York: Allyn & Bacon.

Hayes, S. C., Kohlenberg, B. K., & Hayes, L. J. (1991). The transfer of specific and general consequential functions through simple and conditional equivalence classes. *Journal of the Experimental Analysis of Behavior, 56,* 119–137.

Hayes, S. C., Kohlenberg, B. S., & Melancon, S. M. (1989). Avoiding and altering rule control as a strategy of clinical treatment. In S. C. Hayes (Ed.), *Rule-governed behavior: Cognition, contingencies, and instructional control* (pp. 359–385). New York: Plenum.

Hayes, S. C., Nelson, R. O., & Jarrett, R. (1987). Treatment utility of assessment: A functional approach to evaluating the quality of assessment. *American Psychologist, 42,* 963–974.

Hayes, S. C., & Wilson, K. G. (1993). Some applied implications of a contemporary behavior-analytic account of verbal events. *The Behavior Analyst, 16,* 283–301.

Hayes, S. C., Wilson, K. G., Gifford, E. V., Follette, V. M., & Strosahl, K. (1996). Emotional avoidance and behavioral disorders: A functional dimensional approach to diagnosis and treatment. *Journal of Consulting and Clinical Psychology, 64,* 1152–1168.

Hayes, S. C., & Wolf, M. R. (1984). Cues, consequences, and therapeutic talk: Effect of social context and coping statements on pain. *Behaviour Research and Therapy, 22,* 385–392.

Hayes, S. C., Zettle, R. D., & Rosenfarb, I. (1989). Rule following. In S. C. Hayes (Ed.), *Rule-governed behavior: Cognition, contingencies, and instructional control* (pp. 191–220). New York: Plenum.

Hollon, S. D., & Beck, A. T. (1979). Cognitive therapy of depression. In P. C. Kendall & S. D. Hollon (Eds.), *Cognitive-behavioral interventions: Theory, research, and procedures* (pp. 153–203). New York: Academic Press.

Hollon, S. D., & Shaw, B. F. (1979). Group cognitive therapy for depressed patients. In A. T. Beck, A. J. Rush, B. F. Shaw, & G. Emery, *Cognitive therapy of depression* (pp. 328–353). New York: Guilford Press.

Ireland, S. J., McMahon, R. C., Malow, R. M., & Kouzekanani, K. (1994). Coping style as a predictor of relapse to cocaine abuse. In L. S. Harris (Ed.), *Problems of drug dependence, 1993: Proceedings of the 55th annual scientific meeting.* (National Institute on Drug Abuse Monograph Series No. 141, p. 158). Washington, DC: U.S. Government Printing Office.

Jacobson, N. S. (1992). Behavioral couple therapy: A new beginning. *Behavior Therapy, 23,* 493–506.

Jaynes, J. (1976). *The origin of consciousness in the breakdown of the bicameral mind.* Boston, MA: Houghton Mifflin Company.

Kabat-Zinn, J. (1991). *Full catastrophy living.* New York: Delta Publishing.

Kessler, R. C., McGonagle, K. A., Zhao, S., Nelson, C. B., Hughes, M., Eshleman, S., Wittchen, H., & Kendler, K. S. (1994). Lifetime and 12-month prevalence of DSM-III-R psychiatric disorders in the United States: Results from the National Comorbidity Study. *Archives of General Psychiatry, 51,* 8–19.

Kiesler, D. (1971). Patient experiencing and successful outcome in individual psychotherapy of schizophrenics and psychoneurotics. *Journal of Consulting and Clinical Psychology 37,* 370–385.

Koener, K., Jacobson, N. S., & Christensen, A. (1994). Emotional acceptance in integrative behavioral couple therapy. In S. C. Hayes, N. S. Jacobson, V. M. Follette, & M. J. Dougher (Eds.), *Acceptance and change: Content and context in psychotherapy* (pp. 109–118). Reno, NV: Context Press.

Larson, D. (1998). *Spirituality and health.* Washington, DC: National Institute on Healthcare Research.

Lazurus, R. S., & Folkman, S. (1984). *Stress, appraisal, and coping.* New York: Springer.

Leitenberg, H., Greenwald, E., & Cado, S. (1992). A retrospective study of long-term methods of coping with having been sexually abused during childhood. *Child Abuse and Neglect, 16,* 399–407.

Leonhard, C., & Hayes, S. C. (1991, May). *Prior inconsistent testing affects equivalence responding.* Paper presented at the annual meeting of the Association for Behavior Analysis, Atlanta, GA.

Linehan. M. M. (1993). *Cognitive-behavioral treatment of borderline personality disorder.* New York: Guilford Press.

Linehan, M. M. (1994). Acceptance and change: The central dialectic in psychotherapy. In S. C. Hayes, N. S. Jacobson, V. M. Follette, & M. J. Dougher (Eds.), *Acceptance and change: Content and context in psychotherapy* (pp. 73–86). Reno, NV: Context Press.

Lipkens, R., Hayes, S. C., & Hayes, L. J. (1993). Longitudinal study of derived stimulus relations in an infant. *Journal of Experimental Child Psychology, 56,* 201–239.

Loo, R. (1985). Suicide among police in federal force. *Suicide and Life-Threatening Behavior, 16,* 379–388.

Luborsky, L., Chandler, M., Auerbach, A. H., Cohen, J., & Bachrach, H. M. (1971). Factors influencing the outcome of psychotherapy. *Psychological Bulletin 75,* 145–185.

Malott, R. W. (1991). Equivalence and relational frames. In L. J. Hayes & P. N. Chase (Eds.), *Dialogues on verbal behavior* (pp. 41–44). Reno, NV: Context Press.

Maris, R. (1981). *Pathways to suicide: A survey of self-destructive behaviors.* Baltimore: Johns Hopkins University Press.

Marlatt, G. A. (1994). Addiction and acceptance. In S. C. Hayes, N. S. Jacobson, V. M. Follette, & M. J. Dougher (Eds.), *Acceptance and change: Content and context in psychotherapy* (pp. 175–197). Reno, NV: Context Press.

Matthews, B. A., Shimoff, E., Catania, A. C., & Sagvolden, T. (1977). Uninstructed human responding: Sensitivity to ratio and interval contingencies. *Journal of the Experimental Analysis of Behavior, 27,* 453–467.

McCurry, S., & Hayes, S. C. (1992). Clinical and experimental perspectives on metaphorical talk. *Clinical Psychology Review, 12,* 763–785.

Nesse, R. M., & Williams, G. C. (1994). *Why we get sick: The new science of Darwinian medicine.* New York: Times Books.

Neuringer, A. (1986). Can people behave "randomly"?: The role of feedback. *Journal of Experimental Psychology General, 115,* 62–75.

New York Times. (1993, June 17). Six-year-old commits suicide. p. A12.

Orlinsky, D. E., & Howard, K. I. (1986). Process and outcome in psychotherapy. In S. L. Garfield & A. E. Bergin (Eds.), *Handbook of psychotherapy and behavior change* (pp. 311–383). New York: Wiley.

Page, S., & Neuringer, A. (1985). Variability is an operant. *Journal of Experimental Psychology Animal Behavior Processes, 11,* 429–452.

Pepper, S. C. (1942). *World hypotheses: A study in evidence.* Berkeley: University of California Press.

Poppen, R. L. (1989). Some clinical implications of rule-governed behavior. In S. C. Hayes (Ed.), *Rule-governed behavior: Cognition, contingencies, and instructional control* (pp. 325–357). New York: Plenum.

Pryor, K. W., Haag, R., & O'Reilly, J. (1969). The creative porpoise: Training for novel behavior. *Journal of the Experimental Analysis of Behavior, 12,* 653–661.

Reese, H. W. (1968). *The perception of stimulus relations: Discrimination learning and transposition.* New York: Academic Press.

Regier, D. A., Narrow, W. E., Rae, D. S., Manderscheid, R. W., Locke, B., & Goodwin, F. K. (1993). The de facto US mental and addictive service system: Epidemiologic Catchment Area prospective 1-year prevalence rates of disorders and services. *Archives of General Psychiatry, 50,* 85–94.

Revusky, S. H. (1971). The role of interference in association over a delay. In W. K. Honig & H. James (Eds.), *Animal memory* (pp. 155–213). New York: Academic Press.

Ribeiro, A. (1989). Correspondence in children's self-report: Tacting and manding aspects. *Journal of the Experimental Analysis of Behavior, 51,* 361–367.

Robinson, P., & Hayes, S. C. (1997). Acceptance and commitment: A model for integration. In N. A. Cummings, J. L. Cummings, & J. N. Johnson (Eds.), *Behavioral health in primary care: A guide for clinical integration* (pp. 177–203). Madison, CT: Psychosocial Press.

Rogers, C. A. (1961). *On becoming a person: A therapist's view of psychotherapy.* Boston: Houghton Mifflin.

Rosen, D. H. (1976). Suicide behaviors: Psychotherapeutic implications of egocide. *Suicide and Life-Threatening Behavior, 6,* 209–215.

Rosenfarb, I., & Hayes, S. C. (1984). Social standard setting: The Achilles' heel of informational accounts of therapeutic change. *Behavior Therapy, 15,* 515–528.

Rosnow, R. L., & Georgoudi, M. (Eds.). (1986). *Contextualism and understanding in behavioral science.* New York: Praeger.

Rothberg, J. M., & Jones, F. D. (1987). Suicide in the U.S. Army: Epidemiological and periodic aspects. *Suicide and Life-Threatening Behavior, 17,* 119–132.

Safran, J. D., & Greenberg, L. S. (1988). The treatment of anxiety and depression: the process of affective change. In P. Kendall & D. Watson (Eds.), *Anxiety and depression: Distinctive and overlapping features* (pp. 455–489). Orlando, FL: Academic Press.

Sarbin, T. R. (1986). The narrative as a root metaphor for psychology. In T. R. Sarbin (Ed.), *Narrative psychology: The storied nature of human conduct* (pp. 3–22). New York: Praeger.

Saunders, K. J. (1989). Naming in conditional discrimination and stimulus equivalence. *Journal of the Experimental Analysis of Behavior, 51,* 379–384.

Schneidman, E. S. (1985). *Definition of suicide.* New York: Wiley.

Seligman, M. (1995). The effectiveness of psychotherapy: The Consumer Reports Study. *American Psychologist, 50,* 965–974.

Semin, N., & Manstead, A. (1985). *Social accountability.* Cambridge, England: Cambridge University Press.

Shimoff, E., Catania, A. C., & Matthews, B. A. (1981). Uninstructed human responding: Sensitivity of low rate performance to schedule contingencies. *Journal of the Experimental Analysis of Behavior, 36,* 207–220.

Skinner, B. F. (1953). *Science and human behavior.* New York: Free Press.

Skinner, B. F. (1969). *Contingencies of reinforcement: A theoretical analysis.* New York: Appelton-Century-Crofts.

Skinner, B. F. (1974). *About behaviorism.* New York: Vintage Books.

Skinner, B. F. (1989). The origins of cognitive thought. *American Psychologist, 44,* 13–18.

Smith, G. W., & Bloom, I. (1985). A study of the personal meaning of suicide in the context of Baechler's typology. *Suicide and Life-Threatening Behavior, 15,* 3–13.

Strosahl, K. (1991). Cognitive and behavioral treatment of the personality disordered patient. In C. Austad & B. Berman (Eds.), *Psychotherapy in managed health care: The optimal use of time and resources* (pp. 185–201). Washington, DC: American Psychological Association.

Strosahl, K. (1994). Entering the new frontier of managed mental health care: Gold mines and land mines. *Cognitive and Behavioral Practice, 1,* 5–23.

Strosahl, K. D., Hayes, S. C., Bergan, J., & Romano, P. (1998). Assessing the field effectiveness of Acceptance and Commitment Therapy: An example of the manipulated training research method. *Behavior Therapy, 29,* 35–64.

Titchener, E. B. (1916). *A text-book of psychology.* New York: MacMillan.

Wegner, D. M., Schneider, D. J., Carter, S. R., & White, T. L. (1987). Paradoxical effects of thought suppression. *Journal of Personality and Social Psychology, 53,* 5–13.

Wegner, D. M., Schneider, D. J., Knutson, B., & McMahon, S. R. (1991). Polluting the stream of consciousness: The effect of thought suppression on the mind's environment. *Cognitive Therapy and Research, 15,* 141–151.

Wegner, D., & Zanakos, S. I. (1994). Chronic thought suppression. *Journal of Personality, 62,* 615–640.

Wenzlaff, R. M., Wegner, D. M., & Klein, S. B. (1991). The role of thought suppression in the bonding of thought and mood. *Journal of Personality and Social Psychology, 60,* 500–508.

Wilson, K. G., & Hayes, S. C. (1996). Resurgence of derived stimulus relations. *Journal of the Experimental Analysis of Behavior, 66,* 267–281.

Wulfert, E., Greenway, D. E., Farkas, P., Hayes, S. C., & Dougher, M. J. (1994). Correlation between a personality test for rigidity and rule-governed insensitivity to operant contingencies. *Journal of Applied Behavior Analysis, 27,* 659–671.

Wulfert, E., & Hayes, S. C. (1988). The transfer of conditional sequencing through conditional equivalence classes. *Journal of the Experimental Analysis of Behavior, 50,* 125–144.

Yalom, I. D. (1980). *Existential psychotherapy.* New York: Basic Books.

Zettle, R. D., & Hayes, S. C. (1982). Rule-governed behavior: A potential theoretical framework for cognitive-behavior therapy. In P. C. Kendall (Ed.), *Advances in cognitive-behavioral research and therapy* (pp. 73–118). New York: Academic Press.

Zettle, R. D., & Hayes, S. C. (1986). Dysfunctional control by client verbal behavior: The context of reason giving. *The Analysis of Verbal Behavior, 4,* 30–38.

Zettle, R. D., & Raines, J. C. (1989). Group cognitive and contextual therapies in treatment of depression. *Journal of Clinical Psychology, 45,* 438–445.

Index